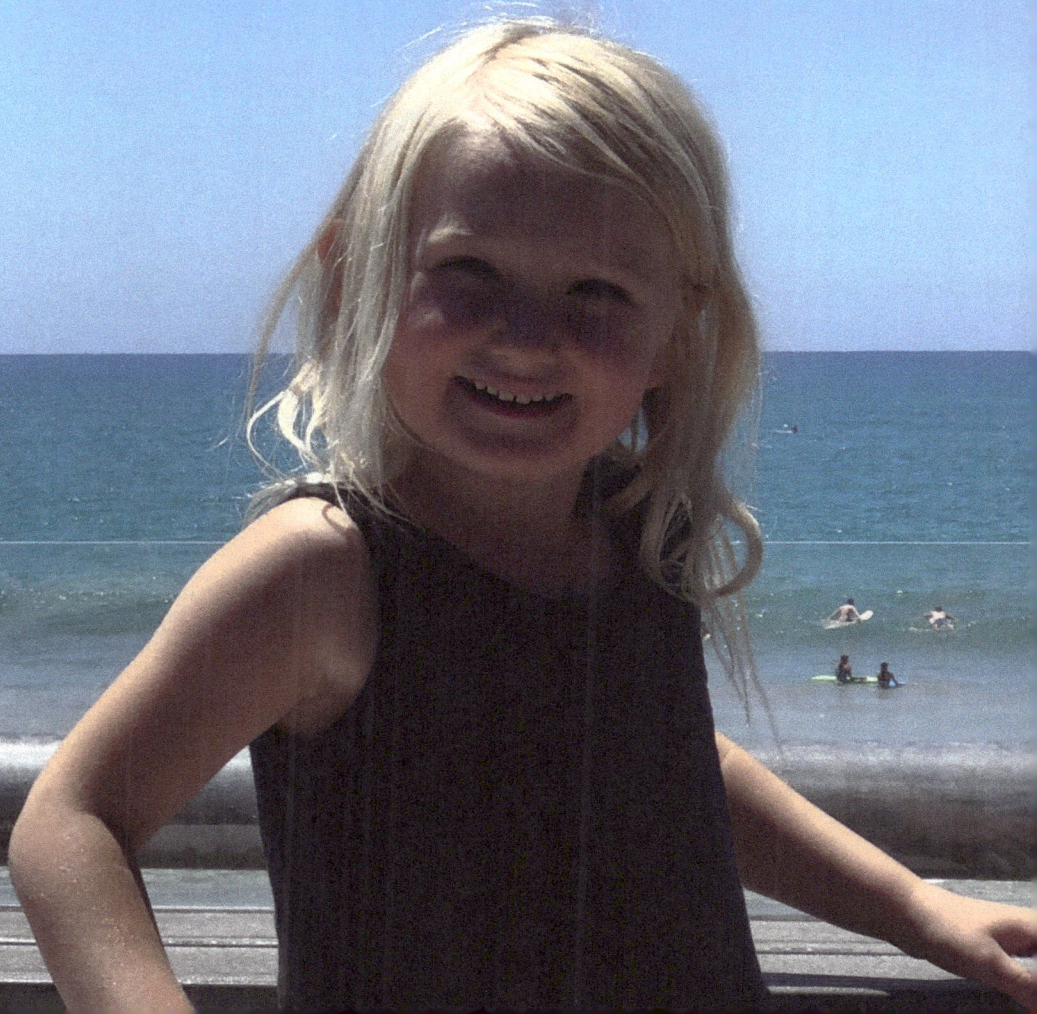

FIN'S MOUNTAINS

Climbing the Seven Summits for Type 1 Diabetes

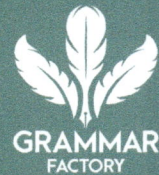

GRAMMAR
FACTORY

FIN'S MOUNTAINS

DAVID MORGAN

Published by Grammar Factory Publishing, an
imprint of MacMillan Company Limited.

Grammar Factory Publishing
MacMillan Company Limited
25 Telegram Mews, 39th Floor, Suite 3906
Toronto, Ontario, Canada
M5V 3Z1

www.grammarfactory.com

Morgan, David
Fin's Mountains: Climbing the Seven Summits
for Type 1 Diabetes.

Paperback ISBN 978-1-998756-46-9
Hardcover ISBN 978-1-998756-48-3
eBook ISBN 978-1-998756-47-6

1. SPO029000 SPORTS & RECREATION /
Mountaineering. 2. TRV001000 TRAVEL /
Special Interest / Adventure. 3. HEA039050
HEALTH & FITNESS / Diseases & Conditions
/ Diabetes.

PRODUCTION CREDITS
Cover design by Designerbility
Interior layout design by Setareh
Ashrafologhalai
Book production and editorial services by
Grammar Factory Publishing

GRAMMAR FACTORY'S CARBON
NEUTRAL PUBLISHING COMMITMENT
Grammar Factory Publishing is proud to be
neutralizing the carbon footprint of all printed
copies of its authors' books printed by or
ordered directly through Grammar Factory
or its affiliated companies through the
purchase of Gold Standard-Certified
International Offsets.

Dedicated to my family, and the countless people I've met, for their acceptance and generosity, wisdom and experience and, ultimately, for helping a father return home.

When challenges such as Finlay's type 1 diabetes come along, we face them together as a family, together as a community. Together we are stronger.
As our children face the world, I want them to carry this strength forward and do so with a little more courage than fear. As one human race, it is my hope we can believe in ourselves and rise to any challenge.

'You must be the change you wish to see in the world.'

MAHATMA GANDHI
The favourite quote of Tanika Pearce,
my beloved sister taken too soon.

01.12.1994—22.11.2013

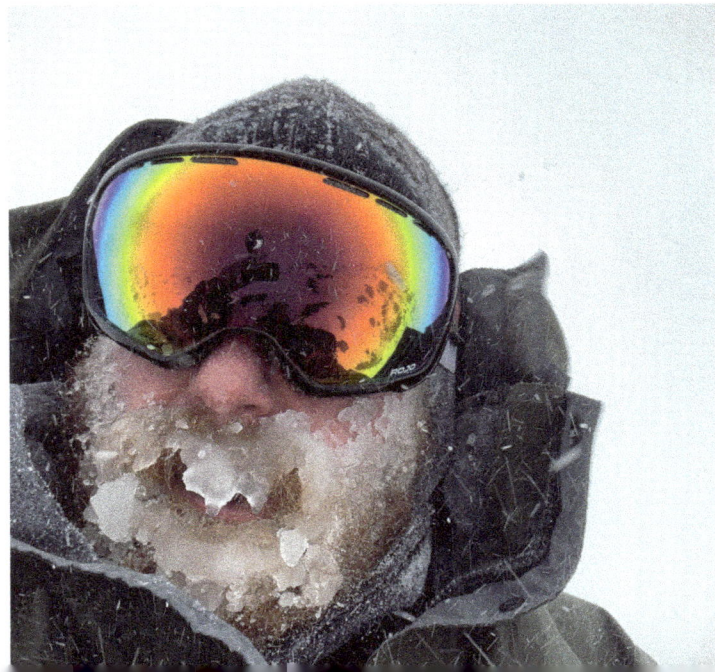

CONTENTS

TYPE 1 DIABETES is a complex health condition that requires 24/7 monitoring, 365 days a year. Once it develops there is no cure. For parents of young children, there are no holidays, no nights off. Diabetes is always there.

When David Morgan's family received the news that four-year-old Finlay had developed type 1 diabetes, they felt like the ground beneath their entire lives had shifted. I talk to many families like the Morgans and I understand how confronting and frightening it can be.

Life will never be the same after a diabetes diagnosis.

But in the face of some of our most difficult challenges, we sometimes draw on reserves of strength we didn't know we had.

For the Morgan family it was actually Finlay's courage and bravery that gave them strength.

David watched Finlay's determination to learn how to manage the condition. He knew then and there that he wanted to do something to honour her strength, raise money for diabetes research, and support the 130,000 Australians living with type 1 diabetes.

The plan he came up with was extraordinarily ambitious: Climb the highest mountain on each of the world's seven continents and run a marathon on each continent.

What David didn't know at the time was that his globetrotting plans were about to be thrown into chaos by a pandemic but, by 2021, he had finally summitted his seventh mountain. It turned out COVID-19 was one of only a number of massive challenges he had to overcome.

This book brings to life not just the mountains that might otherwise remain a distant landscape to many readers, but the journey. Through David's writing and photography, you'll feel like you're climbing alongside him, tracing the footsteps of a man who was committed to doing something extraordinary to support people who do extraordinary things every day.

David's journey is not unlike the journeys undertaken by diabetes researchers who can often find themselves confronted by seemingly unsolvable problems as they seek to reach the summits of their own research. But they don't give up. They run more experiments. They try tackling problems in new ways.

In this sense David's challenge is a tribute to thousands of diabetes researchers who have been working tirelessly for a cure for more than a century. There still is no cure and progress often seems maddeningly slow, but they go on.

Of course, David's challenge wasn't just symbolic. At its heart it was a fundraising initiative to raise vital funds to help researchers continue their search for a cure. He self-funded the entire challenge and all of the donations he secured, from all corners of the globe, were received by Diabetes Australia to support the Diabetes Australia Research Program.

So I'd like to say thank you to David on behalf of everyone at Diabetes Australia, on behalf of diabetes researchers and on behalf of people living with diabetes. Your response to Finlay's diagnosis has inspired us all. I'd also like to acknowledge and thank your family for the sacrifices they made in supporting you.

When I read about how you battled COVID-19 on Mt Everest while climbing with frostbitten toes I understood how deep your commitment to people living with diabetes runs.

I hope the readers of this book are as inspired as I have been.

FOREWORD BY MIKE HAMILL
OWNER & FOUNDER OF
CLIMBING THE SEVEN SUMMITS

THE FIRST TIME I met David, he had just stepped off a Twin Otter prop plane on a barren glacier in the frigid and harsh environment of Antarctica wearing a beat-up contractors hoodie and a worn baseball cap. We were to climb the tallest peak on the continent together. With a firm handshake and an unwavering gaze, the plane's engine roared to life again and I could tell he was unintimidated by the seriousness of this place.

Over nearly three decades of climbing and guiding the tallest mountains on the planet, I have seen many climbers come and go, and have learned to quickly identify who has the will and tenacity to succeed. Upon meeting David it was obvious that he could get the job done. He is no nonsense and dives headfirst into whatever he puts his mind to, whether it be his family, his business, climbing mountains, running marathons or working for a cause. Climbing for a cause is so deeply personal to him, he is unstoppable.

As you will read, David not only got the job done, he did so despite ridiculous adversity; a global pandemic, horrible weather and cyclones, contracting Covid and enduring long periods of time away from his family. Climbing the Seven Summits are hard enough with the best of luck and conditions. David persevered through the worst. The year David stood on top of Everest was the most difficult climbing season I have experienced in my fourteen years guiding Everest.

This is a story about how one man with drive conquered the famed Seven Summits despite incredible hardships. It is an eloquently written account that shows how, with determination and a strong purpose, you can set the biggest of goals and achieve them. It serves as an inspiration to us all.

PREFACE

N 2018 our four-year-old daughter, Finlay—a healthy, active little girl—began to develop an insatiable thirst. Finlay's usually robust appetite disappeared, and my spirited, rosy-cheeked child became increasingly lethargic. Rather than racing around the house with her siblings—Will, Kai and Arlo, now aged seventeen, six and four—Fin spent most of her time lounging on the couch.

Melbourne's Royal Children's Hospital diagnosed type 1 diabetes, a lifelong auto-immune disease that causes the body's immune system to attack part of the pancreas, destroying the cells that produce insulin. Without insulin, the body can't regulate blood sugar levels, which can lead to dangerous complications that affect your body from head to toe, including stroke, blindness, amputations and more. Along with maintaining a careful balance of diet and exercise, a person with type 1 diabetes needs to keep blood glucose levels as normal as possible through a regimen of injecting synthetic insulin. This means that all type 1 diabetes sufferers must inject insulin every day for the rest of their lives, unless a cure is found. Failing to do so can result in death.

Type 1 diabetes should not be confused with type 2, which is a completely different condition. Type 2 diabetes is not caused by an attack from the immune system. Rather, there are several risk factors that contribute to its development—age, family history, ethnic background, weight, diet and physical exercise, which can all be treated with lifestyle change and medication. Type 1 diabetics have done nothing to cause their condition—a fact that is often misunderstood—and anybody can get it.

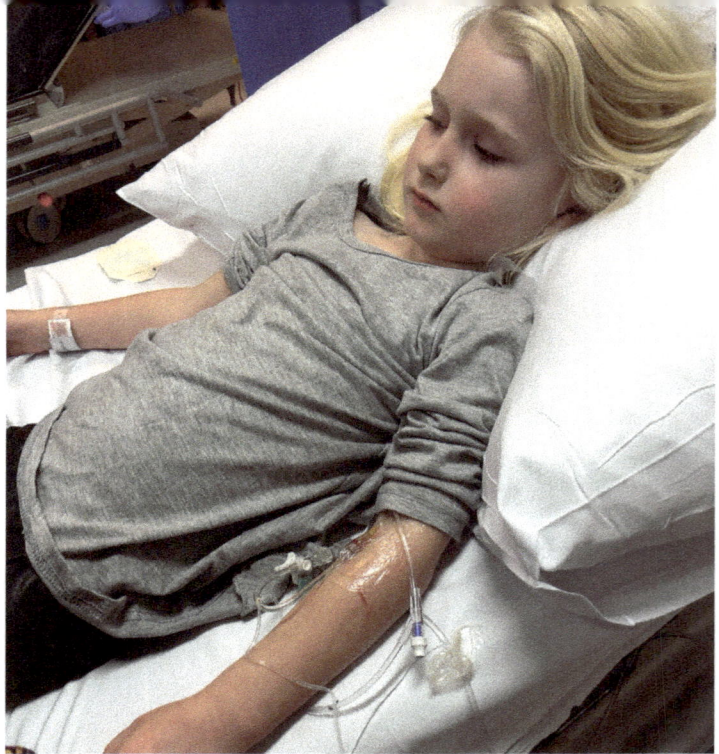

right Finlay awaiting diagnosis

Type 1 usually has onset in childhood or adolescence, and if a child does not receive urgent treatment when symptoms appear, they will become dehydrated, start vomiting and lose consciousness. This is called diabetic ketoacidosis (DKA). DKA is caused by a severe lack of insulin, which forces the body to release chemicals called ketones that turn the blood acidic, and if not treated immediately can lead to coma and death. It is a serious and live-threatening condition.

My partner Heidi and I listened, shell shocked, as doctors outlined the disease Fin had succumbed to with no warning. While type 1 diabetes is thought to be caused primarily by genetic components, it's suggested that there are some non-genetic causes as well. This may be the case with Fin's, as there have been no known cases of diabetes in either my or Heidi's families. But like so many aspects of this chronic condition, we simply don't know. What we do know is that there is no cure.

As parents, Heidi and I knew little about diabetes. When Fin was diagnosed it was a time of fear, anxiety, and learning a regimen of the blood glucose tests and insulin injections essential to manage our daughter's condition. Essential, indeed, to keep her alive.

In the first weeks following diagnosis, a sick and frightened little Fin cried and screamed and fought every time Heidi and I checked her blood sugar levels and administered her life-saving insulin injections. Can you imagine pinning down your small, defenceless child, too young to fully understand what is happening to her, and puncturing her perfect skin with a needle several times a day? To our young daughter, it must have felt like her parents were torturing her. There had to be a better way…

I quickly became immersed in researching diabetes. Who was funding research into prevention and management of type 1 diabetes? Who was looking for a cure? My search led me to Diabetes Australia.

The Diabetes Australia Research Program supports and develops world-class diabetes research in Australia by funding a range of grants across the full spectrum of diabetes research. The program relies on the generosity and support of member organisations, corporates and individual donors. Every single dollar raised by Diabetes Australia is used for this vital research, education, and awareness programs. It was a no-brainer. I would become an individual donor. But not just a run-of-the-mill, chuck some spare change in a tin type of donor. I wanted to make a real difference. I wanted to raise a lot of money for Diabetes Australia research. I didn't want my precious, innocent daughter to shove needles into her body every day for the rest of her life—I wanted a cure for type 1 diabetes.

But how could I do that? I thought about my background, skills and achievements. Was there something there that could help me raise this money? Home is Melbourne, where I'm a builder with a passion for development. Fourteen years ago, from the humblest beginnings, I established Morgan Development Group for the purpose of domestic and commercial construction projects. It's been a hectic fourteen years, full of growth and challenges, during which time we've delivered highly successful projects in premier locations. Our sister company, Morgan & Co, has evolved over the last sixteen years, and together our companies have worked on thousands of projects. Having established two successful businesses from the ground up, I felt confident that I could see through this fundraising challenge, but what form should that challenge take?

During my forty-something years, I've been a bit of an adventurer. I've competed in the Clipper Round the World Yacht Race and the Sydney to Hobart Yacht Race, hiked Papua New Guinea's Kokoda Trail, and been deep-sea diving on the shipwreck of the ss President Coolidge in Vanuatu. Perhaps I could consider being sponsored for some sort of physical challenge? The idea wasn't new. Many individuals have used physical challenges—sailing around the world, cycling some massive distance, or in the case of ninety-nine-year-old Sir Tom Moore, walking around and around his garden. Money can be raised this way—Sir Tom raised an astonishing thirty-three million pounds for Britain's National Health Service.

I have taken on many challenges in building a business, travelling the world and taking to the ocean waves, but one thing I hadn't done—or even mildly considered doing—was climbing mountains. So, you might ask, where did that idea come from? The idea first entered my head when I read of an Australian's record-breaking journey climbing the highest mountain on each of the world's seven continents in just four months (117 days). I was inspired. Here was an idea—an ambitious challenge that started to build momentum in my mind.

So there I was, a forty-something adventurer, sure, but no mountaineer. I'm a little stubborn, however. In fact I've been called dogged, obdurate—even pigheaded. This is a personality trait that perhaps helped when I was trying to establish Morgan Development Group. My lack of relevant experience failed to deter me. As an untrained, unpractised climber not in prime physical condition, and more or less ignorant of the logistics of mountaineering, I decided to attempt the Seven Summits—to climb to the top of the highest mountain on each of the seven continents. While I knew little about climbing these massive geological features, it seemed to be a feat that might be worthy of donations, so I committed to the challenge.

The first question was: where should I start? I made enquiries with businesses I knew that were involved with various charities at a local level. The idea of climbing the Seven Summits seemed ambitious to them, but I wasn't deterred by their lack of enthusiasm for my proposed challenge. Instead, I learnt a lot from them about how to put a suitable presentation together, and went looking for donors.

It quickly became clear that seeking corporate donors required investing a significant amount of time. I say donors rather than sponsors, as I wanted the challenge to both be completely self-funded and serve a higher purpose. Eventually a couple pledged donations and our long-term insurance supplier, Aughtersons Insurance Brokers, agreed to be a represented supporter. Others soon followed.

After talking the talk, now I'd have to walk the walk.

How, you might ask, does one even manage the logistics of climbing mountains? What about the travel, transport, accommodations, equipment, visas? The list goes on and on. How do you navigate all the countries, all the mountains? As I looked into the practicalities of my crazy challenge, I found a whole industry of commercial high-altitude experts. So there was a support network in place, but planning the challenge was still a complicated process. Every mountain seemed to have its own permits and government requirements. Although it took time to seek out local guides, I made engaging the local providers a priority.

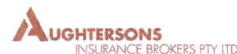
AUGHTERSONS
INSURANCE BROKERS PTY LTD

There were a lot of unknowns to discover, but one thing I was sure about was that I had the emotional support I needed. My partner, Heidi, is an incredibly considerate, understanding woman. She supports me 100 per cent in everything I do—even when the father of her small children decides to embark on a mountain-climbing odyssey to far-flung corners of the planet. What I wasn't so sure about was my body.

I needed to work on my fitness, so I found a personal trainer. I started to run, to use weights. I was motivated. But being out of shape and knocking on the door of middle age, it quickly became apparent that this undertaking would require a superior level of physical fitness. Commitment would be essential.

As every athlete knows, the seed for success is planted in the preparation, training, routine and vision needed to compete. Dedication, and to some degree obsession, is what's required to make this happen each and every day in the lead-up to a challenging event. Type 1 diabetes has the same demands and requires the same dedication from the sufferer each and every day. But for the sufferer of this disease, there is no race day to work towards or finish line to cross. The regimen and dedication demanded by diabetes is lifelong. There are no days off. I needed no further motivation to climb those mountains than to think of Fin's routine, for which there was no end. I had my 'why'.

And so it was in June 2019 that I set off to Africa to climb Mt Kilimanjaro—the first of the Seven Summits. The following month I tackled Russia's Mt Elbrus. Four months later I laboured up the slopes of Argentina's Mt Aconcagua. After aligning with the mountaineering company Climbing the Seven Summits (CTSS), I boarded a Russian plane at a military air base in Chile in January 2020, which took me to Antarctica where I summited Mt Vinson. In early 2020 I climbed Australia's Mt Kosciuszko as part of an ultramarathon event, after which it was time to set off to attempt the highest mountain of all, Mt Everest. At the same time, Covid-19

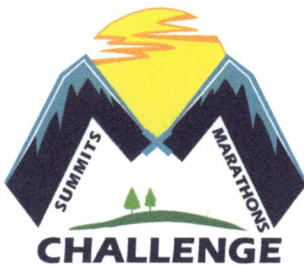

snowballed around the planet and threatened to undo my carefully laid plans. CTSS proved instrumental in providing options and supporting the expedition. And finally, in April 2020, I set off to climb the seventh and final summit, Alaska's Mt Denali.

Fin's Mountains is the story of my climbs. Hopefully, as you read these pages, we can take a journey together. I wrote this book as an extension to my adventure as a novice mountaineer and writer who pushes my perceived limits. It seemed a yarn worth telling. And ultimately, I wrote it so that one day my children can look back and know that I was simply trying to be the best father and human I could.

The symptoms of diabetes

Everyone should be aware of these four symptoms, and seek medical advice if they appear:

- Excessive thirst
- Increased toilet frequency
- Unexplained weight loss
- Extreme tiredness

DENALI
Elevation 6,194m
N 63 06.908
W 151 00.632

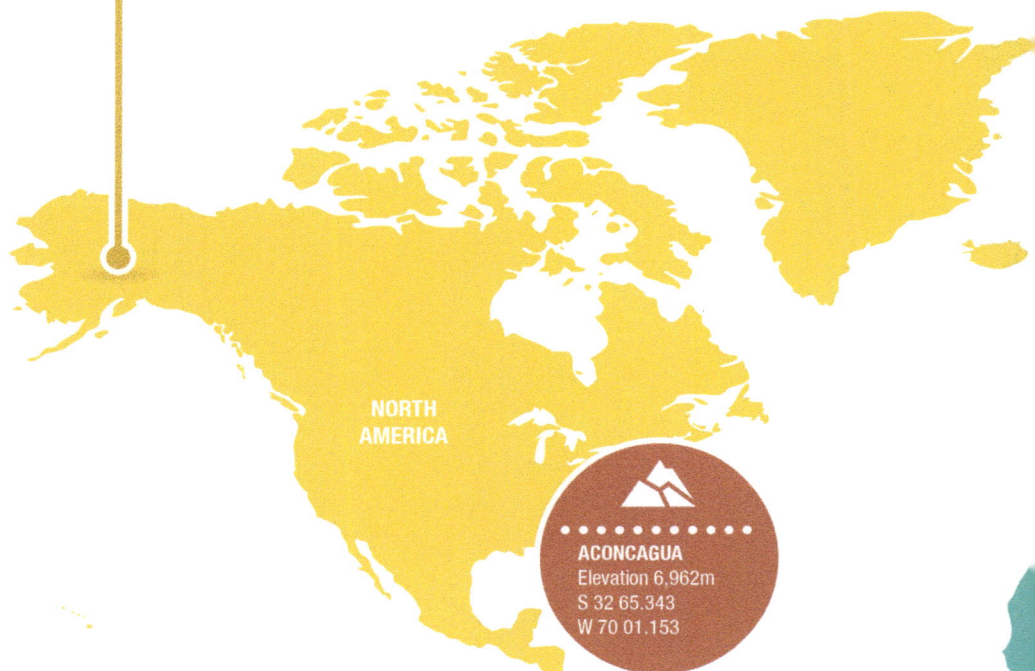

NORTH
AMERICA

ACONCAGUA
Elevation 6,962m
S 32 65.343
W 70 01.153

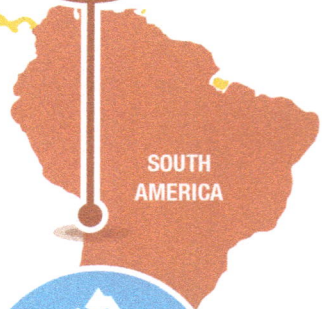

SOUTH
AMERICA

VINSON MASSIF
Elevation 4,892m
S 78 52.548
W 85 61.715

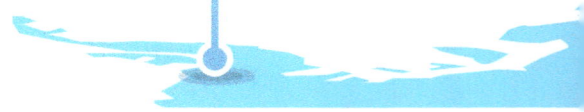

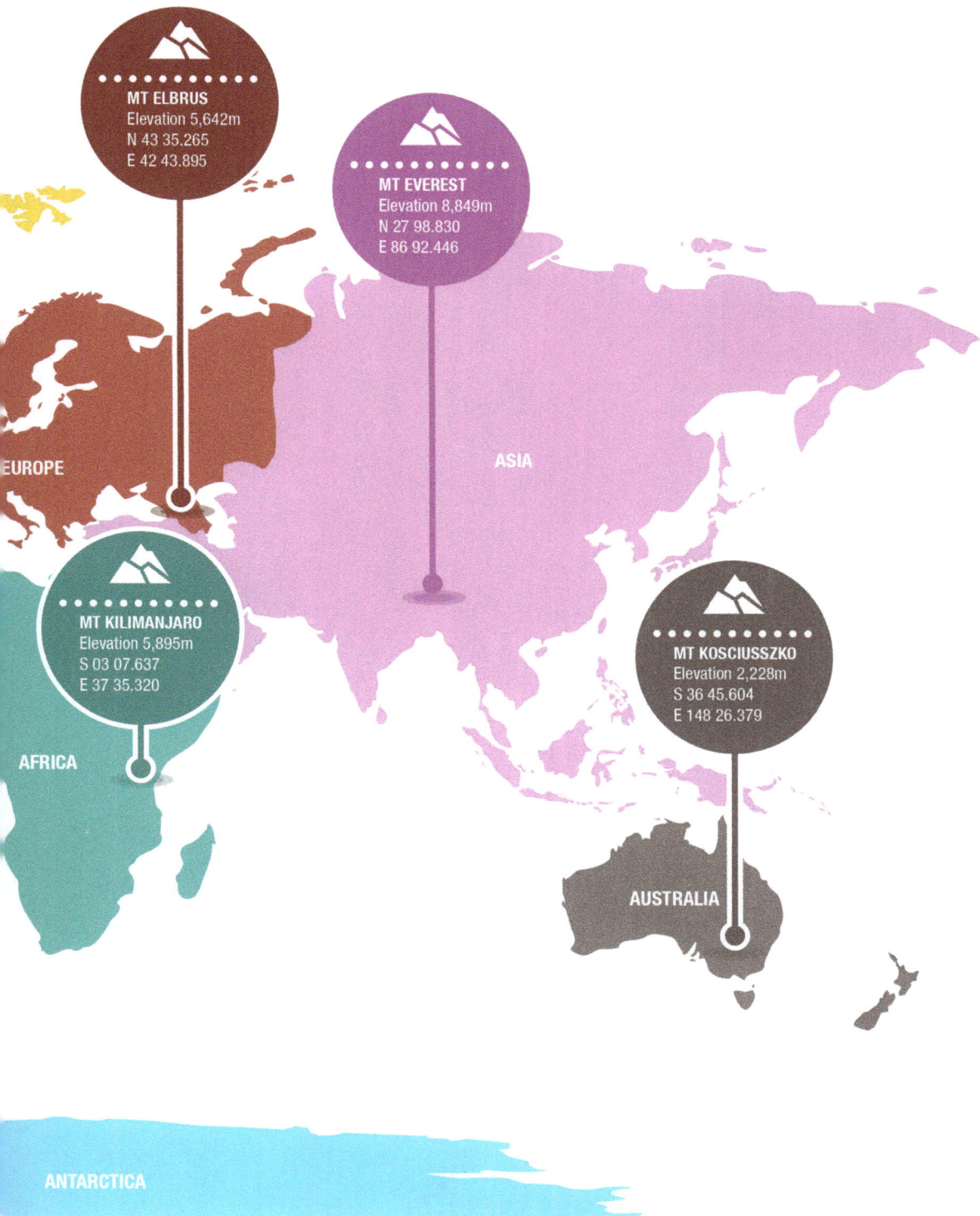

MT ELBRUS
Elevation 5,642m
N 43 35.265
E 42 43.895

MT EVEREST
Elevation 8,849m
N 27 98.830
E 86 92.446

MT KILIMANJARO
Elevation 5,895m
S 03 07.637
E 37 35.320

MT KOSCIUSSZKO
Elevation 2,228m
S 36 45.604
E 148 26.379

EUROPE

ASIA

AFRICA

AUSTRALIA

ANTARCTICA

PART 1

THE
FIRST
FIVE

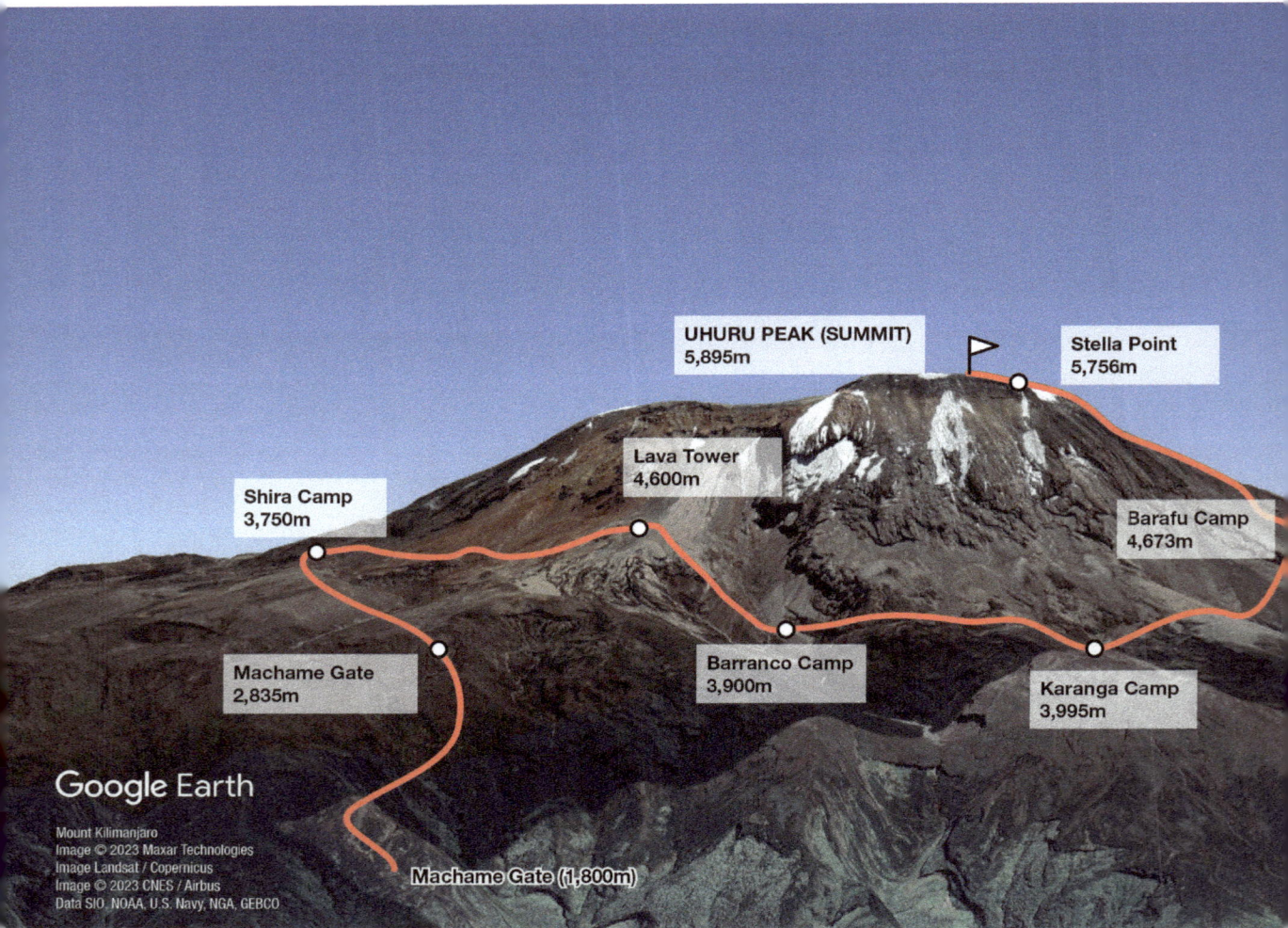

UHURU PEAK (SUMMIT)
5,895m

Stella Point
5,756m

Lava Tower
4,600m

Shira Camp
3,750m

Barafu Camp
4,673m

Machame Gate
2,835m

Barranco Camp
3,900m

Karanga Camp
3,995m

Google Earth

Mount Kilimanjaro
Image © 2023 Maxar Technologies
Image Landsat / Copernicus
Image © 2023 CNES / Airbus
Data SIO, NOAA, U.S. Navy, NGA, GEBCO

Machame Gate (1,800m)

MT KILIMANJARO

11,331km from Home

ELEVATION: 5,895m

COORDINATES:

S 03 07.637

E 37 35.320

17 JUNE—24 JUNE 2019

Mweka Camp
3,100m

Mweka Gate (1,800m)

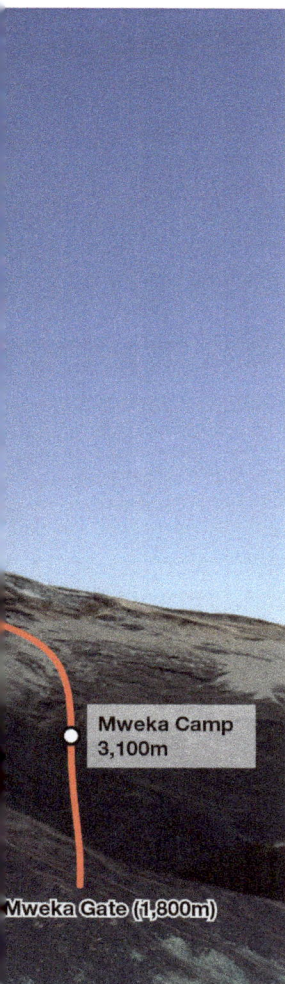

FIRST STOP: AFRICA. Specifically, the country of Tanzania, home to Africa's tallest peak. With a summit 5,895 metres above sea level, Mt Kilimanjaro is the highest freestanding mountain in the world. This makes it a more approachable challenge, and so seemed like a good start for a relatively inexperienced mountaineer and his fifteen-year-old son. I was looking forward to spending some quality time with Will, who I would have by my side as I took my first steps in what would become a life-changing adventure.

'WHERE'S THE airport?' asks Will as the plane begins its descent. Peering out of the plane's small windows at the verdant surrounds, we debate for a moment if the mountain range we saw earlier is where we will find the summit we've come to climb—Mt Kilimanjaro. Africa's highest mountain lies in the north-eastern tip of Tanzania, near the border of Kenya, and is just 330 kilometres from the equator. Will and I have endured just over thirty hours of airports and flying since we left cold, wintery Melbourne, and land at Kilimanjaro International Airport to a steamy, humid twenty-one degrees Celsius.

As far as international airports go, Kilimanjaro might not be vast and sprawling, but it does have a welcome feeling. Situated between the regions of Kilimanjaro and Arusha in Northern Tanzania, the airport is the gateway to the Kilimanjaro region, a major international tourism destination that

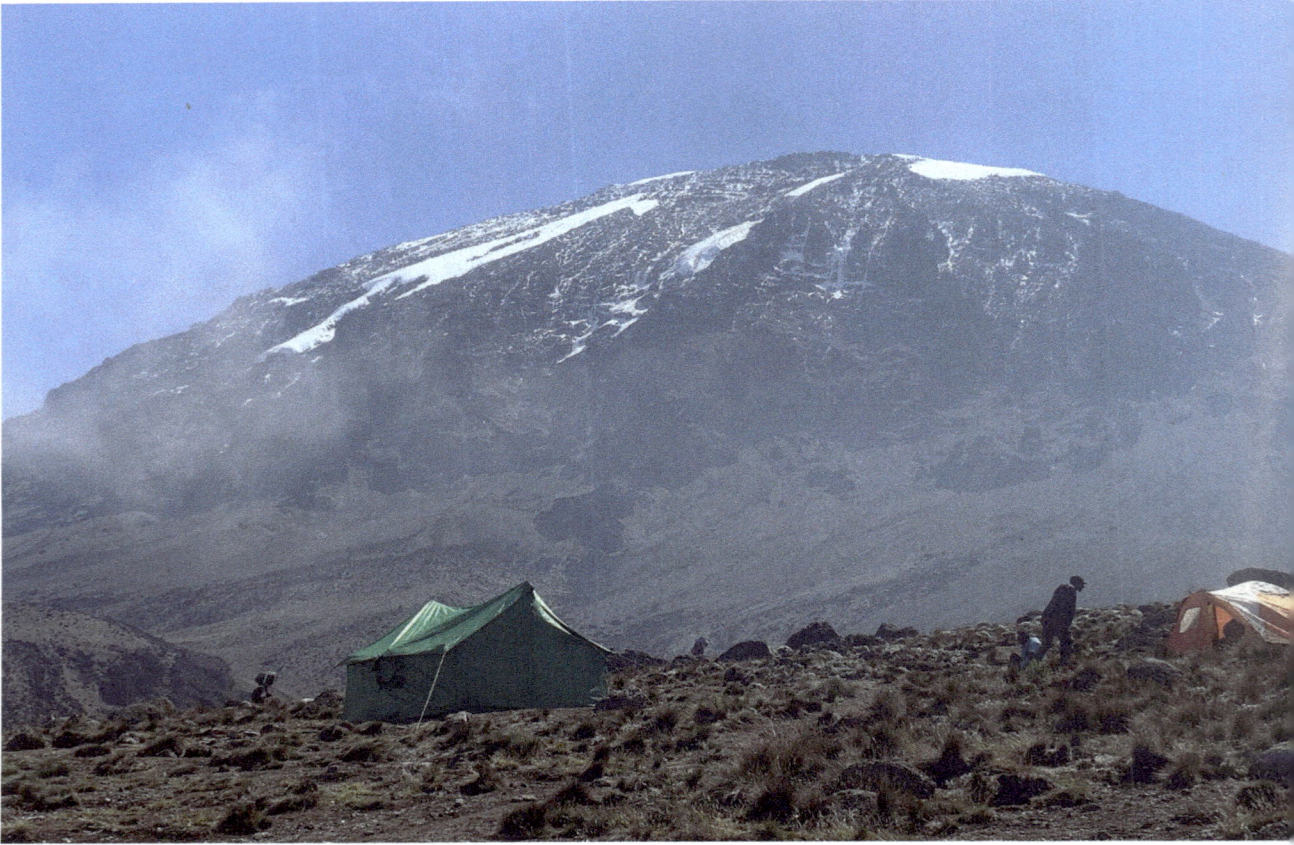

includes Mt Kilimanjaro, Arusha National Park, Ngorongoro Crater and Serengeti National Park.

I brace myself for a lengthy arrival process, not to mention the bureaucracy involved in getting a visa, but my fear is unfounded—it appears we're the only plane arriving today, and in no time we're organised and out the front door, bags in hand, having our first look at this new country. We meet our driver, Ally, and soon we're speeding away from the airport, scanning the distant snow-covered peaks and thinking of the challenge that lies ahead.

Ten minutes into our journey, Ally pulls over on the side of the road to collect Emmanuel, who is waiting in a seemingly random location. Emmanuel has made all the arrangements for our adventure. He looks our way and smiles broadly, acknowledging us as the latest clients who have travelled from afar for his services. If there were any lingering doubts about engaging his small local company to guide our expedition, they disappear with that friendly smile. Dressed in black pants, shirt and collared jacket, Emmanuel climbs into the front seat of the modest, ageing black sedan.

'How was your journey? Pleasant?' he asks.

'Nice enough. It's a long way from Australia, that's for sure.'

I guess Emmanuel to be in his mid-thirties, and definitely educated. His demeanour is pleasant and his conversation welcome entertainment for the bumpy forty-one-kilometre drive to Moshi.

Traffic is light and exposed dry earth frames both sides of the long, straight roads. The landscape is flat, red-brown and dry. Grasses attempting to cover the earth have failed, making for some barren vistas. A slight breeze flicks the browned grass. In contrast, sporadic patches of lush green foliage surround large trees in the distance.

It quickly gets hotter. The road shimmers into the distance, and I'm consumed by the small details: potholes that Ally has to dodge; overloaded trucks struggling to gain momentum; kids with sticks in hand, playing on the sides of the road.

A city with a population of around 200,000, Moshi serves as the starting point for most Kilimanjaro expeditions. Friendly locals walk the sides of quiet, bumpy dirt roads, going about their business. Maybe I was expecting something more hectic, but with the thick clouds above on an otherwise hot afternoon, it's a really relaxed atmosphere.

William, uncharacteristically, hasn't spoken a word. Although he's reasonably well travelled for his fifteen years, he comments, 'This feels remote and certainly different to other countries.'

Will embraced the idea of mountaineering after we successfully scaled Mt Fuji, in Japan, in the off-peak winter season back in June 2018. It had been Will's idea to undertake the challenge, and although that was only a one-day climb, it

opposite A mountain to climb

was a tremendous effort to reach the summit. It was also fun, and I hope we can build on our Mt Fuji experience to make this expedition rich with memories we'll both cherish.

Weaving through a maze of deserted side streets, we eventually arrive at a park. I'm surprised that this is our destination, for there are more barking dogs than people. Passing tall, solid stone walls, we enter a lush garden and realise it's the entrance to our hotel. Two gentlemen sit silently at a small round table nearby, apparently expecting our arrival.

'These are your guides, who will accompany you. I will meet with you once again upon your return,' says Emmanuel.

A gentle handshake, and Emmanuel gestures for us to continue along the thin path made of irregular shaped stones. The sun blasts down, and the humidity is high: there seems no reprieve in sight from the afternoon heat. Hopefully it'll be cool overnight.

'I am Vale. This is Joseph,' says one of the men sitting at the table, momentarily standing to lead the formalities.

'Please, sit with us.'

'G'day. I'm David and this is my son Will.'

Vale offers a welcoming, toothy smile in response.

Both guides were once porters, they tell us. Each has been climbing Kilimanjaro for more than a decade, which has enabled their status and promotion to lead climbers. Softly spoken and thorough, Vale leaves us with no queries to ponder once the briefing is concluded. Joseph, through his limited conversation, comes across as more reserved than Vale, and doesn't really engage in the briefing. I suspect his youthful appearance masks his deep experience on this mountain.

Tomorrow morning, we embark on our seven-day journey to the summit.

I'm surprised that Will and I are the only trekkers on our trip. Yet Vale explains that aside from him and Joseph—our guides—we also need porters, a cook, and assistance to fetch the water. Sourcing water from remote locations can, apparently, be an occupation in itself. This is something I've not even considered in my limited mountaineering experience. Specialty positions add tent-carriers and dishwashers to the personnel list.

Our guides insist on inspecting the climbing gear and equipment we've packed for the mountain. I'm sure I have everything on the list, and almost everything is new or near new. In fact, I have purchased and tried so much new gear there were enough 'doubles' to fill Will's entire backpack too. There's the pair of new boots I purchased for his larger feet, not yet worn in, trekking poles, several jackets, and even snacks from home—just in case. I'm not sure if our guides are impressed, or simply shocked by my compliance.

'Wow—this looks new…' Vale exclaims.

'You are very prepared,' Joseph adds. 'I think you don't need this much.'

Bringing my son along has been a risk, and maybe I have overcompensated with too much climbing gear for the sake of his comfort. Or perhaps it's because I'm a complete novice. Time will tell. It's a relief to know that Will and I are well prepared for our climb, and I look forward to a restful night's sleep.

But thoughts of my young daughter begin to plague me as I settle down for the night. I remember her words as we said our goodbyes back at home.

'I miss you, so I don't really want you to go,' Fin told me. 'But I wish I could go too.'

It's enough to have me tossing and turning beneath my mosquito net throughout the humid night.

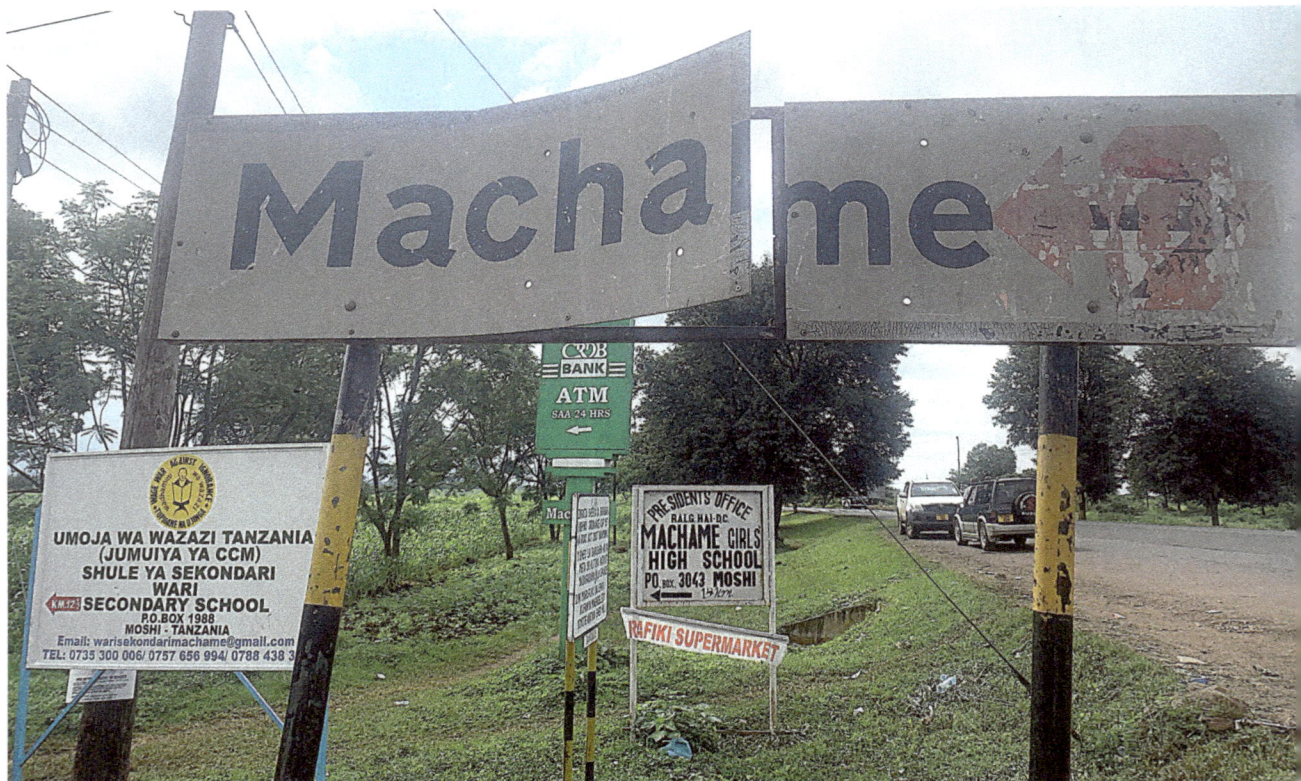

1,800m amsl to 2,835m amsl[1]

DISTANCE: 11km (5 hrs)

HABITAT: Montane forest

---

1   AMSL stands for Above Mean
     Sea Level, which refers to the
     height of a location above the
     average sea level.

Day 1—Machame Gate to Machame Camp

The sun eventually breaks across the horizon, filling the bedroom with light. Dogs have been barking long before noisy roosters join them to signal the dawn.

After a breakfast of beans and vegetables that we don't recognise, the team arrive to collect us in their minivan. We toss our packs on the roof, and then we're off—all fourteen of us. Hiring a local company seemed more appropriate than joining a western expedition, yet I'm surprised by the support staff that's provided just for me and Will.

It's a slow, mountainous thirty-kilometre drive to Kilimanjaro National Park, which covers an area of some 75,575 hectares and protects the largest freestanding volcanic mass in the world—Mt Kilimanjaro—which stands in spectacular isolation above the surrounding plains.

A stop at a local butcher is required en route for our meat supplies. Inside, the small shop's walls are covered in white tiles and the ceiling is slightly mouldy. Three whole carcasses hang on large, exposed metal hooks, plus several others at various stages of dismemberment. Sanitation looks questionable. Wasting no time, the butcher carves the order with his bare hands, then weighs the slabs of meat in a plastic bucket upon cast iron scales with old-fashioned metal weights. I'm fascinated, and a little concerned, by our purchases.

Will chooses not to leave the bus, despite my attempts to include him in the local experience. He's wide-eyed and quiet; I think just looking out the window at this new and very different landscape is a lot for him to process. We're now passing through the village of Machame, located on the lower slopes of the mountain. Next stop, the Kilimanjaro National Park—Machame Gate.

In 1991, the Tanzanian government and Kilimanjaro National Park Authority changed its policy on unsupported treks, and now all trekkers must be accompanied by a registered and licensed guide to trek on Mt Kilimanjaro. Further, the guides must be employed by, or otherwise attached to, a licensed tour operator. Only the tour operator is allowed to purchase the park permits. You can be fined, thrown in a local jail, or deported if caught without a licensed guide, so I recommend following the rules.

At Machame Gate, the process of issuing the climbing permit process is long, though we remain bystanders for the most part. It's a challenge just to identify who is our representative through the crowd of activity and constant introductions. Even though armed guards supervise the area, I can't help but suspect a level of corruption is present. The park fees account for the largest share of expenses, followed by wages for guides and support staff.

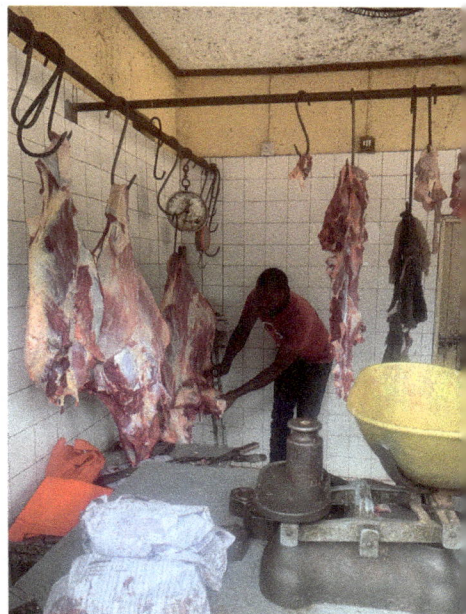

above The local butcher's shop

opposite Let us begin at the start

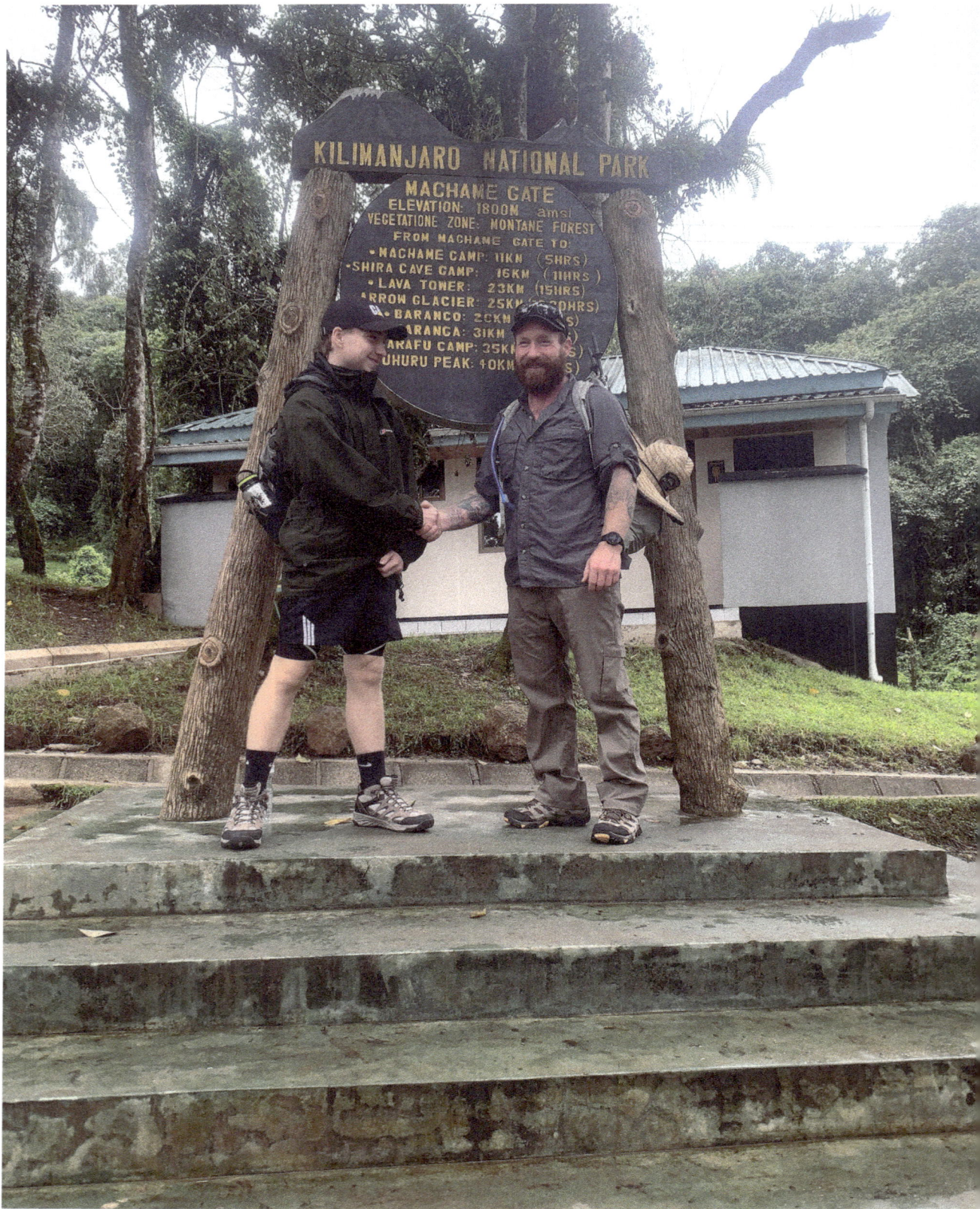

After patiently waiting some time, we're issued our permit and our bags are weighed to ensure they comply with the weight porters are restricted to carry. Twenty kilograms is the maximum. Some companies impose their own fifteen-kilogram limits.

Mt Kilimanjaro moves from gentle slopes to alpine desert with thirty-degree inclines. At the summit there is permanent ice and temperatures are below freezing, we're told. A small safety handbook is passed out from Kilimanjaro Search and Rescue. On the front page, featuring a majestic view of the mountain, it reads 'Karibu Kilimanjaro—Stay Safe'. The back shows a rescue helicopter and emergency contacts.

opposite Machame Gate

Reading the handbook, I'm surprised to learn that acute mountain sickness affects up to eighty per cent of trekkers on Mt Kilimanjaro. There are also serious risks around high-altitude cerebral oedema and high-altitude pulmonary oedema—both life-threatening conditions. I've read this little book twice, thoroughly, and will keep a copy with us. It seems I still have a lot to learn.

Time to saddle up and take our first steps towards a final checkpoint, which literally guards the iron gates we must pass through to reach the mountain. After hours and hours of flying and waiting around in transit, it's finally time to stretch the legs and tackle this mountain with a healthy dose of confidence.

'Pole, pole' is Swahili for 'slowly, slowly', and Vale's mantra, though for today we're invited to hold our own pace.

We're hiking on a windy, well-framed path beneath a thick green rainforest canopy. The brown earth path is sturdy underfoot, and well compacted from the many feet that have trodden it before us. But there are some slick and slippery puddles here and there, inviting the unprepared to test their balance.

We gradually increase our pace, confident and enthusiastic, on the mostly gradual ascent. It's enough to build up a sweat, but not so strenuous as to raise the heartbeat significantly— or so my heart rate monitor tells me. We begin to pass some other groups of climbers and porters. They look professional, while we continue to horse around like we're on a picnic.

Our pace is consistent, and, aside from a short ten-minute break, we arrive after a five-hour climb at Machame Camp and our trekking is complete for the day. The designated ranger checks us in, and then we relax and enjoy some afternoon sun—it's far cooler already. Dense cloud clears momentarily to reveal snow-capped peaks before gradually settling upon us, accompanied by a chilly blast of wind.

With an idea of which ridge is tomorrow's task, and with an easy day's hike behind us, we turn to our generous-sized tent, already set up by the team. They've also set up a mess tent, candlelit, just for two, where we're served soup, spaghetti and chunky meat sauce. I'll be taking some of this local coffee home for sure.

Day 2—Machame Camp to Shira Camp

2,835m amsl to 3,750m amsl
DISTANCE: 5km (6 hrs)
HABITAT: Moorland

'Wear your headlight if you leave the tent during the night, as the ranger has a pistol and might mistake you for a wild animal.' Vale's lingering comment runs through my 4am thoughts as I contemplate rising and walking through the otherwise silent camp. I decide to wait until morning.

After a hearty breakfast of eggs and toast, washed down with yet another cup of the strong and aromatic local coffee, it's hard not to miss the ceremonial singing and dancing taking place in a nearby camp. All the guides, porters and staff are tuned into the entertainment at a large climbing expedition, and more onlookers are curious about the commotion. A male elder, face painted white and wearing ceremonial dress, sings and encourages the dancing. It brings a smile to my face to watch the climbers joining in to dance to local songs.

The most difficult chore remains—finding a drop toilet that is bearable enough to visit. I'm not alone in my quest—it seems

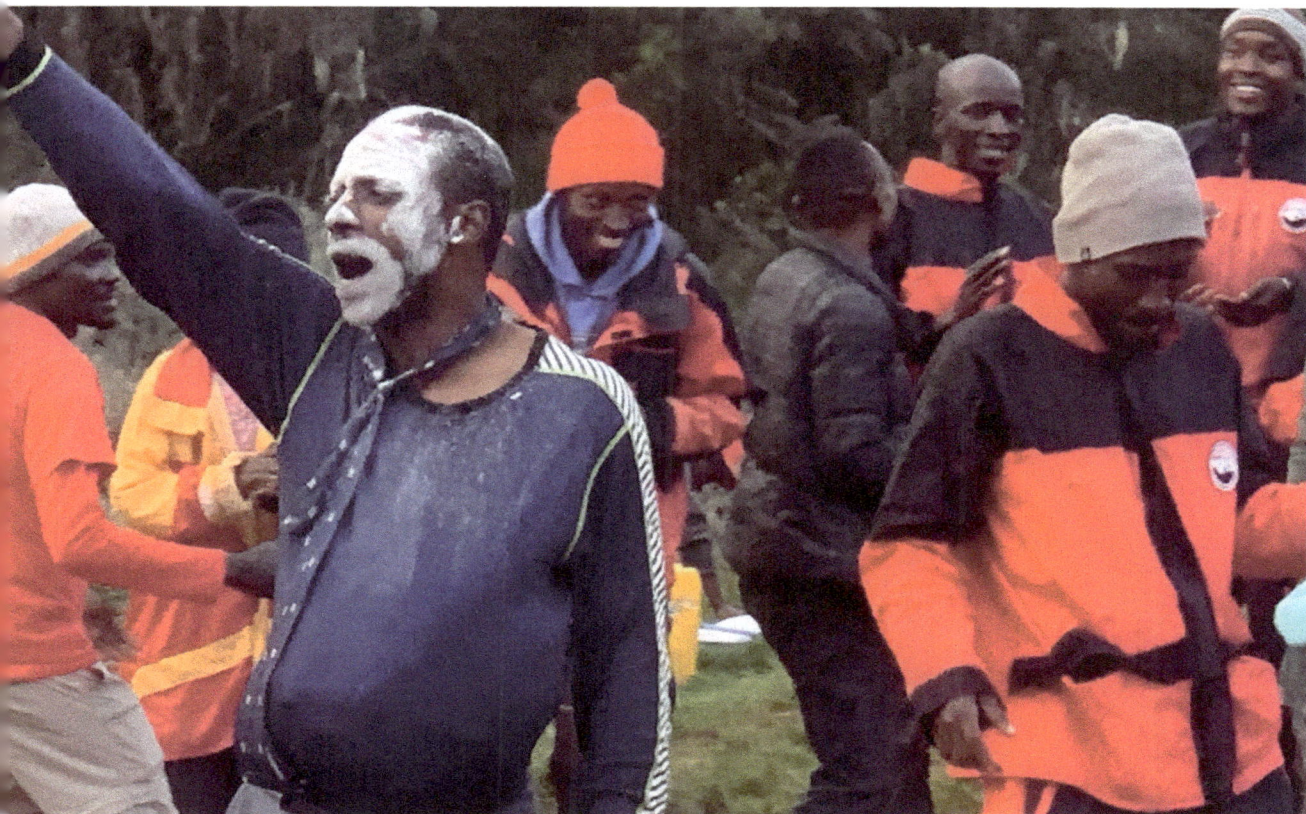

above Good morning vibes

quite a few others have been out on the single tracks that zig-zag between the various campsites, seeking the same relief.

Exiting camp, we leave the shade of the rainforest and continue on an ascending path headed along the Machame route, one of seven main routes leading to Kilimanjaro's summit. The path is hard, compacted earth, smooth but uneven under foot for the many thousands of feet that have defined the route ever upwards.

I feel confident and at ease.

'Pole, pole,' says Joseph as he sets the pace, and we dutifully fall in behind him. It's all uphill now, with a mixture of track and rock scramble.

Along the way, we're encouraged to rest and take in the stunning scenery. At a height that allows us to now look over the rainforest below, hills roll into the distance and give a real sense of how far from civilisation we truly are.

Joseph provides a running commentary on the region's botanical flowers, and insists on photographing each one as we hike. I notice that Will really engages in the opportunity, and both he and Joseph now talk freely.

We cross a small valley, walking along a steep, rocky ridge covered with purple heather until the ridge ends. One rock pass has us clinging to the rock face, choosing our footing with just a little extra care. Otherwise the well-worn trail is easy to negotiate, and the route soon turns west onto a river gorge.

After about four-and-a-half hours of moderate climbing, we arrive at Shira Cave Campsite at an altitude of 3,750 metres. Will says he is getting a headache, but we have the entire afternoon to rest and acclimatise to the increasing altitude. The sun breaks through intermittently as I relax and do some reading. More trekkers arrive, which brings periodic bursts of singing and dancing among the larger parties.

Later we head off for an acclimatisation walk. It's not far, but at one point the clouds break and for a few moments we're treated to a sneak peek of the summit—then it's gone.

'She [Mt Kilimanjaro] is very shy,' says Vale.

On descent we gather in a cave which, we're told, was the guides' and porters' quarters in the early days of recreational climbing. The practice is now banned. It's an education in just how much conditions have improved for these workers. We learn that corruption at the local level was rife for years, but the government of the day is now very strict on standards and compliance . . . including receiving climbing permit monies.

'Progress has been difficult for the locals and their natural laid-back approach,' says Vale.

He also tells us about the receding glaciers at the top of the mountain. 'Due to climate change,' he says.

It is feared that weather patterns have been altered around the mountain and are leading to the collapse of its glaciers. We learn that subtle changes in the glaciers are constant, and at the current rate of decline most of the remaining glaciers could disappear within a few years. Africa's Kilimanjaro massif is just three degrees south of the equator—in the tropics. The fact that glaciers exist here at all is enough for me to wish I'd paid more attention in science class.

Back at camp, hot soup and a rice dish are quickly demolished. Hot water in a basin to refresh ourselves is an unexpected luxury our team has generously prepared. Wind whips across the camp as the sunset paints the sky a breathtaking palette of colours, followed, when the sun sets, by a sparkling canopy of stars. We turn in early to regain some warmth and rest ahead of tomorrow's important acclimatisation day.

Day 3—Shira Camp to Lava Tower to Barranco Camp

3,750m amsl to 4,600m amsl to 3,900m amsl
DISTANCE: 7km (4 hrs) + 3km (2 hrs)
HABITAT: Semi-desert

Will wakes early, not because he's had plenty of rest, but because he's freezing cold. By 5:30am we're packing to get warm and searching for the thermals and comfort of jackets. The colder air temperature combined with howling winds makes it feel colder than it probably is, but this change in weather comes as a surprise. It calls for the feathery layers of a down jacket and the extra protection of a balaclava.

With our breakfast routine behind us, we soon make tracks. Within an hour the sun is visible, the skies have cleared, and for the next three hours we have incredible views of the mountain. We set out with jackets at hand, expecting rain and brisk wind, but instead we're drenched in sunlight.

'Mt Kilimanjaro makes her own weather plans day to day,' says Vale.

We continue to the east, climbing up a ridge and passing the junction towards the peak of Kibo—a volcanic cone in the distance. A fun activity is jumping on one of the large rocks for a photo—there's really not much else to do en route to break up the hiking.

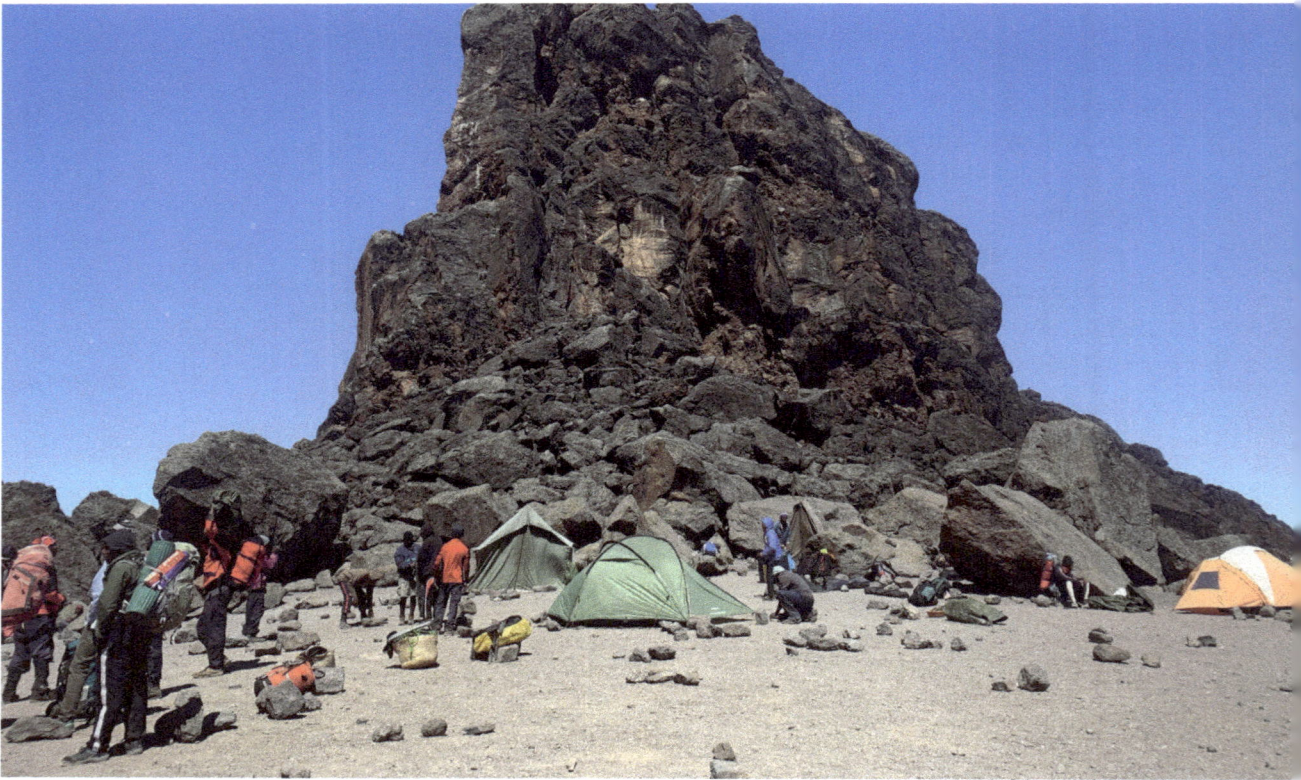

Now, continuing through the rising heat of the morning, our direction changes to the southeast and towards the Lava Tower, called the 'Shark's Tooth'. Essentially, it's an old plug left over from the mountain's active volcanic days.

After a four-hour hike, we arrive at Lava Camp. Positioned in the alpine zone at 4,600 metres, Lava Camp is a rocky and barren high-altitude desert. There is no vegetation here, only rocks, scree, and dust everywhere the eye can see. Flat ground is prime real estate around here, and a cluster of tents spring up on the helipad—apparently the porters aren't expecting any mountain rescues today. There are traces of ice on the ground, and small springs gurgle with sweet drinking water.

Will says he still has a headache. We're told it's generally at around this point that some climbers start experiencing symptoms of altitude sickness—breathlessness, irritability, headaches. He stands at the arrival signage, expressionless, arms crossed, and appears to be suffering. I'm not the only one to pick this up. After some pictures are taken, Joseph places his arm around Will and leads him away. I'm not privy to what's being said, but Joseph continues to lean into Will, arm over his shoulder, offering support.

Words can't express the gratitude I feel for the way this stranger is caring for my son. But there are many kind, empathetic people in the world who genuinely want to help others in need. This is something that Fin's diabetes has taught me. Watching my son feeling unwell and being cared for by Joseph reminds me of my greater charitable purpose, which is now being broken down into days, hours and moments.

The team serve lunch, which is an ideal circuit breaker. After lunch our final leg takes us downhill to arrive at Barranco Camp, at 3,900 metres. But the swifter downhill pace, descending almost 700 metres over about two hours, intensifies Will's headache.

The day has ended at almost the same elevation as our starting point, which feels counter-productive. But that's the way acclimatisation works. You go up, you come down, and then progress upwards to help the body prepare for summit day. 'Climb high, sleep low' is the mountaineering mantra.

We finally reach Barranco Camp, getting some rest and, for Will, some Panadol. Aside from the mess tent nearly blowing away mid-dinner in wild gales, I feel relaxed as I look out upon this incredible landscape of extremes. Behind our tent stands a mountain with plentiful ice, yet in the foreground we gaze upon a tumbleweed bouncing over the stones past wind-worn rocks where conditions keep life to a minimum.

The temperature drops quickly and winds continue gusting through camp, kicking up dust circling in the air. It's time for an early evening, and we cherish the comfort of our sleeping bags. Secretly, I'm hoping I have a built-in resistance to this new concept of actual altitude sickness.

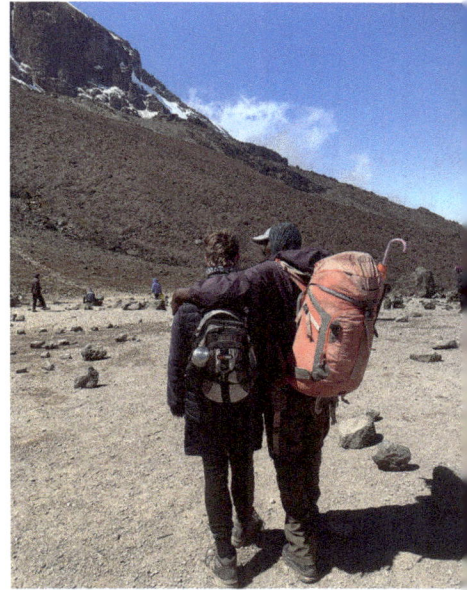

above The kindness of strangers

opposite Lava Tower

Day 4—Barranco Camp to Karanga Camp

It's 1:30am and a fierce gale is howling through the camp. I'm sure some of the clatter of tent poles I hear is the mess tent blowing over and heading directly for our sleeping tent, which is shaking violently. Thank goodness, by dawn the wind has retreated, and we're met with a cool, calm morning.

The Barranco Camp is without doubt the most spectacularly located camp so far, with jaw-dropping vistas of Kibo, one of the three volcanic cones that Mt Kilimanjaro has as a dormant volcano. (The other two are Mawenzi and Shira.)

The Western Breach route, the most challenging and by far the most dangerous way to the summit, is also on view, with the first of the southern glaciers now visible above us. As the name describes, the route leads through a breach in the crater wall and takes you inside the crater itself, whereas all other routes take you only to the crater rim.

Preparing to leave, we watch more and more ant-like figures zig-zag across the rock face adjacent to camp in the incessant pursuit of the summit. I heave my pack onto my back, head down a steep gorge, cross a gurgling, ice-cold stream, and soon become one of the ants.

We leave Barranco behind and continue along a steep ridge. Up and down we climb on the six-kilometre trek to Karanga Camp, gaining 457 metres in four hours. We pass the Barranco Wall—an impressive geological structure some 257 metres high, which is the result of a turbulent volcanic past. Historic collapses resulting in massive landslides down this southern face have created a cliff that, at times, demands all four limbs to scramble across. I'm reassured our guides are ready to assist at all the sketchy spots, but aside from a little physical exertion, no technical climbing is required. We have an ideal photo opportunity on this rough, rocky terrain, with the clear angles of Mt Kilimanjaro behind us and just the rolling clouds beneath. It's simply stunning.

The climb has been exposed in places and narrow in parts, but now opens up to wider passes that allow porters with their heavy loads to overtake and continue on. It's all smiles as we stand shoulder to shoulder on imposing rocks with light blue skies as our backdrop; there's barely a cloud in the sky.

But how quickly the situation changes on a mountain: within ten minutes the clouds roll in and everything is white. So, we press on.

Along the route, small stacks of stones mark the path. It's an old-world system still used to ensure one doesn't get lost. After Vale explains the significance of these stone stacks, and without prompting, I notice Will has taken to re-building some of the ones that have fallen or been destroyed. In his way, he is leaving a contribution to the path. Climbing with our guides continues to teach us about the mountain and the local Chagga culture.

You'll find the Chagga people living on the southern slopes of Mount Kilimanjaro in the middle of banana groves. Fertile soil and successful agricultural methods handed down through the ages have provided their relative economic wealth. An old Chagga proverb translates directly as 'He who leaves a child lives eternally.' It expresses the Chagga belief that people live through their descendants and the value they place on family.

Coming into Karanga Camp, we've reached 3,995 metres, and celebrate with a cooked lunch of hand-cut chips, vegetables and banana fritters. A siesta follows in the warmth of the afternoon sunshine.

Will says his head continues to throb, so I make a call—Diamox (used to prevent and reduce the symptoms of altitude sickness) it has to be. It's not a decision I've taken lightly, and really is a last resort. As your body adjusts to this medication, dizziness, light-headedness and increased urination may occur. Extra hydration is essential. The risks of nausea, vomiting, diarrhoea and blurred vision also exist, which in themselves could turn us back.

With a lazy afternoon behind us it's time for another acclimatisation walk, much to Will's disgust, given the look on his face. Different contingencies are discussed because of Will's headaches and lack of appetite, but he's having none of it—the thought of missing his photo at the summit drives him on.

Being above the clouds, and with the afternoon sun shining as we depart Karanga, I'm in awe of the sunset. Photography struggles to capture the silk clouds and radiant colours stretched across the sky. Life seems simple here. Just the day's passing signalled by tuning into Earth's natural rhythm.

The moment the sun disappears, the temperature plummets. Thermals, beanies—all layers are required until we can seek the sanctuary of our sleeping bags.

opposite A place of environmental extremes

Day 5—Karanga Camp to Barafu Camp

3,995m amsl to 4,673m amsl
DISTANCE: 4km (4 hrs)
HABITAT: Alpine desert

At 2:00 am I wake with a bloody nose, which lasts twenty minutes. Scratching around the tent for something to wipe the blood, I'm worried the bleed may be altitude related. Should I tell the guides or not? Am I overreacting? I decide to see what the morning brings . . .

I wake again at 6:15 am—it's a sleep-in! Will has slept all night and, while not exactly bouncing out of the tent, he's not suffering too much. After reading through the altitude sickness brochure, he says, 'I've got something in every category.'

My bloody nose has returned as I venture to the (very basic) bathroom amenities. I'm not exactly bouncing out of the tent myself, but I contain any personal discomfort for the positivity that I hope will get Will through the day.

We have no appetite at breakfast, but somehow we eat. Enthusiasm is definitely low now. I don't think anybody really knows how their body will respond to a lack of oxygen until you're here at an altitude like this.

But soon enough we're off on foot once more. Before long we're back to the steady, silent rhythm our days often require.

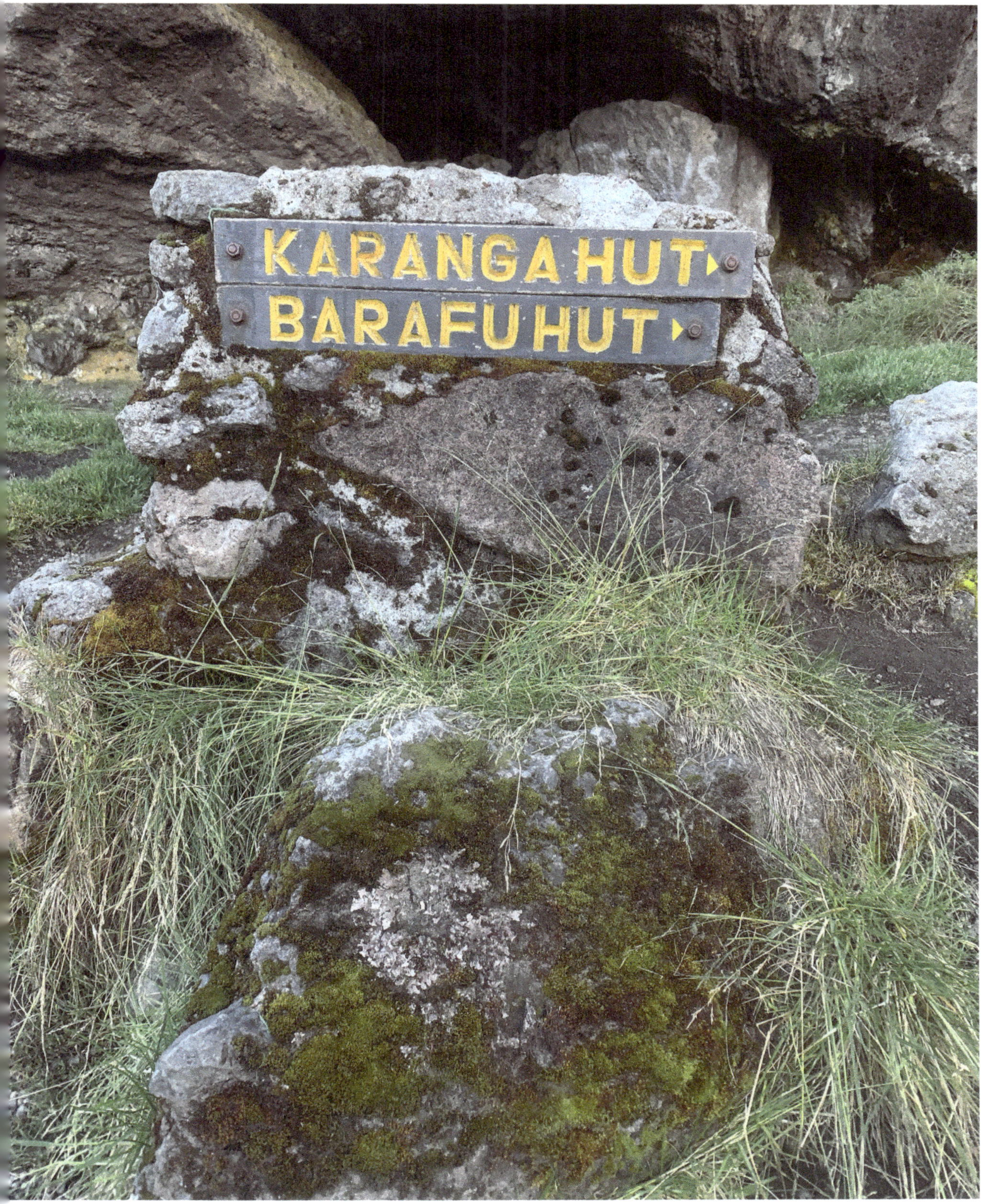

KARANGA HUT ▸
BARAFU HUT ▸

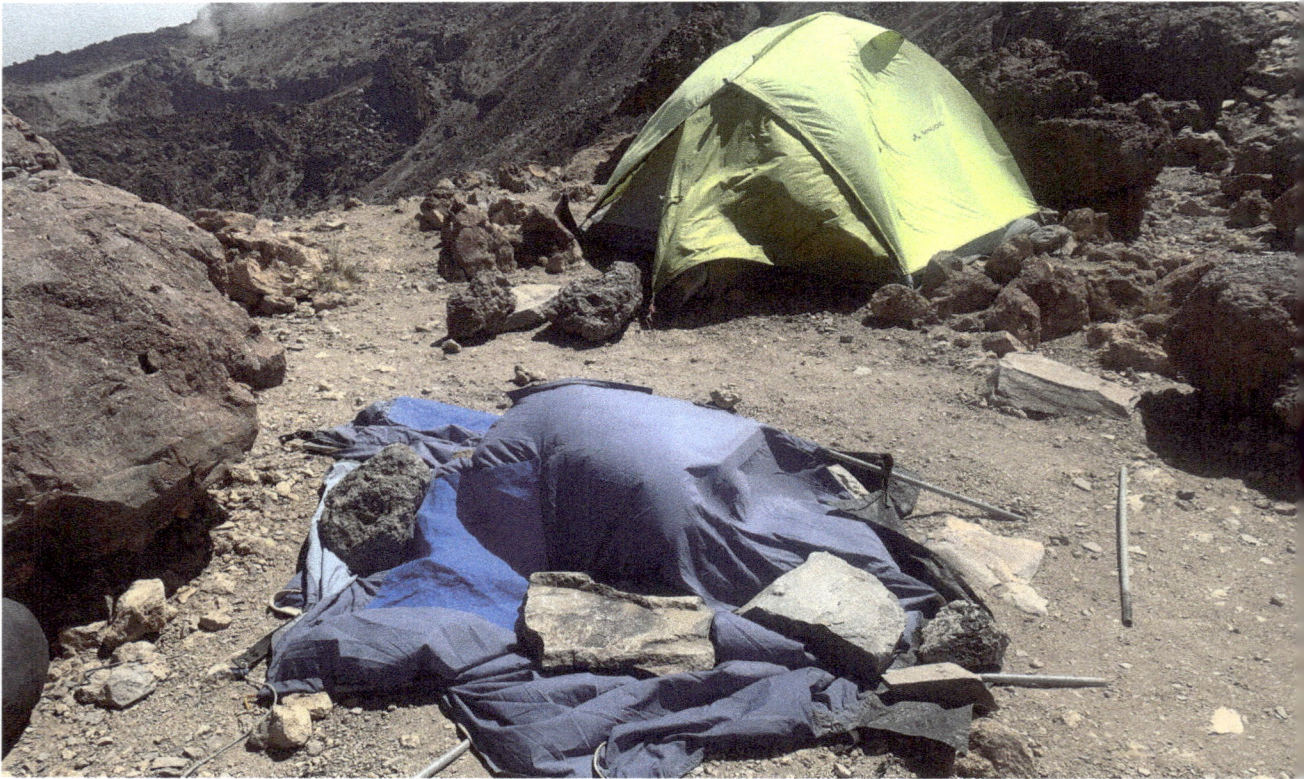

Gone are the views and the amazing scenery; they've been replaced by a dense fog that blankets us in all directions. This is good, our guides tell us. 'No rain, no hot sun!'

There's no plant life as we climb; the landscape consists of rock and slate. It's like a moonscape. The higher we climb, the windier it gets. A couple of hours later we descend off a small ridge, now noticing the next obvious, large ridge in front of us. The final ascent to the ridgeline that takes us to Base Camp is well worn. Fine dust and small loose rocks make up the track surface, with larger rocks interlocked on both sides of the trail.

Finally, we come upon a rock on which sits a simple piece of brown timber with bold yellow letters that spell out 'Barafu Hut'. Barafu is a Swahili word meaning 'ice', and this is one of the final campsites we will rest at before summitting Mt Kilimanjaro.

Will tells us his headache has gone, but has been replaced with slight chest pain and shortness of breath. I too have to focus on breathing at various points. 'Pole, Pole' is a mantra we have embraced. I've got the walking sticks out for the first time to conserve whatever energy I can while still sporting my backpack.

'After an hour walking in the cold and wind from Karanga, I honestly thought I wasn't going to make it to the summit,' confesses Will. 'The climb feels like forever.'

We set out on the final climb amid increasing wind gusts. Clouds around the mountain have cleared, and we soon see shining white glaciers. The summit feels within reach.

The wind really howls, and porters who are descending the mountain tell our guides that some people couldn't summit yesterday because it was too windy. As we make our way to the registration office, the gusts get stronger: there are collapsed tents all over the place. Ours, although held down by rocks, shakes violently. Then the mess tent comes down, hitting the side of our tent with a scary thud. I don't know how our guides get it back up, but when they do it's mostly held down by boulders.

We have an early dinner, the idea being to get some sleep before getting up at 11pm. But with such violent winds flogging the tent sleep is impossible. After a brief rest we're layered-up in our summit gear, ready for whatever the mountain has in store for us.

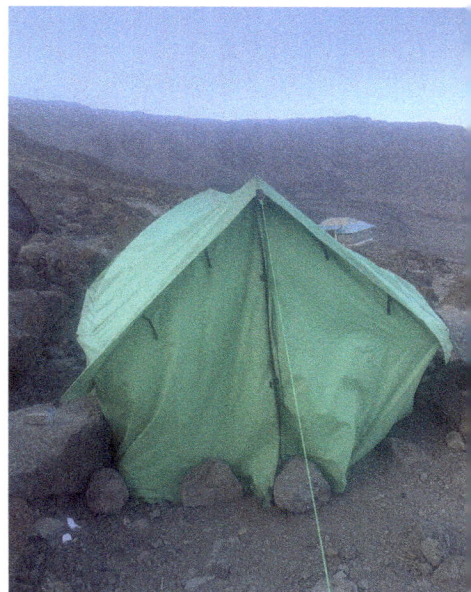

above Our dining tent, hanging on

opposite Wind, making its presence known

Day 6—Barafu Camp to Uhuru Peak (Summit) to Mweka Camp

4,673m amsl to 5,895m amsl

DISTANCE: 5km (7 hrs)

HABITAT: Stone scree and ice-capped summit

At 12:10am we leave camp under the flickering light of headlamps. In the distance are small dots of light from climbers who left before us, and within no time there are rows behind us. This is a popular mountain. It's an anticipated six-hour trek to the summit. Four people are already on their way down, which is a worry.

Rightly or wrongly, and although I've experienced some symptoms, I've opted not to take altitude sickness medication. I've decided that, with all the climbs I intend to do over the next couple of years, I'll see how my body adjusts.

But two hours in, I'm really struggling with nausea. Will says he is feeling the same. Our guides insist on taking my pack, as we have a long way to go. It's a fatiguing slog. I think about a friend who completed the climb and told me, 'Forget that you are strong or young while climbing, because that doesn't matter... what matters is staying positive.'

Before I have the summit in sight, I've hit another problem—strained breathing has given me a chest pain I can only liken to severe heartburn. I slow my pace, grumbling worries and doubts to myself and breaking from the others. For a moment I think I might pass out. Will presses on, and I'm humbled by his perseverance.

Joseph waits for me.

'Copy me,' he says. One foot after the other, I focus on the rhythm of his steps. Then I vomit. 'Don't worry, this is common.'

Just one foot in front of the other. It feels like a dance, and my breathing steadies with his pace. I'm starting to settle back into the climb. Joseph's carefree 'take it as it comes' attitude catches on.

We press on through howling wind and falling snow. The pain in my chest eases, and I know we're going to make it. The sky is clear at times as the sun rises, revealing sparkling glaciers.

Stella Point, at 5,756 metres, is located on the southern crater rim of Kibo, the tallest of Kilimanjaro's three peaks. This is the Arctic Zone of the mountain, a region with no rainfall, high winds, and sub-zero temperatures—the roof of Africa. From here it's about an hour to the summit. At the signage, two figures linger on the approach. It's Vale and Will. I find the sight of them both motivating and surprising at the

opposite, left

Giving thanks

opposite, right

Up here...

opposite, bottom

Where glaciers live

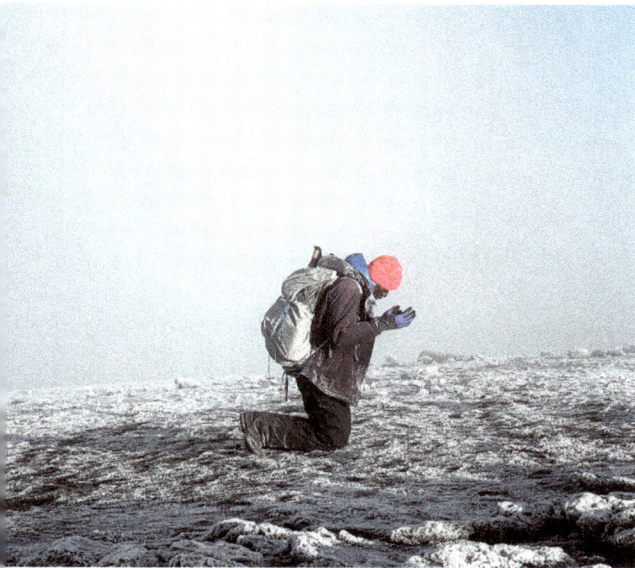
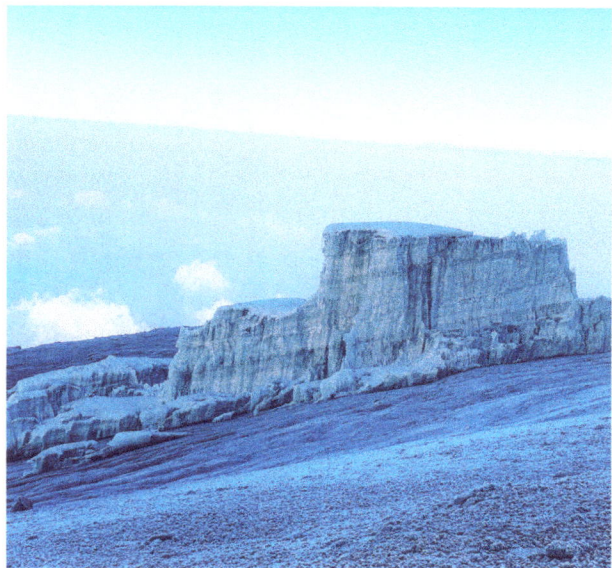
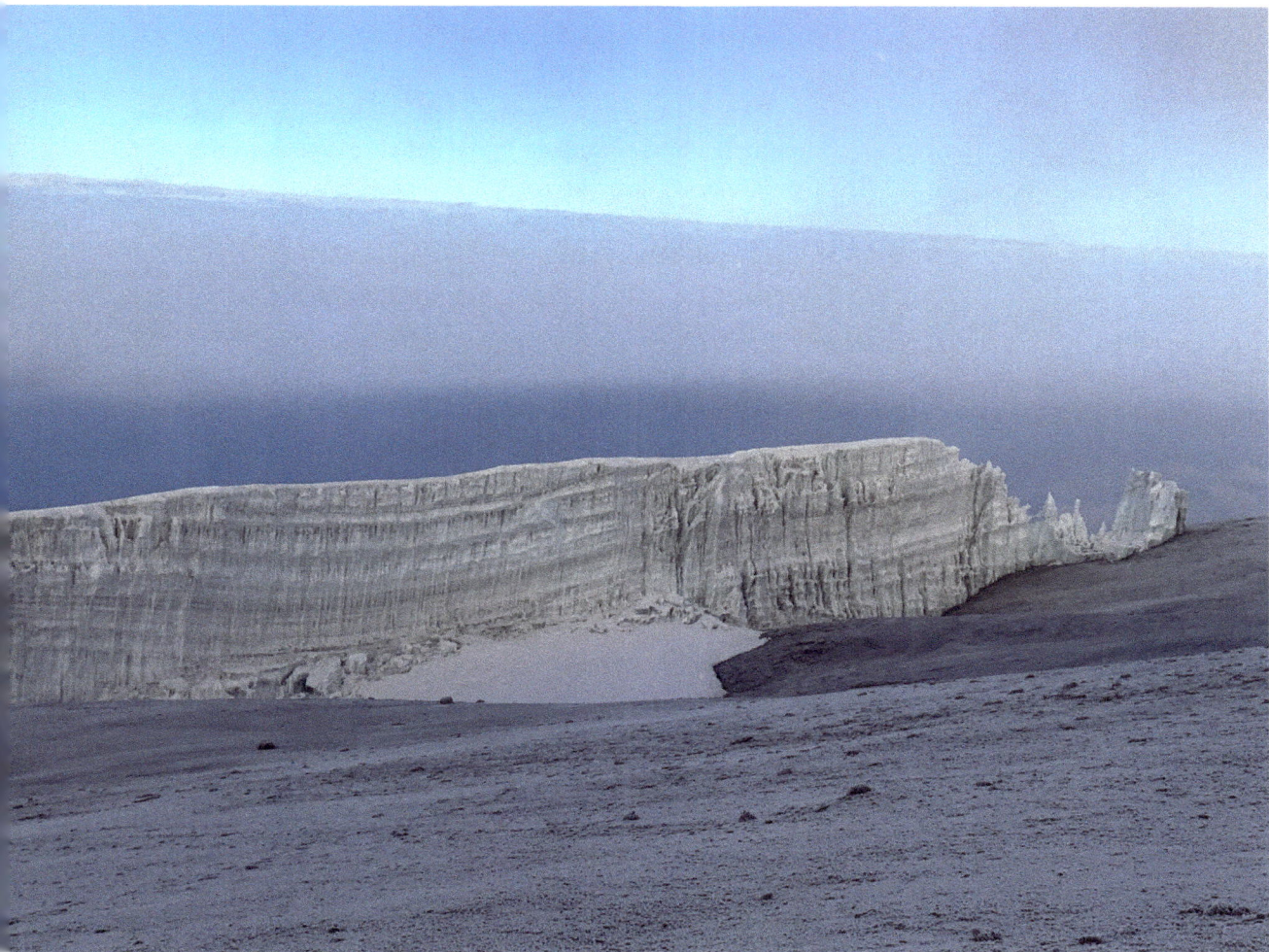

same time. The sun continues rising and with it the promise of warmth for the new day.

While we continue to climb, we pass guides assisting their altitude-affected clients as they descend.

'Just a little further,' and 'Good luck,' call the descending climbers.

opposite Our summit photo

As we approach ever closer, I see Joseph has deviated off the trail into the open fields of ice and snow. Curious, I watch as he drops to his knees, taking a private moment in prayer. Such respect for the mountain and gratitude for the safe passage.

Silent except for the crunching of the ice beneath my steps and the sounds of heavy breathing, I'm in awe, my attention on the dramatic glaciers that surround us.

Summit

In 1889 German geographer Hans Meyer and Austrian mountain climber Ludwig Purtscheller took about six weeks to summit Mt Kilimanjaro. They were the first to do so, and many others have followed.

Now Will and I have also reached the summit that was first conquered in 1889. I imagine the mountain appeared very different back then. Overjoyed and overwhelmed at the same time, my son and I stand on Kilimanjaro's summit, revelling in the simply spectacular panoramas around us.

'Africa's highest point—the world's highest freestanding mountain,' says Vale. Also one of the world's largest volcanoes.

This is the type of view one would expect from the comfort of an aircraft. But here we are in the frame. We stand in silence, staring around us, trying to process our arrival.

In my pack, secure in a clear ziplock bag, there's a precious item that's taken the whole journey with me and never left my side. Brand new, neatly folded with our supporters' logos freshly printed on it, is our flag—the Diabetes Australia flag.

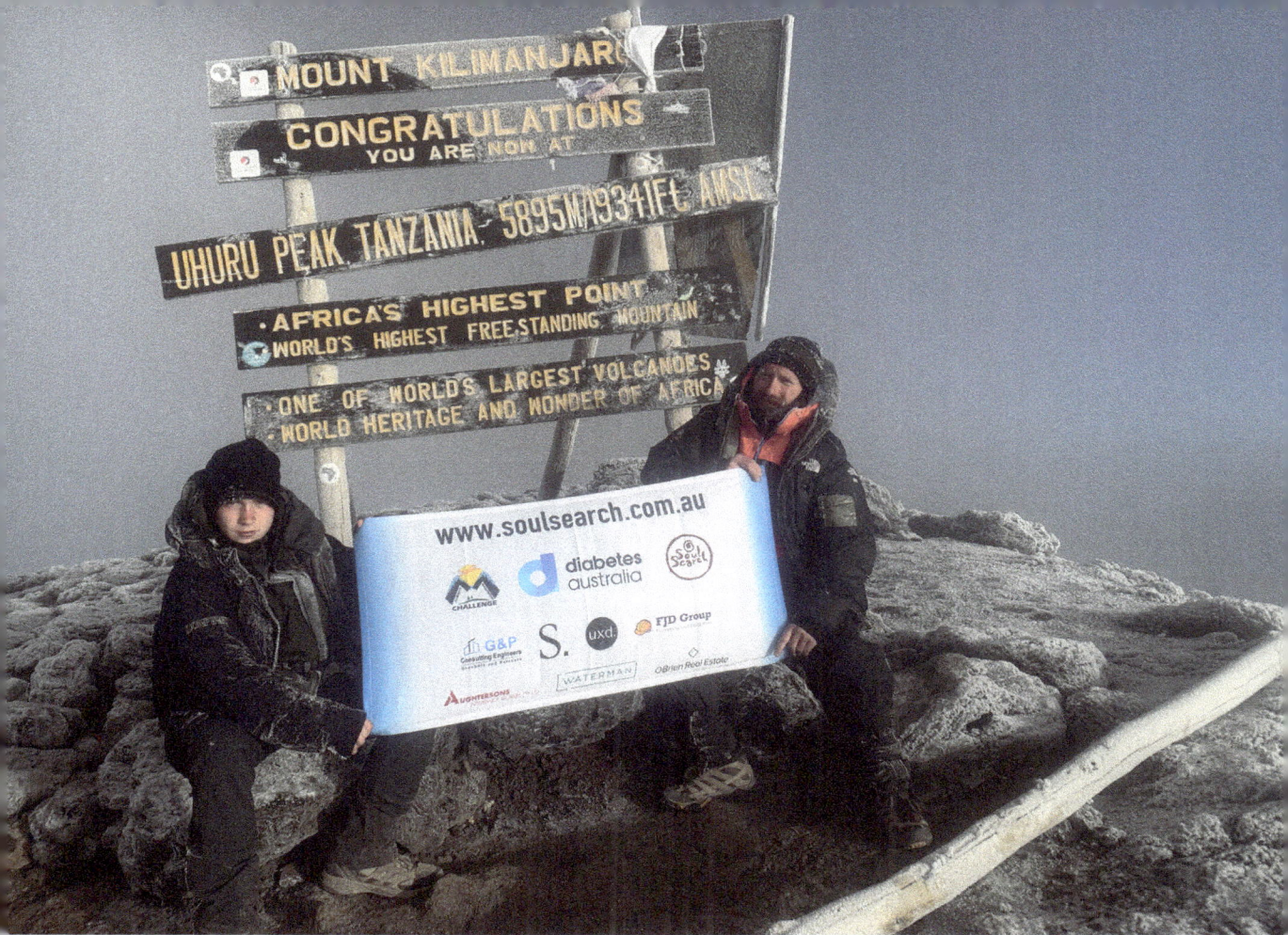

I take pride in unfolding the new fabric that symbolises our hopes and dreams of being here in the moment. We made it, and this proves it. Well, to me at least.

I feel a sense of achievement and relief. I can now relax.

The famous, jauntily angled summit sign that provides our backdrop is a permanent fixture. It's just rough-hewn planks of wood, but signifies more than an arrival point. Here, you have 'made it'. Flying the Diabetes Australia flag at this signpost becomes a high point as we snap pictures and our guides sign the flag. I share some chocolate, and we all share the moment. I'm so proud of Will. I can't believe we are here.

'Today was probably the most physically and mentally challenging thing I've ever done,' says Will.

I see his happiness and the pride in his achievement—not only for reaching the summit, but also for conquering himself and becoming a stronger person in the process.

Carefully, I fold the flag back into a neat shape and place it in the ziplock bag, ready for what comes next.

Uhuru Peak (summit) to Mweka Camp

5,895m amsl to 3,100m amsl

DISTANCE: 12km (6 hrs)

HABITAT: Stone scree

Our celebrations are short-lived; the weather is closing in, and we must descend. With a newfound energy, I throw my backpack on once more, lift my eyes to the horizon and am ready. It's time to get down.

We slog down the mountain, zig-zagging steadily through the loose scree to Barafu Hut Camp, at 4,673 metres, and rest for about an hour-and-a-half. Then we don our packs again for the trek to Mweka Camp at 3,100 metres—four long hours away.

I can feel my lungs labouring hard in the thin, cold air. We're exhausted, and at times I wonder how we're going to make it as we plod along. I have a new respect for the adventure we've undertaken. We've burnt up a huge amount of energy, and at times stop to reflect that we have to just keep moving.

The reality of the dangers of climbing this mountain seem to be around every corner: a woman who has pulmonary problems is being taken down on a stretcher. We enquire why the helicopter hasn't been called.

'No insurance, no money,' we're told.

We finally reach Mweka Camp, where it's time for some reflection, dinner, and the conclusion of our huge summit effort. Five major ecosystems have been transited en route to the summit, and the descent itself is an ecological experience of extremes. At the summit we experienced the Arctic

Zone, then we descended through loose dirt and gravel before we hit the Highland Desert Zone, with its oppressive sun and sub-zero temperatures. All this we experienced within the same day. When we hit the Heather and Moorland Zone, wild grasses and a rocky trail were the discreet signal of our return to air that was easier to breathe. Below us awaited the Rainforest Zone and Cultivation Zone.

At the end of the day, Will was reflective. 'I think the walk back down to camp was harder and longer than the hike up to the summit,' he says. 'Because of how sore and tired we are after only three hours' sleep the night before. Because of the wind, the massive climb, and now the last walk back, which took what felt like ages.'

Day 7—Mweka Camp to Mweka Gate

3,100m amsl to 1,800m amsl

DISTANCE: 10km (3 hrs)

HABITAT: Forest

The deep tiredness of yesterday has gone. The ordeal is viewed in a new, positive memory. I'm looking forward to sleeping in a proper bed tonight, albeit without the absolutely breathtaking nature of the past nights.

It's a quick pace off the mountain, the final trek. Not because there's any sense of urgency, but rather because the legs feel great, the air is easy to breathe, and the track is relatively flat compared to the rocky landscapes of the last week. The flora and fauna are diverse, with ancient trees draped in moss rising majestically from the forest floor. Smooth, compacted trails once again support their travellers and bring them back to the beginning.

We say goodbye to our amazing guides, who made our climb possible. I trust Vale will distribute the tips appropriately to every person in the team—to each and every one of them we are so grateful. They have a parting gift—all ten of our newfound friends sing, clap and celebrate our successful climb. Pure joy and happiness exists in this moment, and the memory will remain long after we leave.

Looking dirty, and smelling worse, there's no indication that we are two novices when we finally descend the mountain. In fact, we look like any hardened mountaineers upon their return from a summit. For Will and me, our next adventure is a safari. For Vale, Joseph and his team, in a few days' time they'll be back on the trek to Mt Kilimanjaro with new guests. What a crucial factor they all were in our success.

In total we completed approximately forty-one hours of walking over sixty-three kilometres, and summited Africa's highest mountain. There's an eighty-five per cent success rate for the seven-day Machame route, and only a fifty-five per cent success rate for the six-day climb, which we chose to undertake. I now know why, and believe our time was just enough to acclimatise and, with good support, accomplish our goal.

Back in the hotel room in Moshi, where we started exactly a week ago, Will grabs his phone. 'It's good to have some wi-fi, catch up with the world, and sleep in a real bed,' he sighs. I'm content to call home and hear some familiar voices. To listen to Heidi and hear about the challenges in her routine, the stories the kids have been waiting to tell me, and the usual chaos that happens within the four walls we call home.

Our leisure time has been a chance for self-reflection as individuals, and for cultivating the important relationship between a father and son, and that of our family. Happiness exists forever in these memories.

BACK AT home in Melbourne, I found the kids camping in a tee-pee erected among the toys littering our messy lounge room. Tucked in among the many blankets was Fin, now six years old and preparing to go away on diabetes camp. (Although at camp we would have rooms with bunk beds, not tee-pees, which would make things easier.)

The camp we were about to attend was run by Diabetes Camps Victoria. These camps are conducted in a private rural setting and designed to help a small child accept their diabetes diagnosis and begin to make progress with its management. It might be difficult to understand how a weekend camp can do this, but over two days a team of educators and professionals achieved progress with the management of Fin's diabetes that I would not have believed possible had I not witnessed it all unfold.

After having many, many reservations about even attending the camp, on day one a beaming Fin proudly held up a pink star cut-out that read, 'I did my injection for the first time—Finlay.' She got to stick it on the board, front and centre of the room, with everyone else's achievement star.

There were also other, more enjoyable activities at the camp, such as patting reptiles and holding snakes. A small crocodile sparked curiosity. Face painting provided the chance to be a vampire. And of course there was lots of education on diabetes and its management. The whole supported program has an emphasis on independence through adventure, and it's an environment of increased freedom that's contagious. The weekend concluded with a chance visit with superheros, complete with a *The Incredibles* themed dress-up party.

At the camp Fin felt she was part of something exclusive as she danced away at the party, yet was humbled by how many other people are living with type 1 diabetes. There are 134,000 people living with the disease in Australia, but until she went on this camp, Fin had not met a single one.

The camp was also vitally important for parents. While we were excluded from most activities, we were invited to discuss parental challenges in a group setting. I've never met a group with such deep-rooted issues that all relate to a single cause—in this case type 1 diabetic children. Diabetes management is 24/7. You never have a day off, let alone an hour. Those days can feel really long when your child isn't well. Every single parent at that camp had a degree of mental health decline at some point. It was a heartbreaking session to take part in, and without a cure there were no real solutions.

I sought permission to tell the kids I was going to climb a mountain, and asked if any of them wanted to draw on my next summit flag. Nearly every single one of them traced their hand and wrote their name. It's all these little moments that add up to mean something—with all those little handprints on my flag, I couldn't not make the next summit.

Arriving home from our first diabetes camp, I was armed with new information and renewed enthusiasm to get on with the project. Every day there was a need to progress towards the goal in addition to the usual work and family commitments. There was so much planning I hadn't considered. More and more training was required. Considerations I hadn't even imagined came to my attention. I thought about the relatively small mountain I had summited, and how high Mt Everest is by comparison. To say I was as engrossed in reading as much as I could about the next six summits as I was about diabetes would be an understatement. But I wanted to raise more awareness and seek more partners and donors. Could this really work?

As well as preparing for my next mountaineering adventure, there was family life to maintain. Heidi and I have always made going away as a family an important priority. We chose to fit a family holiday into our chaotic routines before I headed to Russia, and took a chance to enjoy sunshine, beaches and laughter—our iconic Australian life.

But in preparation for the cold I was reading about, growing a beard seemed like a good idea.

opposite Embracing the real challenge

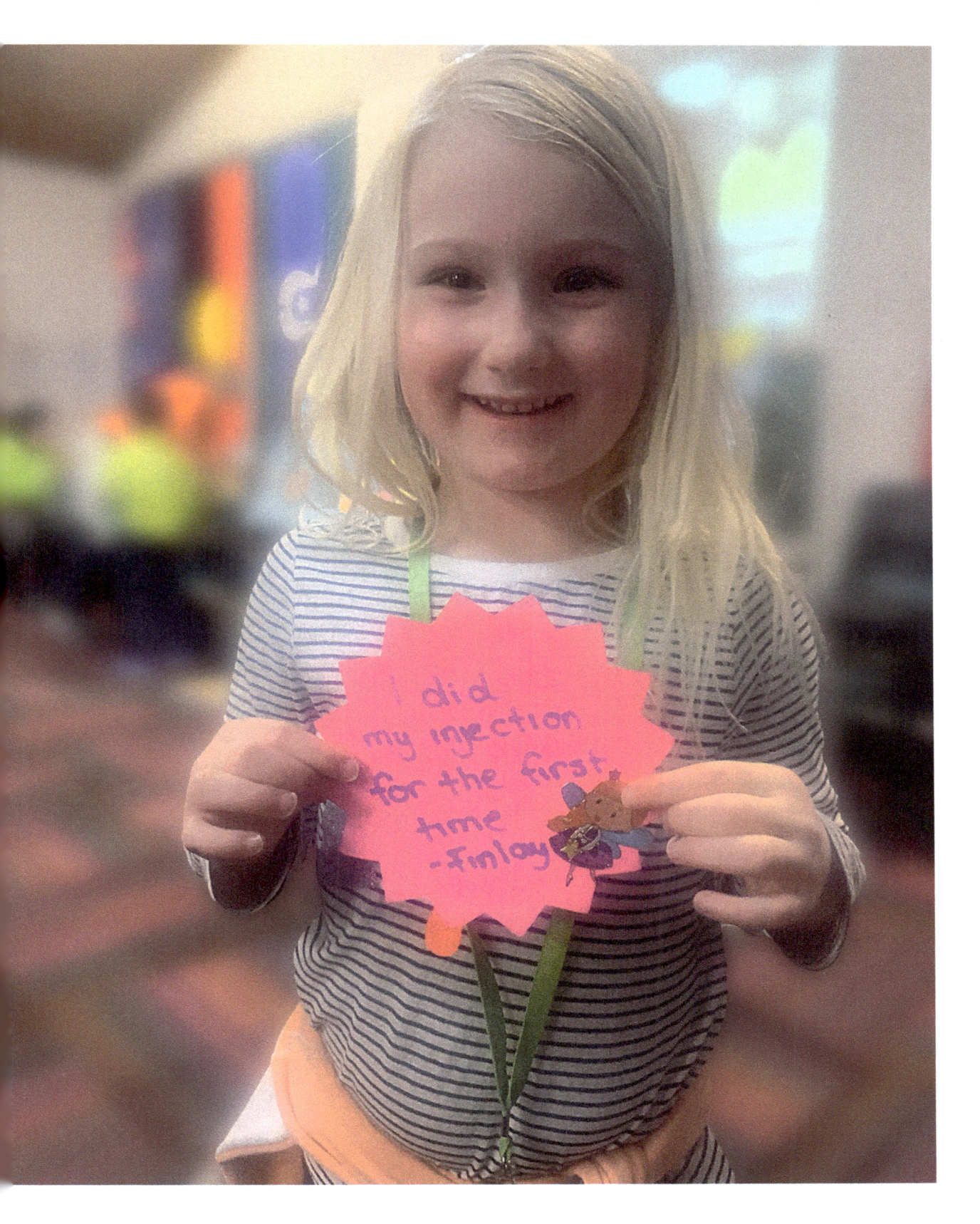

I did my injection for the first time
-Finlay

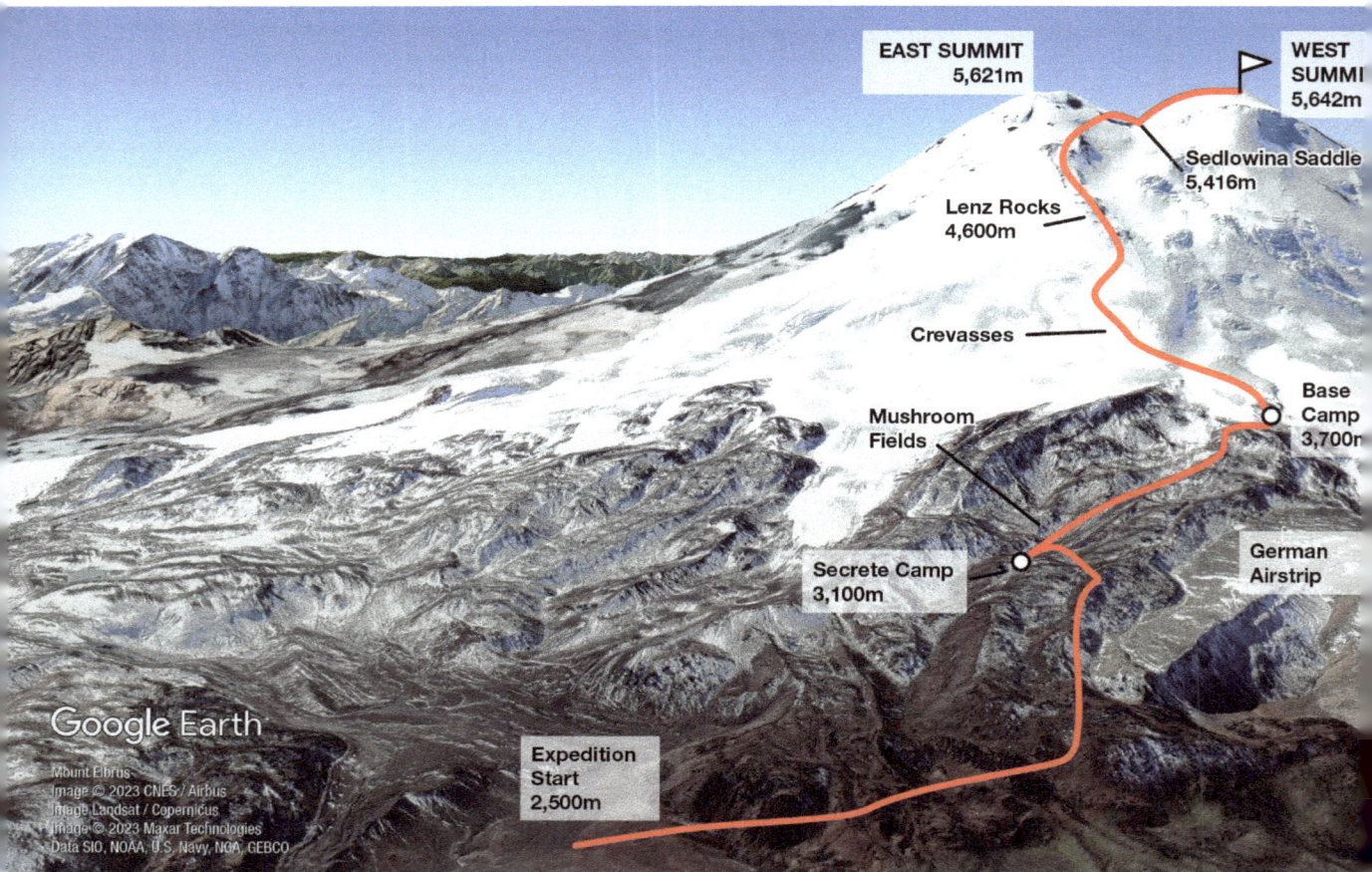

EAST SUMMIT
5,621m

WEST
SUMMI
5,642m

Sedlowina Saddle
5,416m

Lenz Rocks
4,600m

Crevasses

Base
Camp
3,700m

Mushroom
Fields

Secrete Camp
3,100m

German
Airstrip

Expedition
Start
2,500m

Google Earth

Mount Elbrus
Image © 2023 CNES / Airbus
Image Landsat / Copernicus
Image © 2023 Maxar Technologies
Data SIO, NOAA, U.S. Navy, NGA, GEBCO

MT ELBRUS

13,669km from Home

ELEVATION: 5,642m

COORDINATES:

N 43 35.265

E 42 43.895

ELBRUS

18 JULY—23 JULY 2019

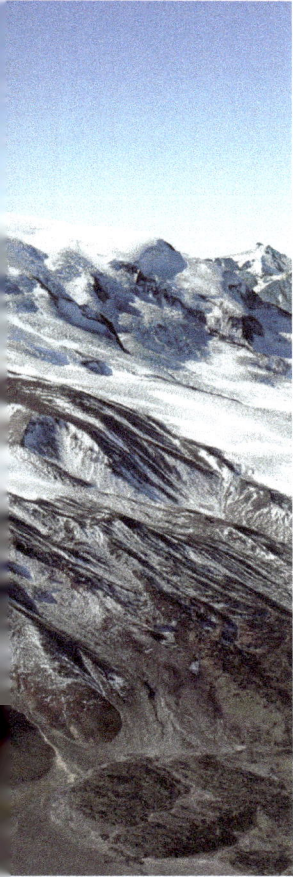

MY RUSSIAN EXPERIENCE starts at Melbourne Airport in my home state of Victoria. I'm seated next to a stocky Russian on a plane carrying me to Russia and Mt Elbrus, a dormant volcano in the Caucasus Mountains that is Europe's highest peak, and one of the coveted Seven Summits. Although said to be technically easier to climb than Mt Everest, the world's highest peak, Mt Elbrus has a higher death toll. On average, twenty-six people die trying to climb Elbrus every year. I'm also told that these 'official' figures are deliberately lowered, and in reality more than forty climbers die annually trying to tag the summit. It's sobering information, to say the least.

The language barrier between me and my new mate means we can barely communicate as we jet to Moscow, which is a fair indication of how this trip might unfold. He knows the word 'whisky' though, and keeps rattling his glass of ice, glaring at the flight attendant when she doesn't fill it as full as he'd like.

During the thirty-three-hour flight to Moscow I try to learn the Russian word for 'thank you', which might be handy over the upcoming weeks. My friend at least has that right in English. 'Whisky, thank you,' he says constantly. Landing in Domodedovo International Airport in Moscow, he shakes my hand and says, 'Thank you.' I don't know what for. He then proceeds to cram airline blankets into his bag before departing. Welcome to Russia.

opposite Yes,
it was 2019

Just getting a visa for entry into Russia was a challenging process, which required local assistance to obtain a 'voucher' for my upcoming climb and accommodation along the way. So I'm surprised it's an easy passage through customs, into the arrival hall, and then straight on to domestic transfers for the two-and-a-half-hour flight south to the smaller Mineralnye Vody Airport.

After disembarking I meet Alex, one of my guides. Athletic in appearance, Alex is around thirty with a youthful, clean-cut appearance. We soon set off for the two-hour drive to Kislovodsk, one of four spa cities in Stavropol Krai, a region in the southwest of Russia. I'm thankful Alex speaks English well. Although I've only just arrived in Russia, I sense that English isn't understood here much, let alone widely spoken.

'Find the joy in everything, everything will be enjoyable,' he offers.

Kislovodsk lies along the Podkumok River in the foothills of the Caucasus, a mountain system and region lying between the Black Sea to the west and the Caspian Sea to the east, and occupied by Russia, Georgia, Azerbaijan and Armenia. Founded in 1803 as a spa taking advantage of abundant local mineral springs, Kislovodsk is one of the largest health resorts in Russia, with seven springs and more than forty sanitoriums and rest homes. Its carbonaceous mineral water, narzan, is bottled and distributed throughout Russia. Alex tells me that Kislovodsk literally translates as 'sour waters', and its natural mineral springs are said to have medicinal powers.

The town is a popular place for Russians to retreat for some R & R. Clustered in a valley surrounded by towering mountains, it features some fine heritage buildings, hotels and spa resorts. The popular Kislovodsk Resort Park is one of Europe's largest man-made parks, Alex tells me as we make our way to my hotel.

I'm staying at a traditional Soviet hotel which, while it's stuck somewhere in the 1960s in terms of comfort and décor,

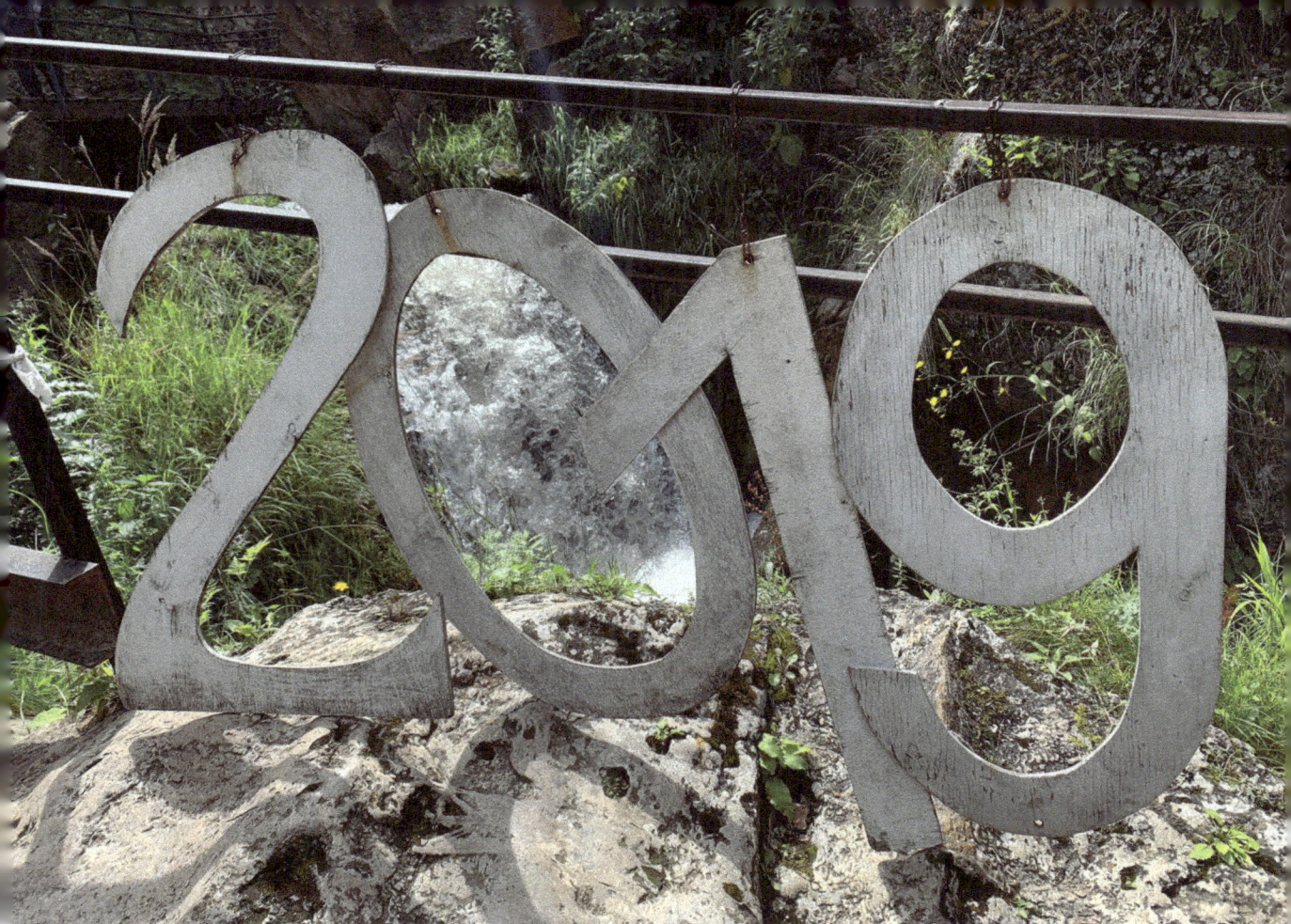

appears to be one of the nicer establishments—yet I note that my fellow climbers and our two guides aren't staying here. Checking in to any hotel in Russia requires an additional layer of compliance to register as a tourist. All nights in the country must be accounted for and a physical card must be stamped and signed off by the staff, which I've never heard of anywhere else until now.

After checking in, a jetlagged Alex re-joins me for dinner, which is a good thing. Without him, I'm not sure how I'll order from the restaurant's menu, of which I don't understand a single word, let alone symbol. After dinner it's time for an early night.

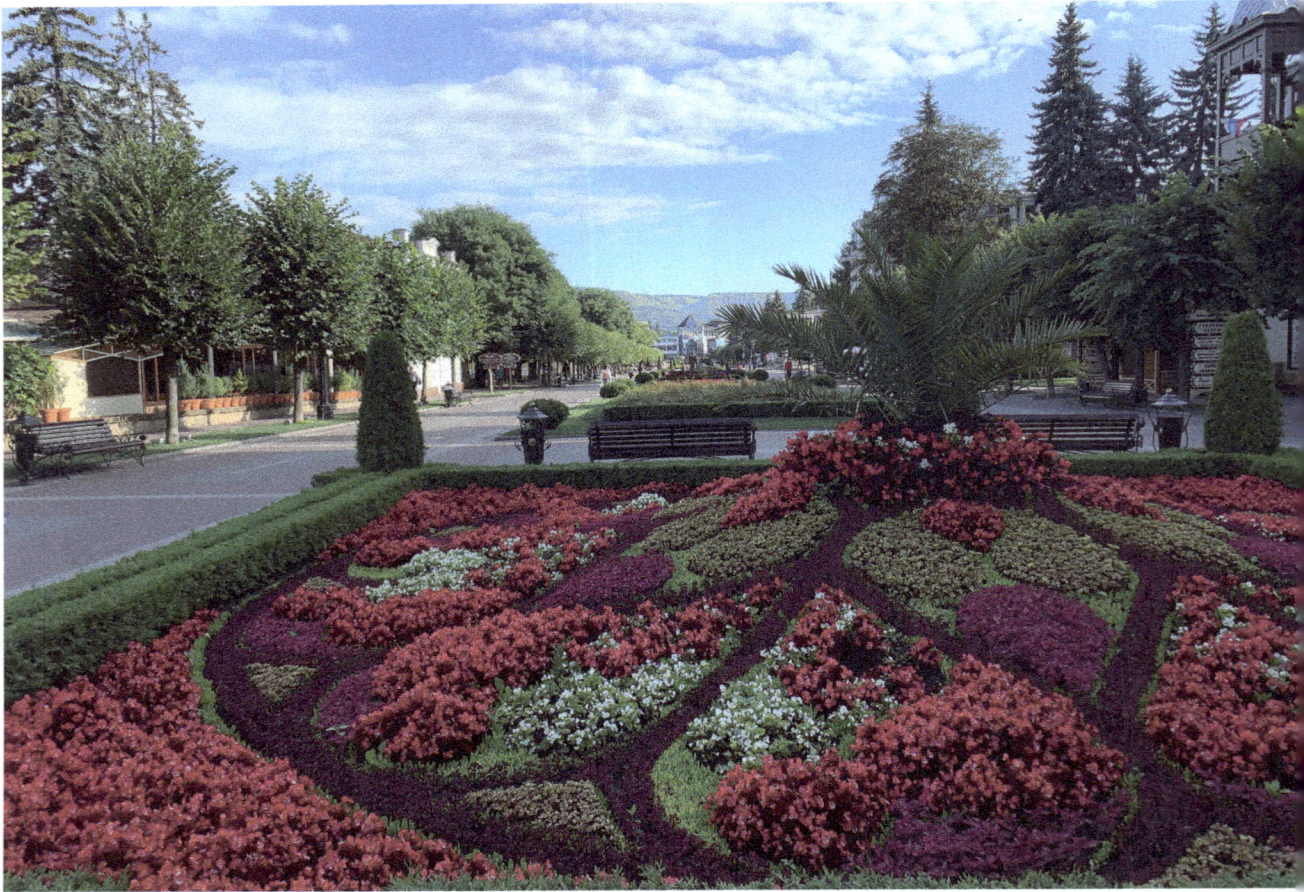

Sunrise is early here in mid-summer, and with light shining into the room by 5am I decide on a walk. The streets are quiet; there's almost no-one about. Heading along a boulevard of manicured gardens, I turn right, heading up a hill to give my legs a much-needed stretch following the long hours of cramped flying over the past few days.

Kislovodsk is all old-world charm, with numerous grand antique buildings, many with domes. Flower-filled planter boxes make vivid splashes of colour along the historic streets. But the further I walk from the town centre, the more the landscape changes. Buildings are more or less derelict, their grounds overgrown with tangles of weeds. While there are more military uniforms than citizens around at this early hour, people start to set up flower stalls and a few wait at bus stops. As I turn back to the hotel, I notice that the closer I get to the city's central area, the more evident are the efforts to keep this part of town in pristine condition for tourists.

Back at reception, I attempt a greeting before being gestured in the direction of the breakfast dining area. 'Good morning,' I say to a young waitress.

'Hello,' comes the reply, to my surprise.

'You speak English?'

'A little,' she says. Which ends our friendly exchange, and the first English I've heard since arriving in Russia other than talking with Alex.

The waitress is kind enough to explain that I'm eating a cottage cheese biscuit. It's a small, slightly sweet, folded biscuit, which I'm not sure I can finish.

I meet Alex in the foyer after breakfast and we set off for another walk around town. Alex proves to be quite knowledgeable about Russian and Soviet history, and gives me a discourse on the various monuments—from writers to war heroes—as we pass them. We venture deep into Kislovodsk Resort Park, which was founded in 1823 and covers around ten square kilometres of winding paths, flower gardens, woodlands and towering trees. I see a sign pointing to a monument with Mt Elbrus in the background, and, while it's quite a hike to reach it, I encourage Alex to trek to the top of a hill to gain our bearings. We soon find the statue and, on the horizon behind it, Mt Elbrus herself—the mountain I've come to Russia to climb, towering 5,462 metres in all her glory.

Snap. Photos done. I'm enjoying being a tourist. So much so that Alex and I almost miss our meeting with Vitaly, my guide from the local company I engaged for this climb, and assistant guide Katia. Vitaly speaks English; Katia doesn't.

'Time is precious, and there is much shopping to be done,' says Vitaly.

opposite Kislovodsk streets

After the shopping trip, Vitaly arrives to check my kit. He appears to be a strong character, and every bit the mountaineer. He speaks good English, which is a relief, albeit with a serious tone. He removes a couple of items from my backpack, and informs me that I'll be carrying my portion of food. And I'll need a better poncho, he says, as it's going to rain.

I'm overwhelmed by how much has to fit into one backpack. And it doesn't, even after many attempts. But there's simply no compromise when it comes to the Diabetes Australia flag, which is the only optional item I've managed to squeeze in. Eventually I rip the pack trying to attach crampons—snow spikes—to the outside. Time for bed; I'm getting nowhere.

Day 1—Kislovodsk to expedition start

The good side of exhaustion is sleeping well. Refreshed, I return to the previous night's failed packing operation. I start to pack, then re-pack, then lash what won't fit inside the backpack to the top and sides. It's very heavy.

For the first time since leaving home I contemplate my motives for this climb. Does Fin really want me to be out here, doing this? Does anyone else really matter or care? I review the route and look to the internet for some assurances. Instead, I find statistics of climbers who died trying to summit Mt Elbrus, and how she is considered a 'challenging' mountain.

Should I have stuck with the easier southern route, rather than the northern? Mt Elbrus's southern route is well supported, with hut accommodation, cable cars and snowmobiles. The northern route is more remote and demanding, and only has tented accommodation.

'Elbrus's north route is like an expedition; we take everything by ourselves,' says Vitaly.

Can I carry all this weight? My pack weighs thirty kilos.

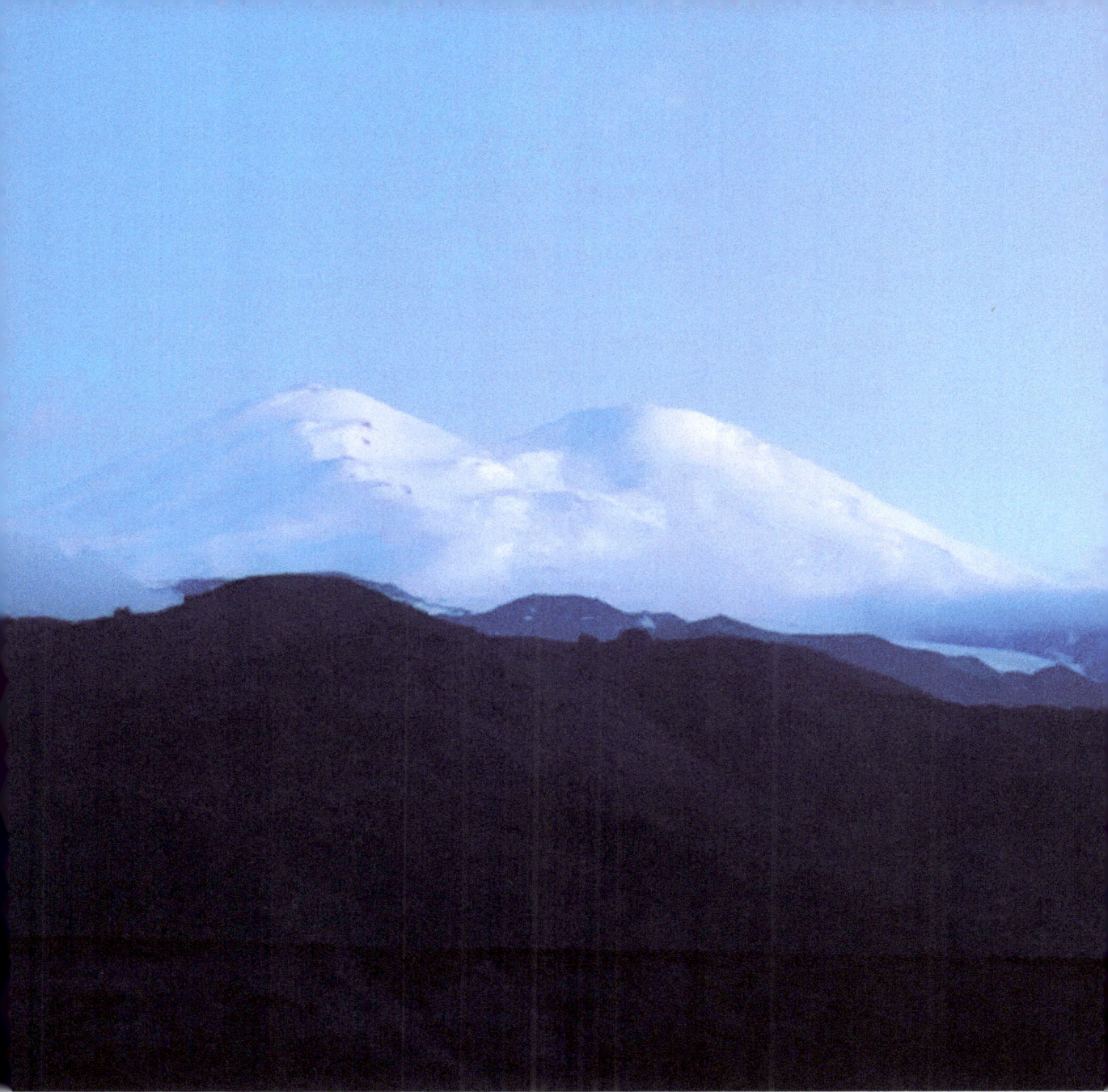

above Elbrus—north route

opposite Start crossing

It's time to leave. Waiting for us outside the hotel are three ageing vans loaded with gear to transport our group of ten to the Mt Elbrus drop-off area. Introductions to my seven fellow climbers and crew are brief, given the absence of English and the fact they're all Russian. They are, however, patient in the exchanges. It's hard to assess appearances without knowing what people are saying, but I think it's how they look me in the eye that feels genuine.

Two women are in the mix: a fellow climber called Valiko, and Katia, an assistant guide. I'm also introduced to Dimitry, who simply nods and then walks off. Two of the other guys are large in stature and dressed in camo gear. I assume they're rather patriotic. Another sways casually. Has he already been drinking? Is this a timely vacation for these guys or a training mission? No-one in the group smiles—at all—and instead maintain concentrated expressions. This shall be interesting. But at least they chat away among themselves, which I take as a positive sign.

The road out of town isn't well maintained; much of it is breaking up, causing us to ride every bump in a low level of comfort. And jolting along the potholed road isn't my only concern in this ageing van—the second van we're travelling with has to stop for a while because it's overheating.

The road's worn surface soon improves though, and we make better time on the four-hour journey to the mountain's northern foot. The lush foothills of the lower Caucasus provide stunning scenery as the van weaves and climbs along the road that's carved into the edge of the mountains.

We pause for lunch at a small restaurant in the middle of nowhere before arriving at the parking area for Mt Elbrus, at 2,500 metres. There are some basic buildings here, and the surrounding area looks like a semi-permanent campsite. Locals go about their business and the odd campfire smokes away unattended. Somehow I'm shuffled into a group photo. Judging by the commotion this causes, I must be something of a novelty.

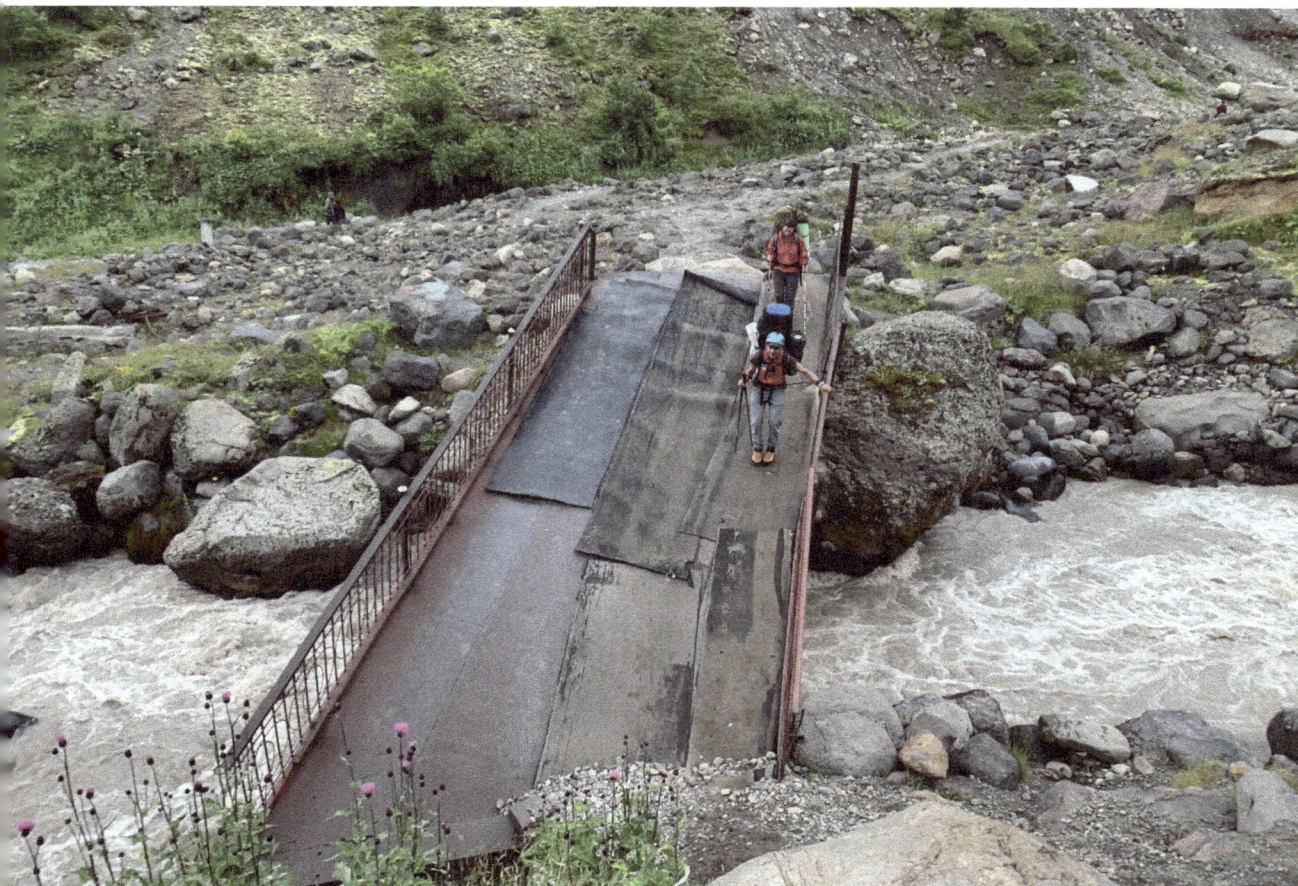

Our backpacks are retrieved from the vehicle, then the food and tents. Additional weight is evenly distributed. My backpack can take no more, yet I still have food supplies to carry, and it's not a small amount. I give up on lashing anything else to the outside of my pack and find a plastic bag with handles to carry my portion of food. My pack is now ripping at the top, and seams I previously couldn't see are now quite wide, presenting a potential problem.

Heave ho—it's time to saddle up with my heavy load and head off for an acclimatisation hike. Within an hour though, while heading up a ridge, I experience a sharp, shooting pain on top of my right glute. I guess my body is complaining about all the weight I'm carrying.

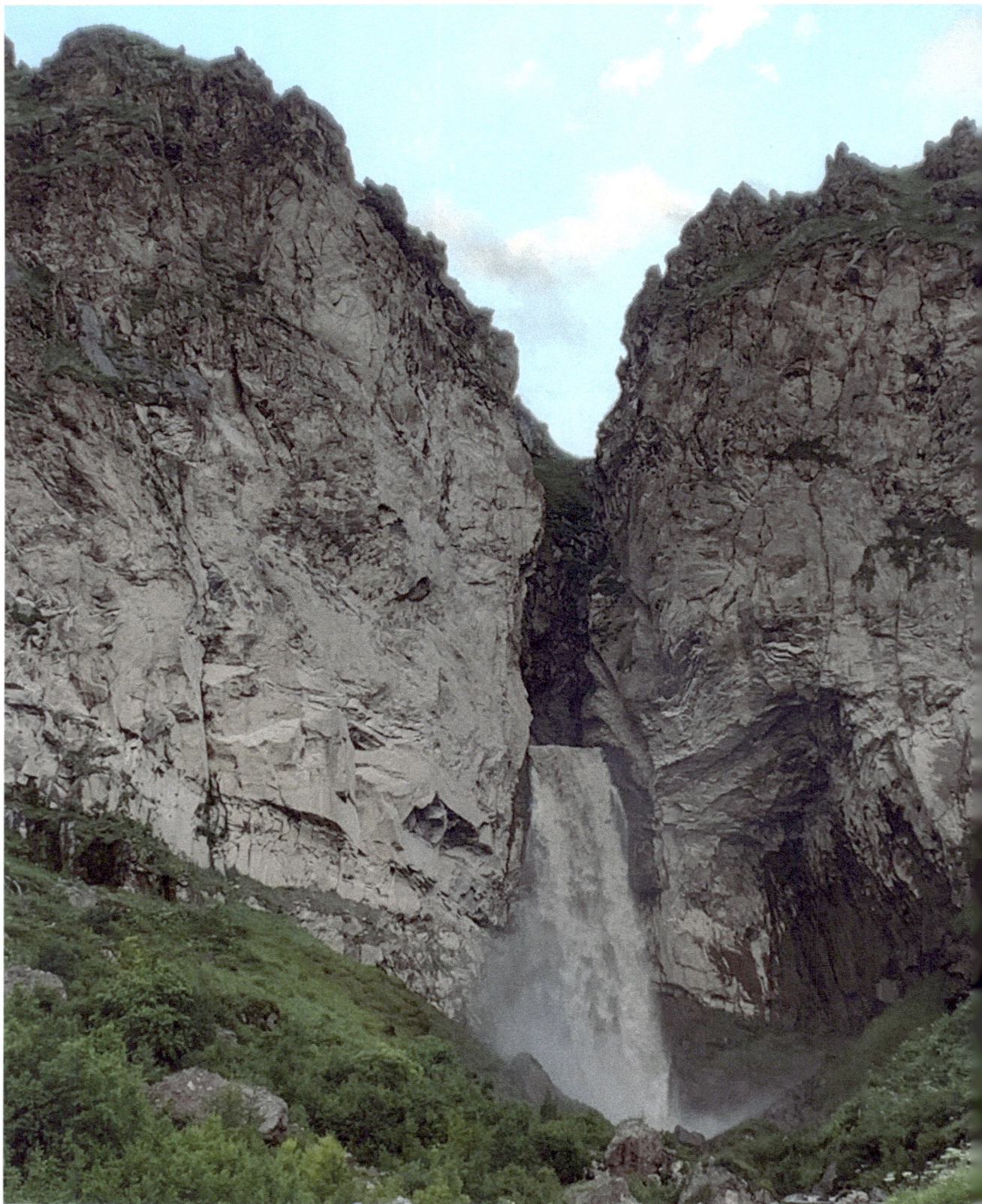

The skies clear of cloud as we round the top of a hill, and Elbrus looms into view in all her towering splendour. We're lucky, says Vitaly, because last time he passed through it never stopped raining. I stop walking with the group, pausing when the clouds disperse to give me the best photo opportunities. Although night is upon us when we finally return to camp, it was worth every shot. I've travelled so far to see this beauty.

Dinner is very simple—a piece of bread with crackers and cheese, and a cup of tea. I'm very glad I brought some nuts.

I'm sleeping in a two-man tent with one other gent, who is already asleep. And there's a problem—my inflatable mattress is dead flat, and attempts to inflate it in the tiny tent with a snoring tent-mate fail. I'll be on the hard ground tonight.

opposite Always looking up

Day 2—Expedition start to Vitaly's 'Secret Camp'

After an uncomfortable night I'm first up, keen to see if there's any visibility from camp as it's already light at 4:30 am. I scramble to get the GoPro camera set up as daylight glitters across snow-covered peaks. I love this quiet time of the day when the sunrise greets me. It's so peaceful. The camp soon stirs to life though and, as I start getting my backpack sorted, my body aches in anticipation of shouldering the load. Breakfast is simple: porridge, followed by bread with cheese and salami.

Packs are soon on and we make tracks. As we trudge uphill, Vitaly informs me that one of our fellow trekkers is Dmitry Yarovov, a renowned Russian artist, who is going to paint a picture on the summit.

With the approaching hill climbs, I decide to press towards the front; hills are something I do well. The mountain has two almost identical peaks: the west summit at 5,642 metres and the east summit at 5,621 metres. Trudging along under the weight of my backpack I contemplate that, without it, maybe— just maybe—I could attempt the double summit. Then again, maybe the altitude is doing something to my brain.

The benefit of arriving somewhere first is additional rest time while the others catch up. I settle onto a nice rock, survey the area, and watch the conga line of fellow climbers approach.

Vitaly soon arrives and we turn off the track to what he calls his secret campsite, which involves scaling another hill through a jumble of volcanic rocks. We weave across the rocks to a small clearing, and at last I can dump my burdensome pack. But happiness is short-lived; it starts to rain, and I'm a man without a tent.

opposite The biggest of mushrooms

Others soon arrive and proceed to set up tents. I wait for my tent-mates to arrive; I've already chosen our spot. I'm told there will now be three of us sharing a small tent.

'This is your new family,' says Vitaly. 'It will be warmer,' he adds.

Two rather large gentlemen present themselves before me. They stand side by side, waiting for something. Given their size, I can guarantee there will not be a spare inch of room in that tent. There will also be no smiling.

With the tent raised, it's time for a rest, but it's not easy as sonorous snoring begins to emanate from the gentleman beside me almost immediately. Adding to the cacophony, thunder starts to roll across the mountains and the rain shows no signs of easing up.

Hours later the rain finally stops, and we prepare for another acclimatisation walk. Vitaly decides this will also be a gear drop.

We trek under clear, sunny skies across what are called the mushroom fields. The fields are strewn with massive boulders, the tops of which stay intact while underneath the rock deteriorates at a faster rate, causing a stem-like feature to emerge and hence the name.

Dense fog rolls in, followed by rain, then wind, and in no time I'm completely drenched. Our trek is cut short at the base of a rock wall we were supposed to scale. Instead, we

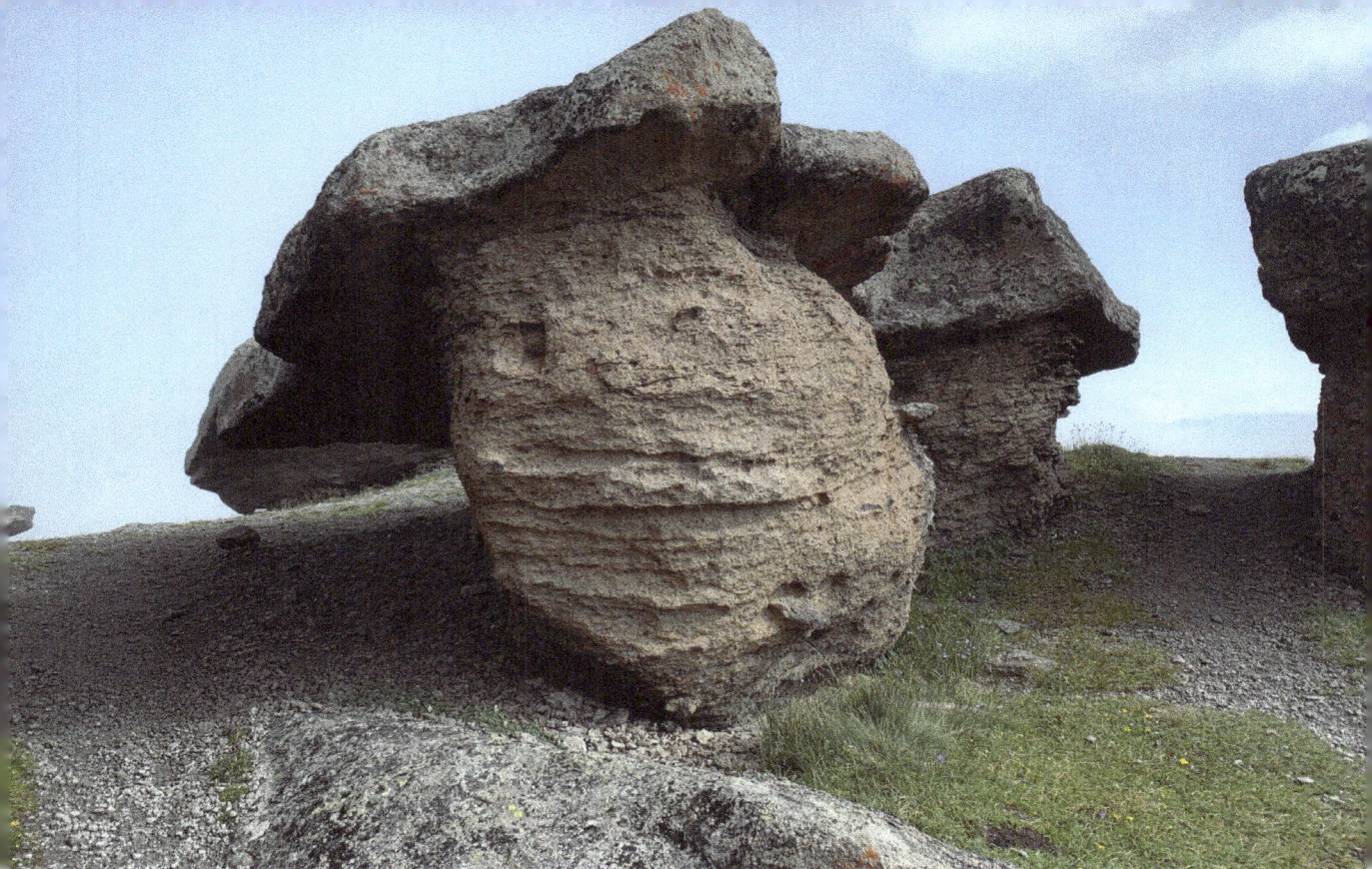

stash crampons, climbing gear and heavy boots beneath some boulders and head back to camp.

Back at camp everything is wet, and fresh ice has piled up against the tent from a freezing hailstorm. I'm offered what Vitaly calls 'Siberian cognac'. It's vodka infused with 'golden root'—the Siberian herb Rhodiola rosea, said to promote energy, stamina and longevity. I drink it because I'm cold.

The rain starts again, and everyone seeks refuge in their tents. Dinner is a bowl of soup and crackers—well short of what I'd consider a square meal. Water is gathering in the corners of our tent, and our sleeping bags are wet. My tent-mates start snoring as soon as I lie down on my uninflated inflatable mattress. Where's the Siberian cognac?

Day 3—Secret Camp to Base Camp

It rains all night, and water has penetrated our tent. Vitaly is right; it is warmer with three of us.

I'm up at 4:30am and disturb the peace by crunching around camp through loose gravel. The mountain is clouded over but soon clears, and everything from boots to bedding is sprawled across nearby rocks in anticipation of some sunshine.

Fresh water is abundant via a free-flowing spring near our camp. The suggestion I purify the water before drinking is met with confusion by my party members. Why would I even suggest it?

'This is mountain water,' they say, looking bewildered.

Re-packing is a process. First, you have to find everything, then re-pack this into dry bags, then get your food allocation and pack that too. On this occasion I offer to carry some tent poles as well, as I now don't have the added weight of the gear we dropped yesterday.

The group is in high spirits as we head back the way we ventured yesterday, up to the mushroom fields. In contrast to yesterday's bleak skies, the morning sun is on us and morale is high. Everyone is climbing and laughing and taking photos. There are twenty-two glaciers around Mt Elbrus, and the scenery is stunning.

I climb up on the boulders, the sun on my face, and enjoy the outlook from the mushroom field. Like a child taking to exploring for the first time, I climb higher, jumping between the mushroom-shaped boulders and crouching under them. I find a lot to enjoy in these simple rock formations. I think of Fin and the unfettered joy that comes naturally to a small child.

Then the fun stops. After re-attaching my stowed gear to my load, I strain under the weight. When I said I'd carry the tent poles, I didn't realise that there would be several rock faces to scale in the next two sections of the climb. My back twinges and my calves feel every bit of the added kilos. I wonder if

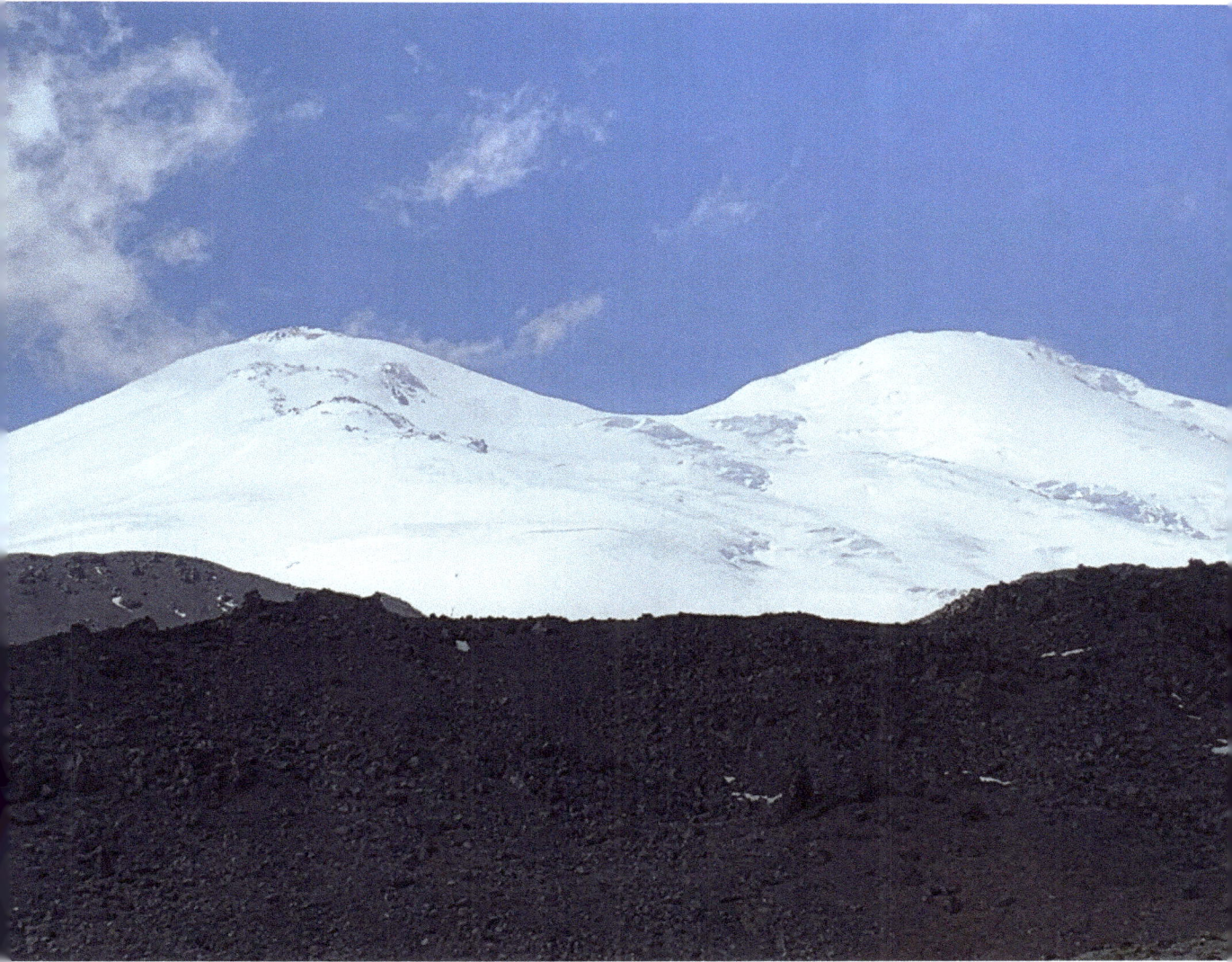

above The distracting view

the shoulder straps will hold; I know I'm well over the weight limits for this backpack. It's a tough climb and, hunched over, I will myself to push forward, step by step. I try all the self-motivation I can muster as I struggle on behind Vitaly.

'We rest here?' I ask.

'No, up there,' he replies as I contemplate the dead weight on my shoulders.

Before long, two more members of our group join us. We climb higher, and soon can dump our burdens. It's a good half hour before everyone else starts arriving, which makes for a decent rest, though now we must press on to camp, up and over another rock section, and this time traversing snow as well.

Briefly out of the snow, with wet boots, I slip on a rock and slam my knee and elbow as the full weight of the backpack thuds against me. I grit my teeth and curse myself. Could this happen at a worse time? My knee aches. But it could be worse, I suppose; nothing is broken. I slow my pace, and take extra care scaling jagged rocks and tramping through the snow.

Nobody is in sight now. I'm sure they would have come in this direction, but I've lost the track. I step carefully. There are still rocks to scale. Where did everyone go? Eventually one of the guys doubles back to point me in the direction of camp. I'm thrilled at the idea of getting this pack off my back. Base Camp, at 3,700 metres, can't come soon enough, and my back yells at me to hurry up while my shoulders cry.

I think this is it.

'Welcome to Base Camp,' Vitaly confirms.

Doesn't look like much of a campsite. Just a couple of big rocks separating what could be some areas big enough for a tent. Maybe. Vitaly and I throw up the main tent, and he helps me level an area for our sleeping tent. What our platform lacks in space it makes up for with spectacular views of Elbrus. We're on the edge of the snow line, so from here on we climb with crampons.

The toilet situation here involves finding a rock big enough to crouch behind in the surrounding area, and a rock small enough to stop any toilet paper blowing around. Nature will take care of the rest. Sanitary facilities are clearly an issue here.

Trying to blow up my mattress again—in vain—I find the hole. In my misguided wisdom, to save on weight, I didn't bring a repair kit. So I stick on a Band-Aid and hope for the best.

Our lunch is a piece of bread, torn off a cob loaf, two small cheeses, and a slice of unidentified meat washed down with a cup of tea. It's not enough for my hunger, but everyone's portions are equal. And I wouldn't want to carry any more weight for the minor complaint.

Vitaly delivers a briefing in Russian, then provides a quick translation to bring me up to speed. At 5pm—in a couple of hours—we must be ready for an acclimatisation hike across the snow.

This hike turns out to be more of a lesson in crampon climbing, but first I have to work out how to get these things on. This is my first time in crampons, which are essentially metal plates with spikes that are fixed onto your boots. It's definitely a worthwhile exercise, albeit all delivered in Russian. The group spends time practising the 'rest step' and general team-line work that will be required. I try to make sense of the Russian language, to no avail, and can only copy the actions of others.

We climb slowly, which is a lot better than scaling rock hills with my loaded backpack. I'm also happy with my breathing, and the exercise itself feels achievable. Conserving energy in the long run seems to be the aim of the game.

Once we've reached the top of the intended rock line, an example is given on descending foot placement, in Russian, but I'm used as the example, so I get the concept.

Heading back down, Vitaly tells me he's happy with this group because we're all good descenders, which is important— he's had some plodders in other groups, he says. Shouting 'like this' as he completes the actions of a plodder is quite amusing. Or is it just the accent?

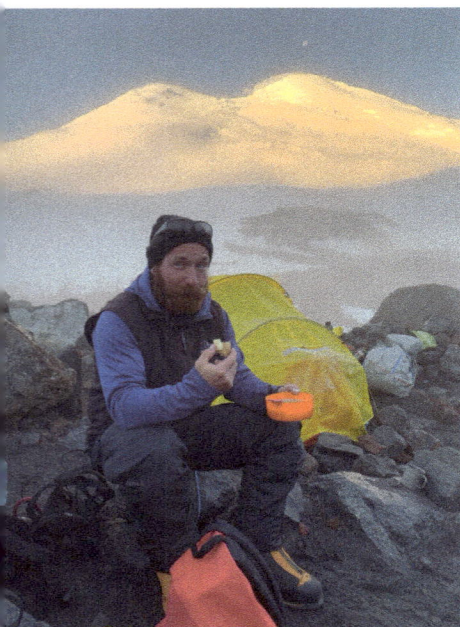

above Camp life

opposite Above
the clouds

Although all seems to be going well, the dangers of mountaineering are always present. I learn that seven people died, or went missing, presumed dead, trying to summit the week before we arrived.

'Keep an eye out for them,' I'm told. The information is chilling.

Thick fog closes in, and we head back to camp. Sitting outside in the light rain, dinner is soup, bread, a small piece of ham and a piece of garlic. My companions are certainly not big eaters, and I oblige by finishing any scraps.

Day 4—Base Camp to Lenz Rocks

It's 4am and everyone is up. I'm filthy that my Russian buddies have again snored and wriggled throughout the night. It's hard to adapt to being leaned on while trying to rest. As the sun appears over the horizon one of them yells to me to bring the camera over the ridge. Sunrise turns the clouds into a breathtaking kaleidoscope of colours. I set the GoPro and admire the view as my sleep-deprived self adjusts to a new day.

It's a rush to gobble down breakfast (porridge) and pack my backpack. In no time we have to leave and head off in single file for another acclimatisation hike, this one a six-hour stretch. Stops are brief, and the crampons tire the feet. After the first stop, Vitaly asks that I fall in behind him. Our pace is slightly faster, which divides the group over time.

Alex catches up with us for a while, and I enquire how everyone is going. 'Some are really struggling,' he says. I ask if it's because of altitude, and his answer is to the point: 'If you come to the mountain you must train. You cannot blame the altitude or say it's this only. You must be fit and prepared.'

Now high above the cloud line, I gaze out over the thick fog hovering below. The temperature is enough to warm me, and here I can take a jacket layer off.

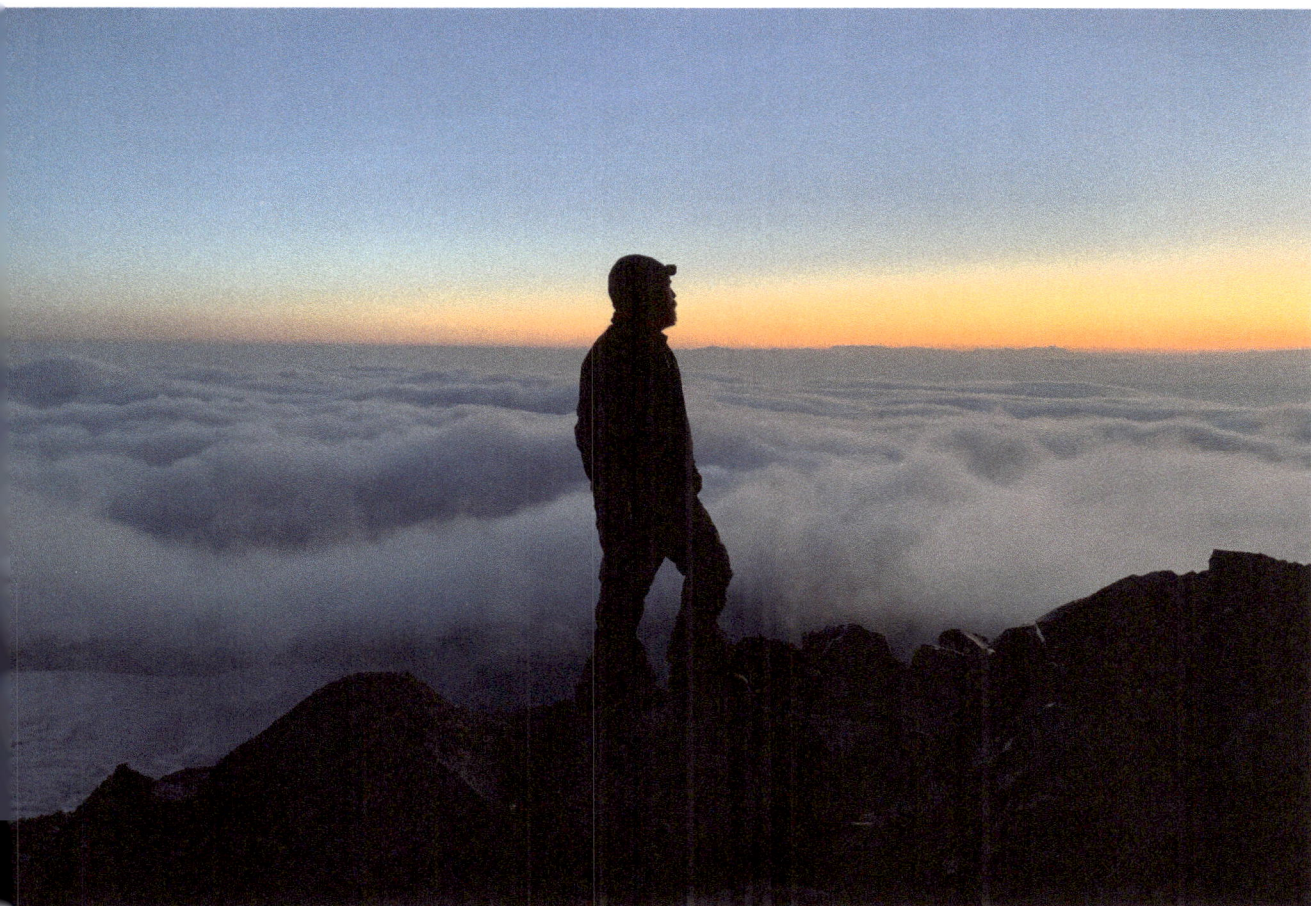

The mountain's highest camp, snow-covered Lenz Rocks at 4,600 metres, is the next welcome stop. We pause long enough for photos and some respite from the pack, but it only lasts until the group catches up. Then we press on. Lenz Rocks is the minimum acclimatisation for today, but as the weather is favourable we trek for another couple of hundred metres and rest for an hour or so to really breathe the air. For Dmitry, the artist, it's a chance to put a brush into action. We're all impressed.

Vitaly pulls me aside to offer some techniques in ice-traverse and descending. While we stomp around, he tells the story of a military helicopter that tried unsuccessfully to land here on the mountain. Apparently the military had to send Special Forces up here to dismantle and retrieve all the expensive hardware from the Mi-8 helicopter—hardware reportedly worth ten million dollars. It took more than a year before the fuselage was even able to be dismantled and evacuated by another helicopter, says Vitaly. The remains that either couldn't be retrieved or weren't valuable enough to warrant retrieval are still visible.

Heading back down the mountain, the continued downward impact leads to a blister on my big toe, taking the shine off an otherwise successful climb and descent. Every foot placement is now accompanied by pain. I contemplate the fact that, weather permitting, I could be going back up again in twelve hours with the blister. While the weather is favourable now, winds of up to fifty kilometres per hour are forecast in the morning.

Back at camp, it's become routine to dry out gear while the sun shines. If it's not wet from rain, it's being saturated from sweat. Changed gear, new batteries and an organised kit is required in case the weather turns and we have to descend in a hurry or, instead, we get the go-ahead to push for the summit.

Day 5—Summit

I've slept through my tent-mates' thunderous snoring and wake just before midnight feeling recharged for the task ahead. Thank goodness, as just getting dressed is a challenge—thermal leggings, fleeced outer hiking trousers, waterproof pants, thick mountaineering socks, two thermal tops, jumper, jacket, waterproof jacket, hat, gloves, goggles.

Today my tent companions have left the tent before me. Now I can look at this toe that is sore to the touch. All I can do is tape it up for now and delicately slip on a thick sock. On goes my inner boot, followed by my insulated technical mountaineering boot. Nothing to see here. Out of sight, out of mind. Hopefully.

I'm soon organised, it's just gone 12am, and it's time to hit the snow.

Strapping my crampons onto my boots, I take the first steps cautiously, waiting for the pain. It's a relief that everything feels normal in these initial steps. The ice is, however, harder underfoot with the night's lower temperature. To my surprise, this makes traversing just that little bit easier. When everything is going well my thoughts wander, time moves faster, and the distance builds behind us as we tramp through the snow.

Dmitry and I are right behind Vitaly on the ever-upward push. He says the next stop is 'The Rock', then falls back to assist the rest of the group while Dmitry and I press on. We're very pleased with ourselves, and take photos of an incredible sunrise beaming vividly across the horizon as we wait for the others. After a short rest I ask Vitaly if we can keep going.

'You must stay with the group,' is his sharp reply. But along the way the inevitable happens, and the group becomes two; Alex is now leading my tent buddies far below us.

Fellow mountaineer Valiko, who is climbing with our group, is tiring and she moves behind Vitaly. After retrieving my biggest jacket to reduce the cold exposure, I trek behind her to help shield her from the increasing wind gusts as we plod upwards. After climbing for about ten hours, I become concerned about Valiko. She seems exhausted, and there's a long way to go.

There's a planned stop to hydrate before our next push upwards. I try for a little conversation, 'Hey Vitaly, what's the name of this rock?'

'It's Nameless Rock!'

That is now its new nickname: the Nameless Rock. Joking about it lightens the mood.

The oxygen density in the air at 5,000 metres is half that of sea level. There are many stories of people who underestimate this and then suffer severe injuries or even die due to altitude sickness. Which brings home the magnitude of the challenge.

Against the howling, freezing wind, Vitaly makes an announcement—every person who has made it this far has, in his statistics, summited. It's a surprising comment. Maybe he can foresee that not everyone will make it the whole way?

The summit appears closer than it really is, although we're close enough to watch the dirty weather building and our visibility deteriorating. Vitaly's speech is good timing, as it brings me a sense of imminent success. I've been taking in carb bars, snacks and fluids every hour to ensure I've got something left in the tank when it counts—which is now. No altitude sickness, back pain or blisters will stop me now, and I'm raring to go.

The wind increases as we tackle the long slope to the top. Valiko is short-tethered to Vitaly, and everyone huddles close as we face violent winds and gusting snow. As we wait for more of the group to catch up, a blast of wind knocks Katia, one of the guides, to the ground.

Trudging along in single file, the tether-line inches closer to the summit. We struggle against unbelievably strong wind gusts, which force some of us to drop to their knees. Penetrating snow hits us like needles. My clothes are frozen and feel like they could snap in half.

The situation starts to deteriorate. Katia falls to the ground, and when I help her up I see she is having difficulty breathing. I grab her backpack and pull her to her feet, but she falls again. 'Up, up,' I shout, and up she gets.

I hear a yell from Vitaly—'One hundred metres to go!'—and feel that, while this will be touch-and-go with such ferocious weather, we might make it. I want to capture the summit on the GoPro, and try to set it up in the wild wind as the group inches forward.

Catching up with the group again, I see that many are getting blown about, some have been thrown over, and others are crouching near a rock to avoid the onslaught. Vitaly is now

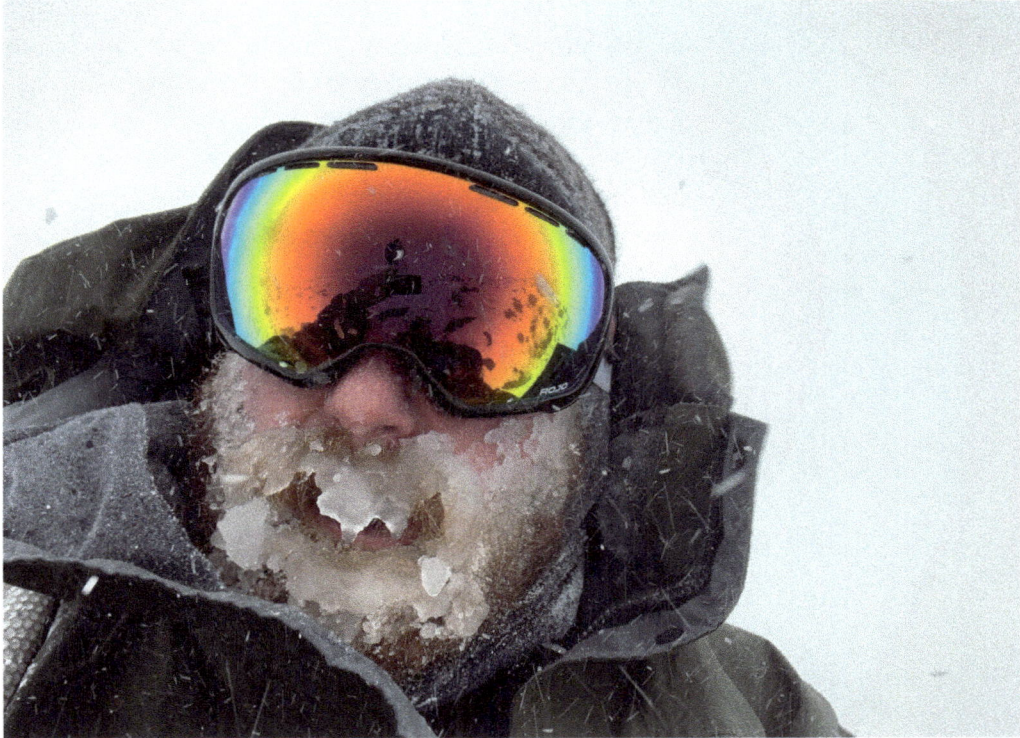

shouting constantly in Russian. Valiko slumps to the ground, unconscious. Vitaly proceeds to slap her face, and luckily she regains consciousness. I don't perceive the severity of the situation; it's later that Vitaly tells me that she was 'close to death, actually.'

The GoPro has died, and I'm now focused on putting it back in my pocket while inching forward amid the blasting winds. The snow feels like icy cold needles hitting my face.

Then I hear Vitaly yelling, 'Go David—it's just there!'

I plant one foot after the other, forcibly, deliberately stomping my way forward, upward towards my goal. I suck in the thin air through gritted teeth. I'm alone, yet it's far from quiet. The winds are howling past at a deafening pitch.

Ice is building on my cheeks, covering my beard. I can no longer breathe through my nose for the ice that fills my nostrils. Once, I look back, and everyone is gone. At least, I can't see them through the swirling snow. It's a whiteout, but the terrain ensures I know which way is up. Step by step, if I'm going up, I'm getting closer. That's my theory, anyway.

Peering through the driving snow I see the summit, and in a burst of energy—I don't know where it comes from—I aggressively stomp my way... one foot after the other... to the top.

I am alone on the summit. On hands and knees now, as there's nowhere further to climb. The relentless wind rips into my face. I'm here, I've done it.

Through the impossible visibility, Dmitry comes into view, dropping to the ground near me. I can't believe it at first. One moment there's nobody, nothing but the weather, then another human being arrives. No words are said; our beaming faces capture the moment. I'm elated.

Crouched on my knees, I wrestle off my backpack, which is almost ripped out of my grasp by the wind, and scratch around to find the Diabetes Australia flag. I peel it open against my backpack.

'To all the kids from the diabetes camp: stay strong, keep being awesome!'

All those little handprints have made it to the summit with me. As the wind threatens to snatch the flag out of my grasp, it's as if those hands are waving in triumph.

We're done. I wrestle the backpack on again as the wind tries to wrench it from me. The cover fly is ripped off and ricochets into the distance, lost. I have everything in that pack, and hang onto it for dear life amid the raging tempest.

We have to get off the summit, urgently, before we're blown off. The task ahead now seems perilous. While we compose ourselves to descend, a father and son team emerge from the whiteout to summit. We make our way over to them,

opposite Dmitry (Dema) makes the summit

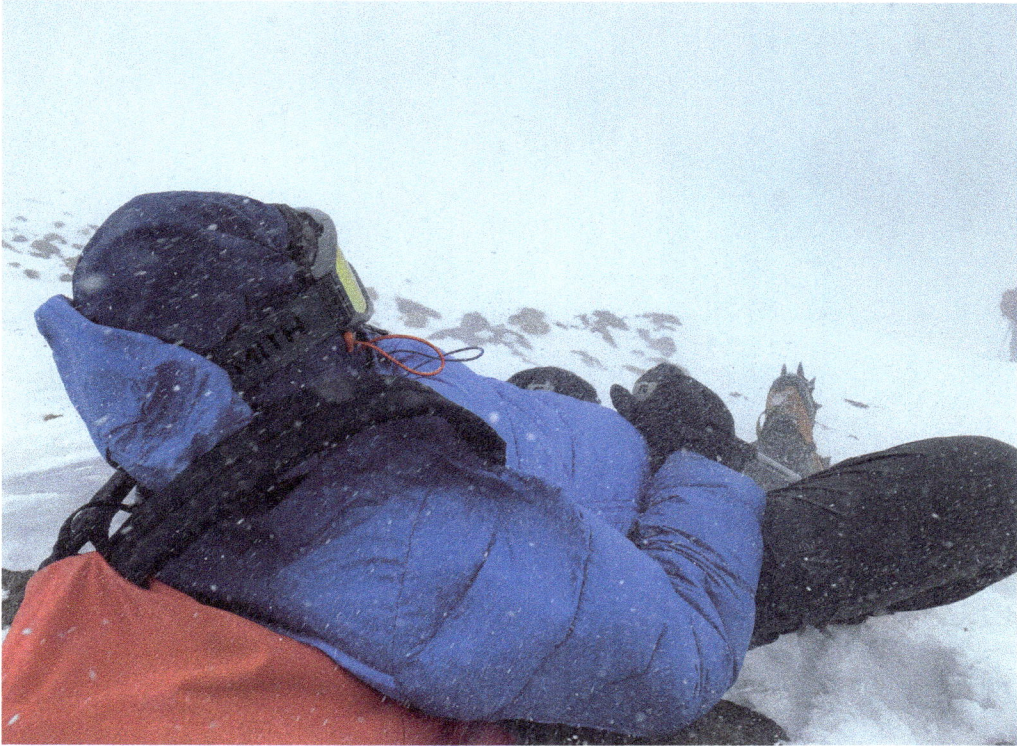

a loop-in rope is thrown my way, and we are all tethered together, ready to descend.

I'm first off the ridge, and I stumble: a ferocious gust of wind lifts me and my heavy backpack fully into the air, then dumps me back on the ground. Descending as quickly as I can manage, step after step, I look back. Although we're all joined together, the others seem a long way behind me. But I press on; a rapid descent is a good descent. I feel on top of the world—I suppose I am at the top of Europe, after all—because everything has gone so well. It's only later I realise that the reason everyone is so far behind me is for safety. I've been put at the front of the tether on what's called a 'crevasse line'—if I fall into a crevasse, the others can haul me out. A good twenty

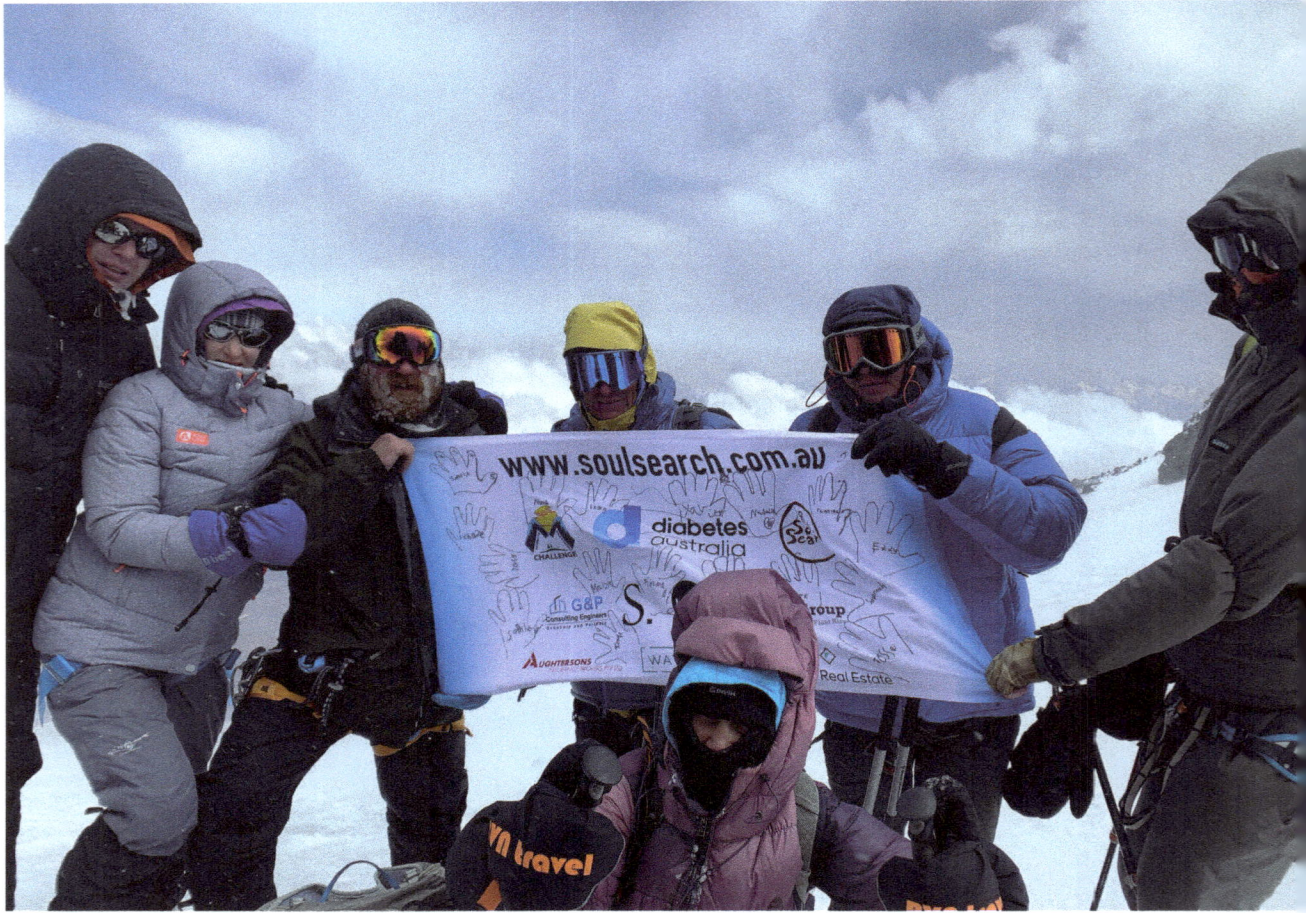

metres of rope is between me and the others. This essentially ensures the ice is okay for everyone to pass. Food for thought as we press downwards.

After a few hundred metres the violent wind gusts subside to high winds, and it feels like the danger has passed. The four of us soon come together to unclip from the tether so we can make independent descents. With the visibility improving, I note the tracks in the snow and eventually spot others making their way to Nameless Rock. With newfound direction, it seems the worst of the weather is behind us.

Vitaly has led the remainder of the team to this same rock after aborting the final push to the summit's peak. While they were very close, the rest of the team didn't get to stand on the very top of the mountain.

'Has anyone taken summit photos?'

I explain how hard it was trying to hold the flag.

'Let's do it here, again, everyone in,' Vitaly says.

So, we capture this moment in time. A moment filled with relief, happiness and a sense of accomplishment. Mt Elbrus is done, and will always be remembered.

It took a sixteen-hour slog to summit Mt Elbrus, and will take me three hours to descend to Base Camp. The descent is mostly undertaken in isolation, with plenty of time for reflection as I trudge through the snow. My legs are shaking involuntarily under my weight. Perseverance is the only constant: the elation of the summit has deteriorated into something else—utter exhaustion. What time would it be back home right now? And wouldn't it be nice to be in bed? I'm past fatigued.

Back at Base Camp, I find it unusually empty. I'm the first trekker back. After quenching my savage thirst, I head to my tent and make no waste of the free tent space, crawling into the comforts of my sleeping bag. It's serenity and relaxation I've earned.

opposite Reunited with the Russian team

Day 6—Descent from Base Camp

Thunder, lightning, wind and rain; the night is an eventful one to spend in a tent. My Russian tent buddies have kept up the snoring, but this shocking weather now competes for my attention. The tent can't withstand the storm, and water leaks inside as the little structure shakes violently in the wind. It's impossible to sleep.

When the rain finally stops, I crawl slowly from my sleeping bag. I feel the strain in my muscles and a stiffness in my back. It's quiet in camp. After draping the Diabetes Australia flag over a rock to dry, I head off in search of the elusive phone service I'm yet to find, and discover it's still elusive. I sit, defeated and sore, on the highest rock in camp. Then, some ten minutes later, my phone beeps.

The elation of hearing my family's voices brings pure happiness to my morning. Heidi has been taking the kids to the park. Fin is enjoying the routine of her first year at school. Arlo is excited for her upcoming third birthday, and I get to hear what cake she would like. It was the lift I needed to get back into camp, pack my gear and embrace the strenuous hike out.

Waiting for the team to muster, I notice that the father and son team in a camp below us are also readying for departure. The son is overwhelmed with excitement to have reached the summit, or maybe it's the chocolate I just gave him that causes a wide smile to spread across his suntanned young face. Either way, his father insists, in Russian, that I drink his homemade golden root vodka. Which I do. With an incredibly tired and aching body, yet another icy cold morning, and a long hike ahead, I opt for seconds.

Our time here is done, and we slowly depart in the direction we came. Big days such as the one I'm now facing are unforgiving on the body, but the thought of a real bed and escaping this tempestuous weather is motivation enough. One push to go.

Dmitry strides along next to me for company. Though we can't verbally communicate, I get that he wants me to call him Dema. Facial expressions and short gestures form our interactions, and a new bond has blossomed from our summit ordeal. It's a unique friendship—what other experience in the world could possibly bring the two of us to this point?

The river waters are now raging, the fog that surrounds us is thick and feels like it's permanent, and the rain comes down sporadically as we tramp on and on and on. A natural spring provides the opportunity for a cool, refreshing drink. Water on my face is invigorating. A sense of relief washes over me; I know we're nearly there, and we must continue.

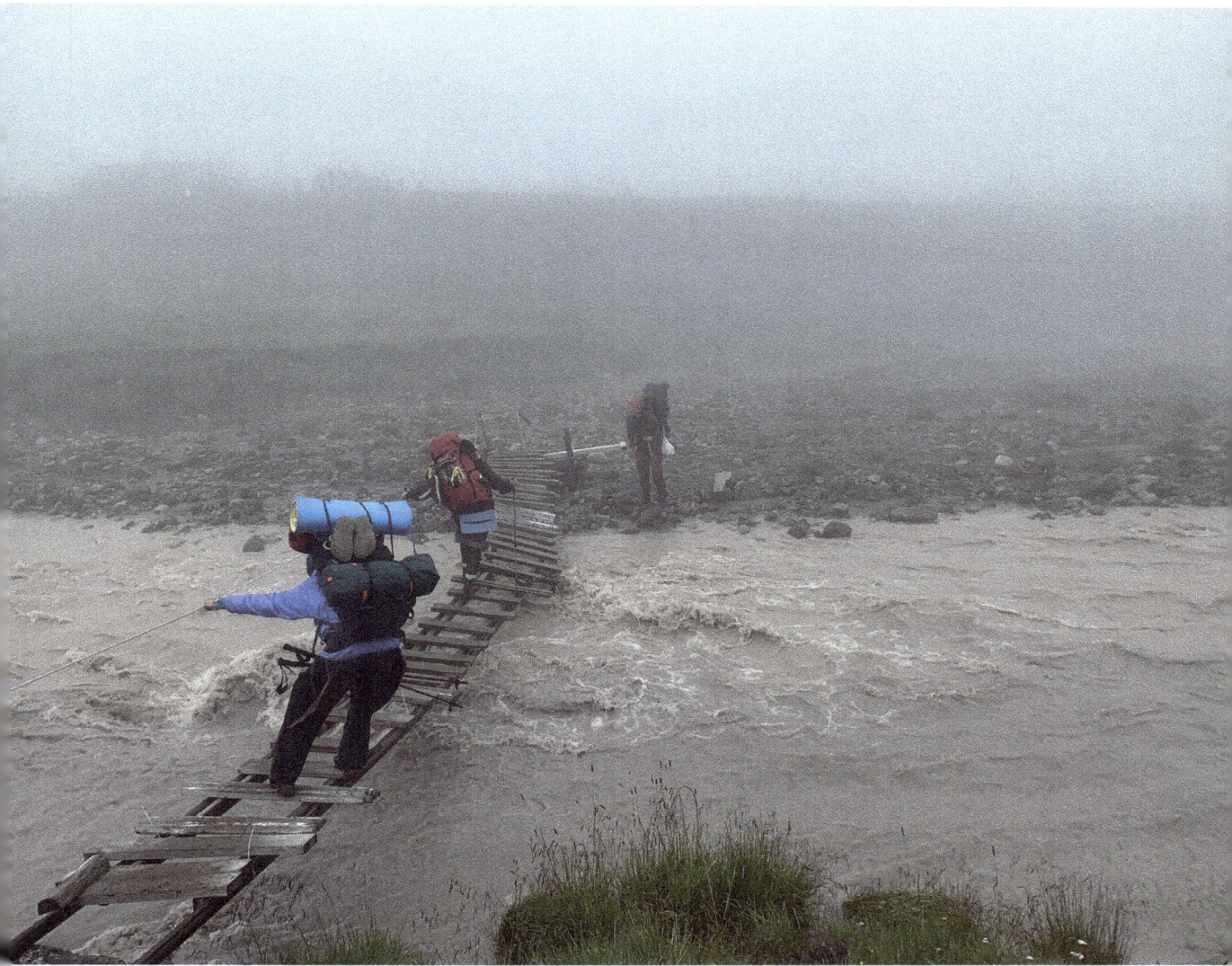

above Time to leave

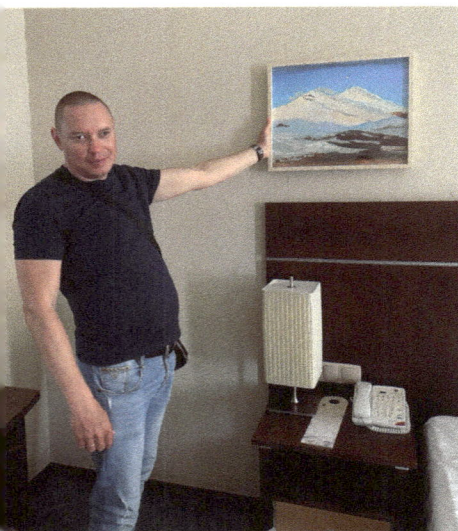

above My friend, Dema

It's an anti-climax as we climb the final hill, totter down to a collapsed bridge and onto a man-made road. One last hill, and I've arrived at the manned checkpoint boom—right where we started. I'm done with the burden of my backpack and throw it to the ground. Well, at least for now.

AFTER TOUCHING down at Moscow airport, I see a middle-aged woman wearing a short black dress and a long black overcoat holding up a placard that bears my name.

'Hello,' I offer.

She replies in Russian, so I have no idea what she says before she turns and walks away. I simply follow her, without speaking a word, through the airport and outside to a central pick-up point.

We stand in silence for ten minutes before a black SUV hurtles around the corner at great speed, and the lady shrieks and waves at the car. The SUV stops and backs up, then the driver leaps out, grabs my bags, and tosses them into the back of the car. The lady in black looks my way for the first time, and gestures for me to get in. I oblige. She then turns quickly on her black heels and walks away. The driver's door slams, and we speed off, hopefully to my hotel.

En route, the driver speaks to me in Russian while waving his hands in a flurry of strange gestures. I can only plead, 'English—sorry.' This feels like something out of a movie. After a short drive we arrive at the hotel, where the doorman, thankfully, speaks English, and I'm soon ensconced in the comfort of my lavish room. Going from a thin, shaking tent on a mountain amid a raging tempest to five-star luxury accommodation is quite an adjustment. But not an adjustment that takes long to achieve.

On my final day in Russia, Dema, whom I shared the summit with, arrives at the hotel. During the night he has painted a personalised interpretation of Mt Elbrus as a gift. I have no words, just the greatest admiration.

I ARRIVED in Melbourne to find there was no chance of any down time, as work commitments had piled up in my absence. I had to finish a commercial build that was no more than concrete panel walls when I left. Concrete floors needed pouring before a roof could go on and winter took hold. A new house build was starting, while another project was ending. Numerous other work projects needed my time. I was physically still exhausted, but that wasn't going to stop me. Some of my workmates joked I was half the worker they once knew for all the weight I'd lost.

In my office, Dema's painting, now framed, was hung in pride of place. Just looking at this art still humbles me, and I miss my friend.

But not as much as I missed my family as I slogged through the tempest to the summit of Mt Elbrus. After I returned home I found the joy of an ordinary domestic scene more precious than the most magical and magnificent vistas that I had the privilege to witness as I climbed the highest mountain in Europe. Arlo's big third birthday arrived. The house was in full chaos with balloons scattered across the floors and *Peppa Pig* cartoons blaring in the background. A pink swan cake was the request and certainly a treat. Kai danced around the lounge room with a box bigger than he is sitting on his head—complete with eye, nose and mouth cutouts. It was a joy to gather with the whole family at the park around the corner to play, talk and unwind.

But there was still work to be done. I embarked on the Seven Summits challenge to raise awareness and money for Diabetes Australia, and my commitment to that cause didn't wane just because I wasn't slogging my way up a mountain.

My friend Tarn arranged a Diabetes Australia fundraiser evening at Marybrooke Manor to raise money in support of my efforts. I couldn't believe the effort she personally contributed to make this evening a success. While images of my journey thus far were on display and a silent auction was in progress,

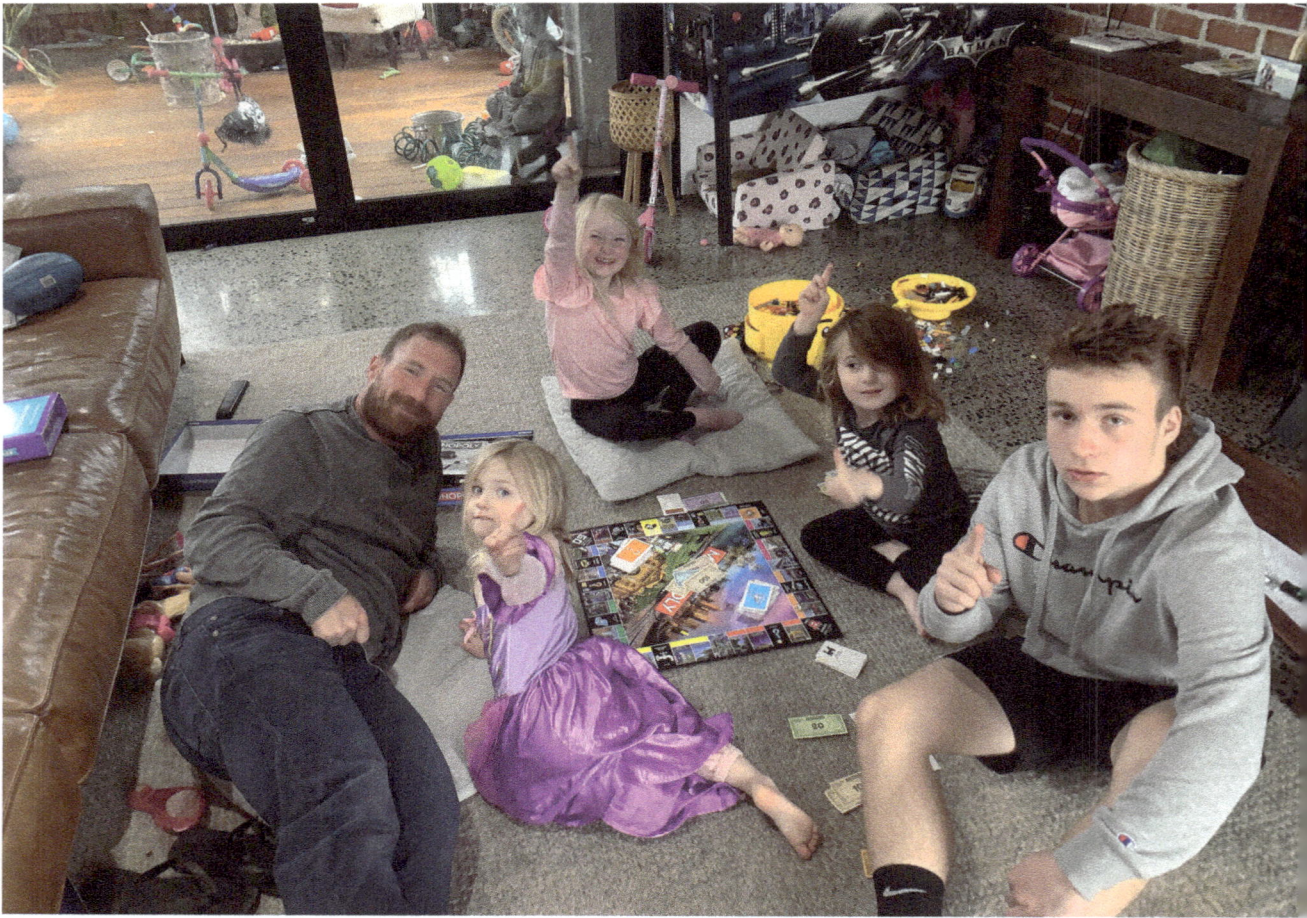

it was the speeches and information on diabetes we presented to the audience that was the biggest hit.

I started my speech by trying to explain why somebody would seek to climb big mountains. Mine is not a story of an important historical event, nor is it informative in a way that might meaningfully change the lives of my audience, but still they listened—intrigued.

In the background was a photo of my face packed with ice, taken on the summit of Mount Elbrus in Russia. The image freezes me in the moment and sums up the conditions and experience better than I could ever convey. Reaching the summit was almost secondary to the experience of getting there.

Carrie Keller, Deputy Director, Development (Clinical and Biomedicine Research) at Monash University generously provided information to our audience on the topic of diabetes. Her dedication to, and experience with, the topic allowed her to deliver an informative speech and also describe the new technologies and innovations in the field. It was a class act, and you could tell the subject is meaningful to her. To say I appreciated Carrie generously giving her time to us that evening is an understatement at best.

opposite Who won?

Of course, the star guest was Fin, who bravely stood beside me on the stage. A small child, so shy in front of the crowd, yet the reason we were all there.

When the formal part of the evening concluded, we stayed on for a long time, discussing the impacts of diabetes in the community.

Family, work and the Seven Summits challenge. These were the three things consuming my time. Life was busy, but I wouldn't have it any other way.

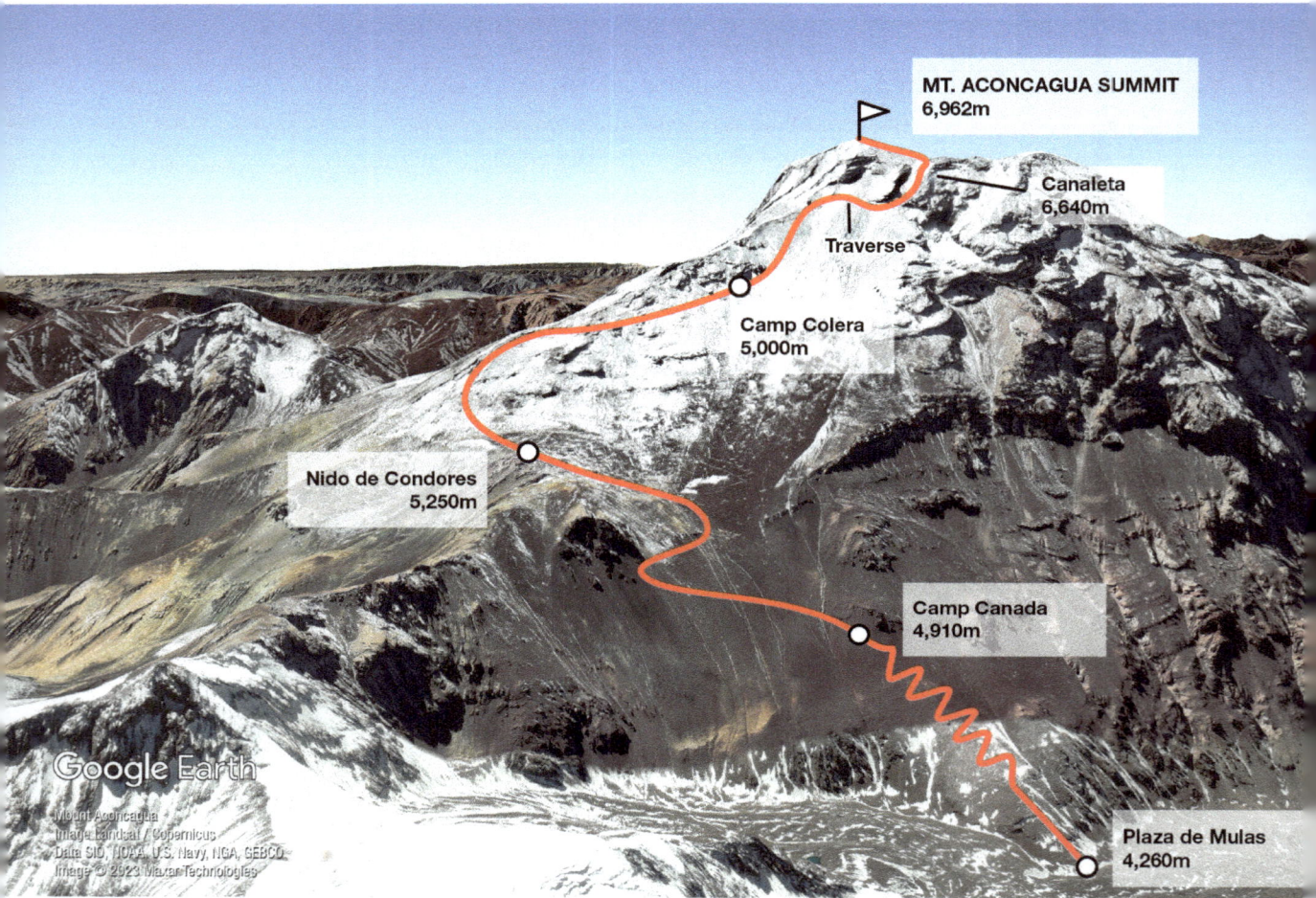

MT. ACONCAGUA SUMMIT
6,962m

Canaleta
6,640m

Traverse

Camp Colera
5,000m

Nido de Condores
5,250m

Camp Canada
4,910m

Plaza de Mulas
4,260m

Google Earth

Mount Aconcagua
Image Landsat / Copernicus
Data SIO, NOAA, U.S. Navy, NGA, GEBCO
Image © 2023 Maxar Technologies

ACONCAGUA

11,404km from Home

ELEVATION: 6,962m

COORDINATES:

S 32 65.343

W 70 01.153

ACONCAGUA

23 NOVEMBER–10 DECEMBER 2019

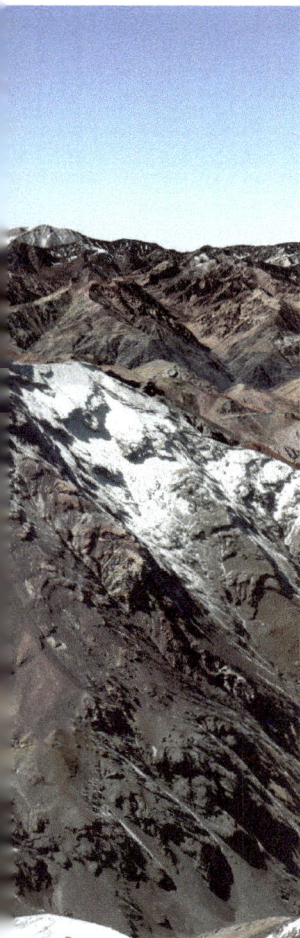

3

I'VE ARRIVED AT Mendoza City, just over 1,000 kilometres west of Argentina's capital, Buenos Aires, to meet Mt Aconcagua. Its jagged, snow-clad peaks seduce every traveller who gazes upon it, and with a summit of 6,962 metres, Aconcagua is Argentina's answer to Mt Everest. It's the highest mountain in the southern hemisphere, the highest mountain in the western hemisphere, and the highest mountain in the Americas.

In a couple of days I'll meet a team of fellow climbers and our guides in anticipation of a twenty-day expedition along what's known as Aconcagua's 'normal route'. Around 3,500 people undertake this climb every year, but only about forty per cent reach the summit. Every year sees an average of three deaths on Aconcagua's slopes.

Digesting these statistics, I set off to explore Mendoza, a cosmopolitan city with a population of more than one million that lies in the Cuyo region, part of Mendoza Province, in the heart of Argentina's wine country. The area is renowned for its Malbecs and other reds. It seems appropriate that, while I adjust to time zones, I take the opportunity to visit some of the best wineries—which is where I head first.

Later I walk to the top of Cerro de la Gloria—the 'Hill of Glory'—to find a monument commemorating the Army of the Andes, a military force of 3,500 soldiers organised by the South American independence leader José de San Martín in

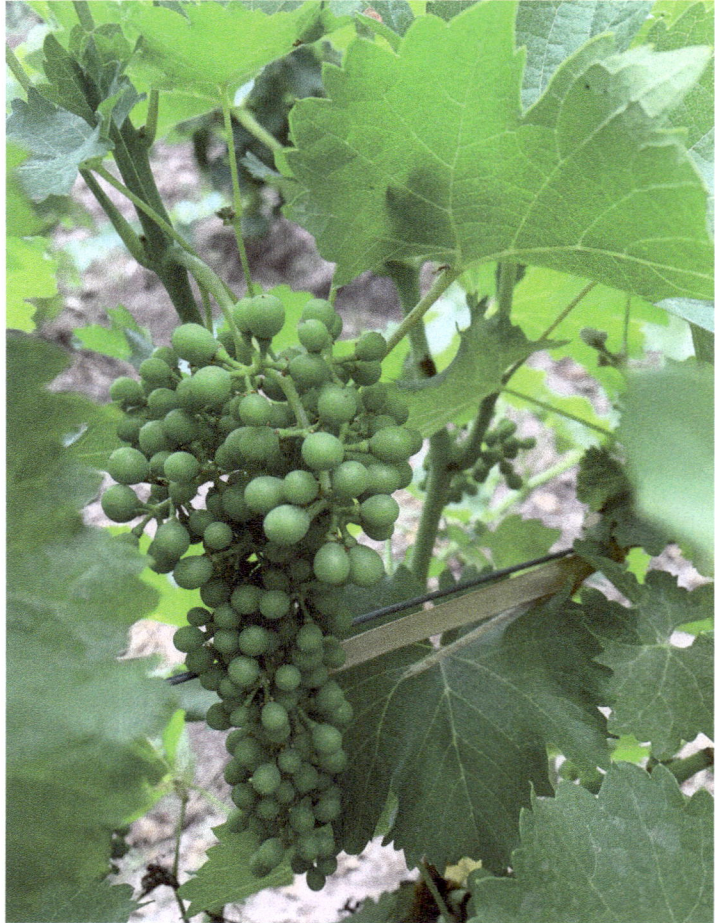

right Admiring
the produce

1817. Hiking up Cerro de Gloria to a height of 980 metres, I want to run, but know I shouldn't: denial isn't sufficiently masking the pain of my ITBS (iliotibial band syndrome) injury, acquired by pushing my running capabilities back in Melbourne. Unfortunately, it appears that no amount of stretching, training or positive reinforcement will heal this one in time.

Day 1—Mendoza (760m)

Technically, today is day one of my Argentinian adventure. I meet Diego, our lead guide, as well as climbers Grant, Sam and Vicky, who have flown in today from Britain. Ashley from the USA is to join us tomorrow. Our afternoon is reserved for equipment checks and last-minute preparations.

Mendoza is highly regarded for its steak, as well as the wine I have already sampled, and Estancia La Florencia restaurant doesn't let the city down. The chef hits steak perfection with a medium-rare lomo (fillet or tenderloin). It's pure flavour; juicy and tender without being raw. On top of that, sipping extraordinary wine, I learn that Estancia La Florencia is also the centre of the Malbec universe.

Day 2—Mendoza to Penitentes (2,725m)

I make use of the last opportunity to call home before we depart Mendoza for the 185-kilometre drive to Aconcagua Provincial Park, near the border of Chile. I have to ring early, because Mendoza is thirteen hours behind Melbourne and it's already getting late at home. We have plenty to discuss. I hear about the full day of activities that have taken place, what was for dinner and who everyone played with. In turn, I can tell everyone what I'm up to for the coming day before wishing them a good night's sleep. It's not the same as tucking Fin into bed and reading her a bedtime story, but at least I get to hear her voice.

On the way to our destination we travel through areas where Brad Pitt filmed *Seven Years in Tibet*, and take in views of the snow-capped volcano, Tupungato, before arriving at Los Penitentes, a ski resort made up of a few buildings—including our quaint hotel, Ayelen—and some chairlifts that criss-cross the mountains.

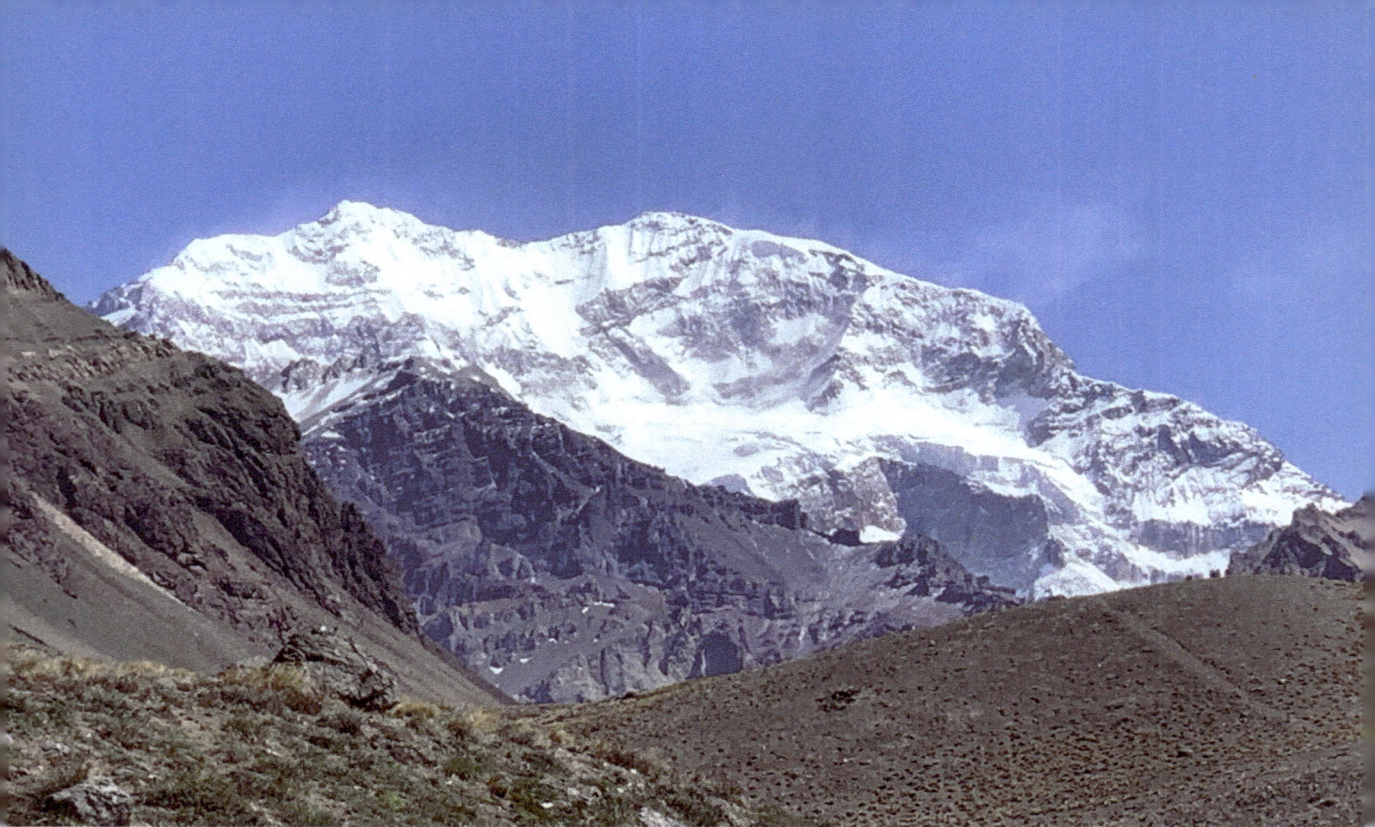

Grant and Sam join me to stretch our legs in the surrounding area. We cross a bridge, wander along an obsolete rail line and scramble up some rocks. The air is a little thinner, and the temperature flickers between moments of warmth and chilly blasts. Time to retreat to the comfort of our lodgings as the weather rolls in.

Nearby, at the Depot at Los Puquios, the mules' loads are being prepared for tomorrow.

Day 3—Penitentes to Confluencia (3,400m)

Diego has us signing our climbing permits as we set off towards Aconcagua by minivan. Just moments into the drive we get a full view of the mountain's south face; it's seriously impressive.

Along the way we stop at Puente del Inca, Bienvenidos, a rock formation that forms a natural bridge suspended some twenty-seven metres over the Las Cuevas River. It's an unusual shape, with walls of colour varying between shades of orange, yellow and ochre stretching around forty-eight metres long.

Our journey begins in earnest at the park ranger's station at Horcones (2,950 metres), where we lodge our permits. From here we're on foot. 'Good luck, and look after yourself,' are the park ranger's only comments.

After leaving the Horcones lagoon, walking along a well-defined path, we cross the bridge over Horcones River, which was built during the making of *Seven Years in Tibet*. Our path forward remains visible on the right riverside. Although the day is clear, wind whips around us.

'At least it's not snowing,' says Diego as we adjust our walking sticks on the well-worn, picturesque trail. Walking is not too difficult. I'm starting with my pack at fifteen kilos today, to prepare for carrying some weight and to test out the knee. It's a new experience to see mules being herded through as carriers, a lifeline of supplies for all the operations up to Base Camp.

It's a three-hour trek up the gentle yet steady slope to our first camp, Confluencia (3,400m above sea level) for our first night and that all-important acclimatisation.

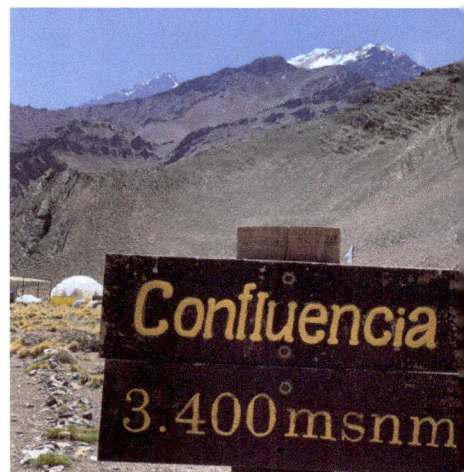

above Confluencia

opposite Aconcagua's south face

Day 4—Confluencia to Plaza Francia (4,000m) to Confluencia

Dawn arrives after a broken sleep, and I'm first to be up and about. I set up the GoPro to capture the new day amid the incredible beauty of the Andes.

Enthusiastically, I pack my gear—I've increased the pack weight to nineteen kilos, and it feels comfortable—and proceed to pull down my tent. Which was a mistake ... Whether it was a lack of listening last night, or critical information lost in translation, I hadn't taken in the fact that our program has us return to this camp tonight after a daytime acclimatisation hike. The tent goes back up, which humours my fellow climbers no end.

From Confluencia, the trail leads to the bridge over lower Horcones River, and after crossing the trail follows the left riverside of lower Horcones River to an area of old moraine—soil and rock left behind by a moving glacier. We trek through riverbeds that are cracking due to the absence of water; at this same time a few years ago, this was a flowing river, Diego tells us.

'Every year the river is a bit drier, the glaciers a bit smaller… soon Mendoza might have big problems—not enough water.'

The government, apparently, measures and monitors the situation—a tale I've heard before.

'There's not enough snow now,' says Diego. Which signals a new problem for us—the prospect of carting water from Base Camp to Camp 1.

We lunch at Plaza Francis (4,000 metres) near the halfway turnaround point of the fifteen-kilometre round trip, where Aconcagua looms large in the background.

Not long into the return trip, Vicky suddenly collapses and is nauseated. Diego helps her to sit before she starts vomiting. In the process she's also slipped and cut herself on a sharp rock. Out comes the medical kit. Eventually we move on, unsure how much the meds will help.

After climbing a steep section of loose ground, we see a pack of mules mustered in the same direction behind us. The sun is shining and the wind is blowing at twenty-five to thirty kilometres per hour as I film these beasts of burden powering up the hill.

Back at camp, the conversation is around Vicky's health. We're told the park usually hosts doctors who undertake mandatory medical assessments at a couple of checkpoints. As it's so early in the climbing season though, none seem to have been appointed, leaving Diego to check our blood oxygen level and heart rate.

Our second guide, Tito, hasn't joined our party yet. He's escorting a late inclusion to the program who is attempting a speed ascent. The merits of this have consequences for us all.

The camp kitchen provides a dinner of tasty pizzas that satisfy my ravenous appetite before I turn in for the night.

Day 5—Confluencia to Plaza de Mulas (4,260m)

Our bodies are working overtime to counter the environment. There's the fact that we've flown from different parts of the world with different germs, the altitude is forcing our bodies to make more red blood cells, and different food and water is entering our systems. All of which makes you wish the toilets were better.

We pack our gear, pull down the tents, and prepare for our next move to Plaza de Mulas—Base Camp. Exiting Camp Confluencia, we head in a different direction from yesterday's trek, this time following the Horcones Superior River. All around are jagged peaks and snowfields.

'Plaza de Mulas 8 Hours' says a sign as we descend onto the now-dry river flats, which are surrounded by towering mountains, some of which have never been summited due to the danger of sheer cliff faces and rock falls. The wind blows at very gusty thirty to thirty-five kilometres per hour as we press directly into it, stopping for a five-minute break on the hour. Packs of mules occasionally stream past, herded by their masters. Breathing through a buff covering my mouth and face proves better than consuming the vast amounts of dust blowing around here.

Arrival at the halfway point signals both lunch and a massive rock for shelter at the end of the river flats. Currently we're at 3,748 metres. The dominant backdrop is the mountain Cerro Cuerno at 5,380 metres.

We're climbing from the flats when Diego spots some mules headed our way. The track isn't wide enough for the mules to pass us. I crouch on a crest to film the animals approaching. It's rocky underfoot and steep enough to be impressed by how they manage in this unforgiving environment. After the mules pass it's our turn to navigate the narrow track, which hugs the mountain.

The terrain becomes steeper the closer we get to Base Camp, which lies at the base of Aconcagua's western summit. It takes the eight hours indicated on the signage to get to Base Camp. All up, we've trekked 22.5 kilometres, with over 1,350 metres going up, around 450 metres back down and ultimately 900 metres of altitude gained.

Plaza de Mulas is a small city of tents. Camping spots are related to the different companies that provide different services. There is phone service here, and everyone is soon shooting messages home or checking in on the rest of the world. During our Base Camp stay, we're entitled to one shower in a tent complete with hot water and a timber floor. I'll choose my shower day carefully; today it's wet wipes again to remove the dust.

As the day nears its end, I pitch my tent ready to escape the elements. Shivering now from the cold, the warmth of a sleeping bag is welcome indeed.

Day 6—Rest day

Glancing around the breakfast table, everyone looks like they need this rest day. It was cold and windy last night, making sleep a challenge.

At Base Camp there is little or no vegetation, and it's dry and cold. I warm up by walking up a nearby ridge to take photos of some fantastic-looking ice formations. These thin blades of hardened ice, randomly spaced closely together, are only found at high altitudes and point towards the sun.

Upon returning, there's little to do. I'm learning that it's better to keep moving to remain warm. There's a plaque nearby that Grant and Sam are setting off to find, so without hesitation I join them for the walk. The plaque eludes us, however, and eventually we return to camp and a warm pie for lunch.

Diego explains that last year the whole mountain face we're viewing was covered in 'penitentes'. These spires of snow and ice range in length from a few centimetres to more than five metres, and grow over all glaciated and snow-covered areas in the Dry Andes above 4,000 metres. There are fewer now, and they are melting faster, he says. Diego adds that this is the first time in all his years here that there's been no snow at Camp 1.

'Climate change is a big problem for the mountain,' he says.

Day 7—Plaza de Mulas to Mt Bonete (5,100m) to Plaza de Mulas

A helicopter stirs the camp into life as it delivers supplies near the ranger station before loading rubbish to take back, its rotors sending dust bellowing across camp. The morning sky is clear blue, with only a cold breeze now. Perfect for flying—and climbing.

We're off early, aiming to reach the summit of Mt Bonete (5,100 metres), which doubles as an acclimatisation day. Early into the trek we stop at an abandoned hotel, a huge place built in the middle of nowhere that closed some eight years ago. The hotel's grounds are used as the principle rescue headquarters, complete with simple outbuildings and rocks marking a helipad.

We navigate through a section of large penitentes grouped together, which is unlike anything I've seen before. Beyond these it's zig-zagging up the scree track on the mountain, where you must be ultra-careful with your footing. It's a hell of a long way down. How does one self-arrest in the event of a fall? I don't particularly want to find out.

The loose surface is unforgiving and requires plenty of effort as we climb upwards. It's a scramble up the last section

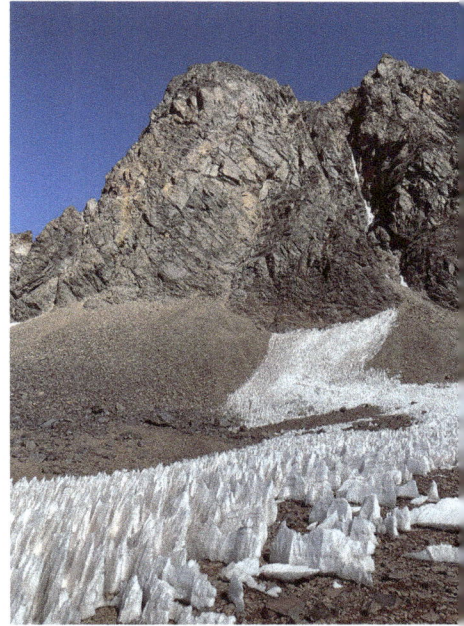

above Receding penitentes

to finally reach the summit of Mt Bonete, which is marked by a metal cross. From here we can track the valleys we've travelled across, admire the landscape, and trace our upcoming route on Aconcagua, which looms majestically before us. Though visible, Base Camp appears as a small speck in the far distance.

The loose gravel makes for some fun sliding downwards. After the odd bum slide and a laugh at each other, we begin the trek back to Base Camp. Water crossings that were manageable this morning are now raging rapids. This is a sure sign the fragile environment is disappearing. Diego contemplates how much ice will be left at the end of the climbing season.

'All the mountains are normally covered in snow at this time, but there is very little this year,' he says.

An Andean condor, the world's largest flying bird, glides majestically overhead. The sun today has afforded us some afternoon warmth and we enjoy the display. Before the evening is out we've distributed weight for the communal gear, for those of us without porters, and packed what extra gear we can drop in for the haul to Camp 1, called Camp Canada, at 4,910 metres. I'm going to be carrying twenty-three kilos, which is manageable, although the route is almost entirely vertical.

Day 8—Plaza de Mulas to Camp Canada (4,910 m) to Plaza de Mulas

There's no gradual introduction to this climb, and within moments we're all huffing as we haul ourselves and our heavy packs directly up a steep route, before following a series of switchbacks that continue to lead us steadily upward. After three challenging hours we reach Camp Canada—and not before some of the team are becoming spent. Gear and belongings are dropped in the communal tent before we turn around for the trek back to Base Camp.

The trip back down, though, is fast and fun. We follow a series of switchbacks and pass through a field of penitentes.

It's refreshing to have the backpack free of weight. Back at Base Camp, after days of dust and sweat, I've decided to go for it and head for the hot shower.

Julian, our speed ascent hopeful, has arrived at camp in his quest to complete another of his Seven Summits. Everyone becomes acquainted over a pasta dinner. The compulsory health check doesn't eventuate when the doctor doesn't arrive, so we call it a night.

Day 9—Rest day

A weather system has rolled in, bringing clouds and snow. I join Grant and Sam for a walk to find the plaque of Mattias Zurbriggen, a Swiss mountaineer who, in 1897, was the first person to successfully summit Aconcagua.

The doctor has arrived to check our health. It's a brief but thorough examination, and I'm cleared to climb. But Julian hasn't made the altitude adjustment as hoped: altitude sickness has incapacitated him. After an eleven-hour hike in, he's booked to endure a three-hour mule ride out. After having just flown in from Tokyo, I can only imagine how devastating this outcome must be for him.

A memorial plaque in camp translates to: 'The only fight that is lost is the one that is abandoned.' Which seems relevant to the day's events.

Day 10—Plaza de Mulas to Camp Canada

The porter packing the tents feels my bulging pack. 'Good luck, you can have a job as a porter after you've climbed the mountain,' he laughs.

This morning is feet-numbing, hand-tingling cold. The sky is heavy with cloud, and 'graupel snow'—a mix of snow and hail—begins to fall. The weather might beat us on this climb; the snow becomes heavier as we push the last rise for the safety of Camp Canada's common tent, where I happily dump my twenty-five kilo-plus pack.

Time to pitch our tents, which we do in the howling wind as a snowstorm sets in. Inside the tent I dig out every bit of down gear I have; there are icicles blowing through the gaps between the tent's two zips.

opposite After the storm

With thirty-five-kilometre per hour winds accompanied by powerful, freezing gusts, I make a dash for the common tent, where ice-melting has begun. Everyone takes turns huddled around small gas burners, melting snow in one pot, then boiling it in a kettle before it's stored in large thermal containers. We check the weather, eat some dinner, and laugh about how miserable it all is.

Camp Canada is now completely white, in stark contrast to yesterday's gear drop—about fifty millimetres of snow has fallen in a few hours. It hasn't been a great day to summit for those climbing before us: some trekkers have abandoned their attempt just 500 metres from the summit. One climber is so unwell she's descending, while a male climber has fallen and hurt his knee and elbow. And yet I watch two climbers press on through the snow, headed for Camp 2—Nido de Condores— at 5,250 metres.

The storm passes in the late afternoon, and from this vantage point I can witness both the storm front and clear skies side by side, in stunning contrast. Our plan is to leave for Nido de Condores tomorrow morning, when the winds, hopefully, will have dropped.

Day 11—Camp Canada to Nido de Condores (5,250m)

Overnight was a howler: wind gusts blew so hard that mist pressed through my tent's zips and formed icicles on my sleeping bag. I'm thin on energy, so this morning it's one chore at a time. Toilet with ice particles whipping off the snow: check.

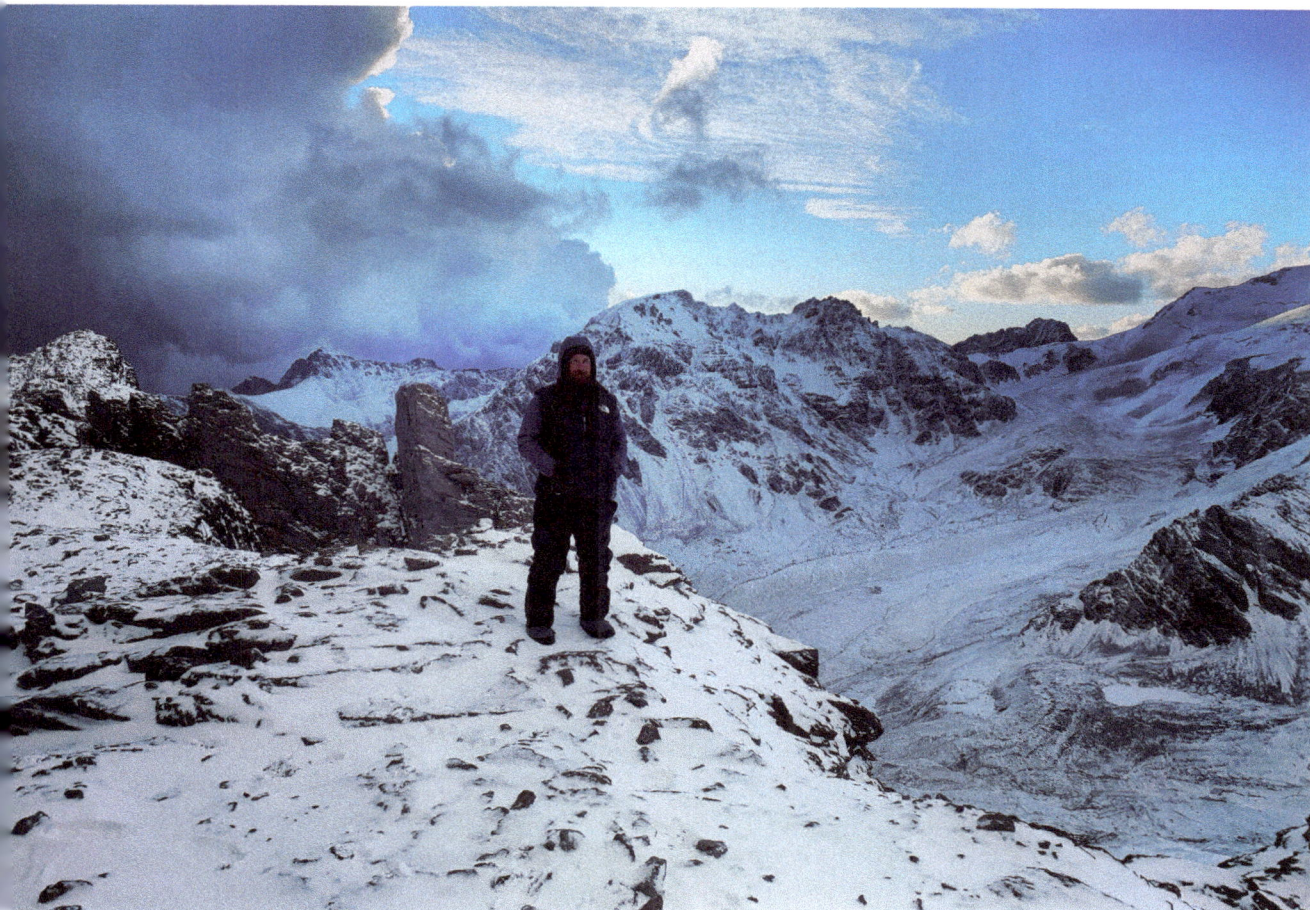

Roll up wet sleeping bag: check. Lie back down, exhausted: check. But I can't lie here all day...

Eventually the tents are down, packs are filled, lunch is handed out, and we're ready. Adding boots, jacket and crampons to my pack has pushed it somewhere near thirty kilos. It's an effort to lift; I'm bracing for a long day.

With a head as clear as they come, my mind moves past thoughts of the immediate demands to thoughts of home. I've already surrendered to the mountain. Can I ever be at peace with Fin's diagnosis? The hindrance of this disease upon the innocence of my beautiful daughter is something that is difficult to accept and hard to push out of my thoughts. But I think of how strong Fin has to be as I carry my thirty kilos—a mere trifle compared to my daughter's lifelong burden—along the path that will eventually take me to the summit, and a strong resolve develops deep within myself. I visualise the moment I will unfurl the Diabetes Australia flag.

'You'll be right,' I mutter to myself.

opposite A sunset to remember

The mountain is covered in snow. Fresh air blows past constantly, unhindered. Given the steep terrain, every foot placement is critical and occupies most of my concentration. And while we warm up while climbing, we shiver in blasts of icy wind when we stop for a break. There's a rescue team of two ahead who are training for the season. Passing us, they offer well wishes. I'm impressed as I watch them forge ahead at pace.

Struggling through the fresh snow, ever upward, this is a really tough day. When we eventually have a break, I drop down and momentarily see stars. I'm spent. But we must push on. I keep putting one foot in front of the other. My entire back feels like one huge knot, my right hip like it's carrying the entire load, and the straps dig in.

'It's the beast!' the porter from the camp yells as he passes me. It's a welcome distraction to the suffering. But I certainly don't feel like any kind of a beast. Certainly not one evolved to exist in these harsh conditions. If I have any special quality, it's the thought of my darling daughter and the inspiration she has given me to undertake this quest.

As Nido de Condores Camp comes into sight after more than three hours climbing in terrible conditions, my pack hits the ground along with me in front of it. I'm so relieved. There is an area here made up of rocky peaks of unusual shapes that can provide some shelter from the strong winds, which don't let up for a moment. After taking some photos, I struggle to pick up my load again and move it to the common tent.

Vicky arrives half an hour later, and she's exhausted. She has had enough.

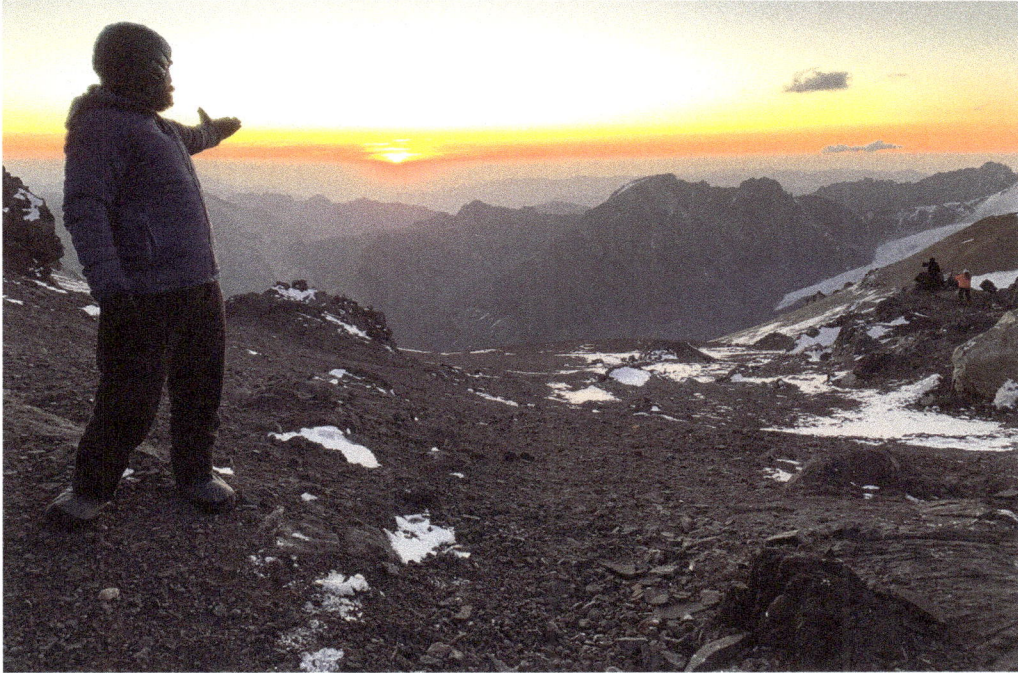

The wind is against us again as we look for tent sites. Wrestling the flimsy tents into place and securing them with rocks is an arduous task. Everything is a chore, including breathing and walking. Once I finally get my gear into the tent I lie down for a while, pondering where the next bit of energy might come from. Maybe chocolate will help.

Dinner is burgers, which sit okay in an otherwise depleted body. Over dinner Vicky tells us she is descending tomorrow. Grant will see how he pulls up in the morning.

Diego checks in on me. 'You feeling tired today?'

'Yes, a little. My back is tight.'

'Ah, so you are human! I am tired today, too.'

The wind dies down as the sun sets across spectacular mountain peaks in an array of blazing colours. I decide I must not motivate myself a little longer to catch this sunset on film.

Day 12—Rest day

The chance to gain more acclimatisation and recover somewhat is appreciated. But health deteriorates rapidly at this altitude. Tito, our assistant guide, is unwell and needs to descend. He's tried to rapidly acclimatise in line with Julian's ambitious program, but altitude sickness has struck again. Vicky says she has had a reasonable night's sleep and has decided to stay on. I respect her determination, yet hold concerns for her ability. In a surprising turn of events, both Grant and Sam have quit and will head back down the mountain with Tito. Just hanging out with these guys has been fun. I'll miss their good humour.

We're reduced to three climbers and one guide for our summit attempt. Of the descending climbers, I find out that about half have made the summit. Not the most encouraging of updates.

Day 13—Nido de Condores to Camp Colera (6,000 m) to Nido de Condores

The side of my knee feels like it's been torn all over again, presumably from the way I slept. Doubts about my knee plague me; I worry it could prevent me summiting. My stomach is churning and my head feels like it's swelling. All I can manage is coffee and two pieces of dry bread for the morning. Chewing slowly, I eat outside the tent in case I involuntarily vomit. For now, I can only focus on one small task at a time.

Shared gear is split four ways for our communal drop at Camp 3—Plaza Colera (6,000 metres), a five-hour climb. Heading off at a slow pace, there seems to be less oxygen. Trying to get into a rhythm, both in breath and body, requires putting the negativity of the morning aside. We're heading northwest, and when we take a break I look back at the incredible vistas of Chile to the left and Argentina to the right.

Surprisingly, I start to feel better as we climb higher. But the climb has proven too much for Vicky, despite her consistent effort, who at this point concedes her summit attempt. Our team narrows to three—me, Ashley and Diego, our guide.

I can see the summit of Aconcagua in the near distance, and it's inspiring to know we're so close. Any fears of acute mountain sickness and the knee are swept aside—I'm breathing a little easier and have regained my enthusiasm to push on. The route continues eastward on its way up to a group of rocky hills.

After acclimatisation and lunch, we trek back down to Camp 2 as the clouds gather. Wind and snow are probable, but our summit window is looking okay at this stage. I spend the afternoon organising gear; I'm ruthless about carrying minimum weight. While I'm sure I'd smell a treat climbing and sleeping in the same clothes for several days, with constant wind and my own tent, who cares? It's time to focus on the finish.

Day 14—Nido de Condores to Camp Colera

Packs are out, our communal weight distributed, and tents come down. Porters carry tents, but we carry everything else: water storage, pots, pans, fuel. We move at a reasonable pace, probably because we did this same walk yesterday, traversing the jagged mountain face back up to Camp Colera: a three-hour climb.

Camp Colera is a dramatic place to camp, with exceptional views across the Andes. It's windy, and the camp is more exposed than others. Getting the tents up is again energy-sapping work. It's vital to know where all my climbing gear is at all times in this hostile environment. Again, I take inventory of my gear. A pair of gloves is missing, which can have unforeseen consequences on a summit push. Though I have my summit gloves, now there's no back-up in the event one is lost in various scenarios.

A serving of powdered mashed potatoes isn't what I would recommend for our last dinner before our summit attempt tomorrow, but that's what we have.

Day 15—Summit day

opposite Look for the pyramid shadow

Sleeping at 6,000 metres is terrible. I hoped to wake on this special day—summit day—rested and motivated. But it's more a case of broken sleep and a pounding headache. My heart's beating out of my chest with the exertion of getting ready. I need to settle a bit. No way have I come this far to do anything other than reach the summit. My daughter is surely counting on me. Diego says he saw snow on the summit last night, and advises us to pack crampons for safety.

I emerge from the tent at 5am with little enthusiasm. But this is it. I wanted to do something challenging to increase awareness around type 1 diabetes and let my daughter believe in a future of possibilities. This mountain is giving me the chance to dutifully fulfil that ambition. It's time for me to live in the moment.

Bottles are filled with hot water as we wrestle jackets and gloves over all our other layers of clothing before it's time to take the first step. The three of us barely speak as we trudge upwards, our head torches shining in the dark. We climb for several hours before the sky starts to show the promise of a new dawn.

With a clear route and nervous anticipation, we continue among rock formations to an area known as Piedras Blancas, where the route has us on the northern edge of the mountain. With the sun rising, I snap a photo of the horizon, which distinctly shows the mountain's almost perfectly triangular pyramid shadow. This natural phenomenon is the result of the perspective effect when looking along a long corridor of shadowed air that extends to the horizon. Amazing.

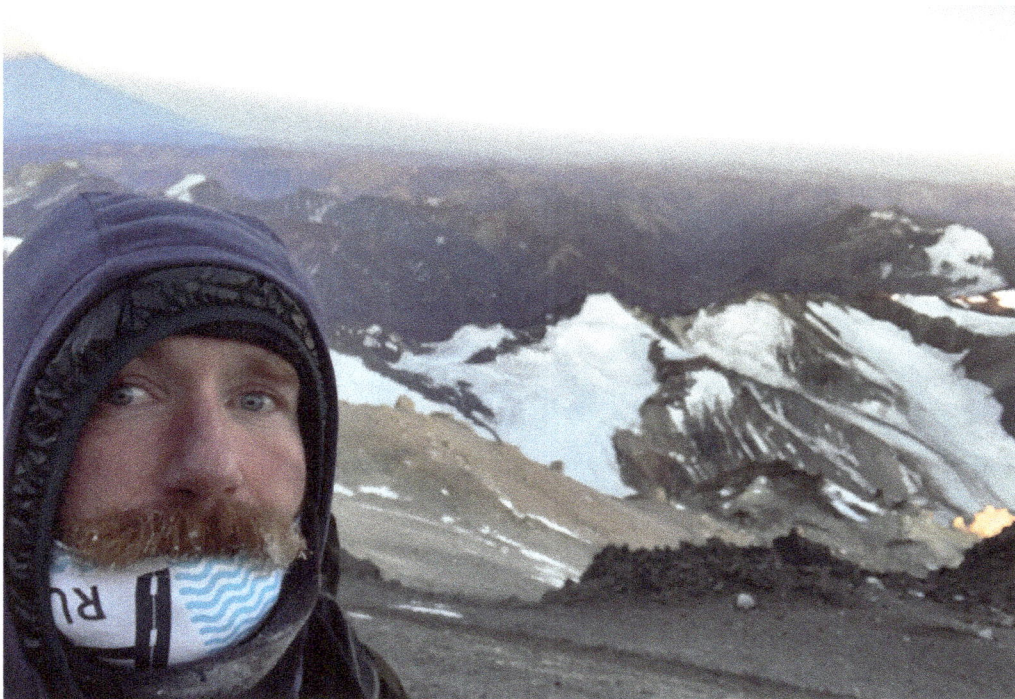

We take our first rest at a huddle of small makeshift huts. Refugio Independencia (6,380 metres) gives us a chance to add another jacket and pants. Heading south-westerly through a pass known as Portezuelo del Viento, the next long and arduous slog is in the shade of the mountain, above the Gran Acarreo from east to west, with violent, freezing wind as our companion.

Fear of frostbite and hypothermia creeps in, as first one finger, then two, and then my entire hand, goes numb. I stop to put on a handwarmer. Strong gusts persist up from the valley, adding to the miserable wind chill. The ascent is around thirty degrees and rocky, and snow hides the gravel, which collapses with each foot placement.

'Time for crampons,' yells Diego against the wind.

We finally reach La Cueva—The Cave—which is the base of the long, rocky gully known as the Canaleta (6,640 metres) and begins the steep climb to the ridge separating Aconcagua's north and south summits. We've now been underway for six hours.

The Canaleta gully is choked with boulders and is unremitting hard work. Energy is running low, so I try to eat some chocolate. I don't know if I can stomach it, as breathing has become increasingly difficult, and I feel nauseated. But after fourteen days, with around just three hours to go, it's impossible to give up. That said, I understand anyone who does: at La Cueva, so close to the summit, a man lies flat on his back, unable to walk any further. Behind us a Frenchman struggles to push on in his second summit attempt.

Our small party presses on. The path up La Canaleta is incredibly steep. I try to take some photos of the breathtaking views around us whenever we pause to drink, and the effort just to do this cannot be underestimated. Ashley, although struggling to continue, remains focused.

'I'll crawl to the top if I have to,' she says.

Coming out of the gully, the route traverses the top of a large amphitheatre and ends up on the final ridge to the summit. Diego ties a rope around Ashley's waist for safety as the unforgivable terrain becomes increasingly difficult to climb. Pressure to keep moving has us taking one energy-sapping step at a time. Progress is slow.

I feel exhausted, and start to contemplate the 'why' of the last two weeks as I trudge up the mountain. I'm immersed in an individual journey right now, but believe that one day my efforts will benefit Fin, and possibly the whole type 1 diabetes community. This somehow calms my mind and spirit for now.

Ashley is really struggling—somewhere in between crying and vomiting, she warns us. I feel her pain, and Diego and I do our best to motivate her ever upward. Some of the longest hours of my life pass as we climb and climb—this is suffering. We keep an eye on the blackening sky: there's a change coming, and it doesn't look good.

At the final stages of the Filo del Guanaco, just before the summit, there's a stack of huge boulders to navigate. The mental and physical conditioning are tested one more time.

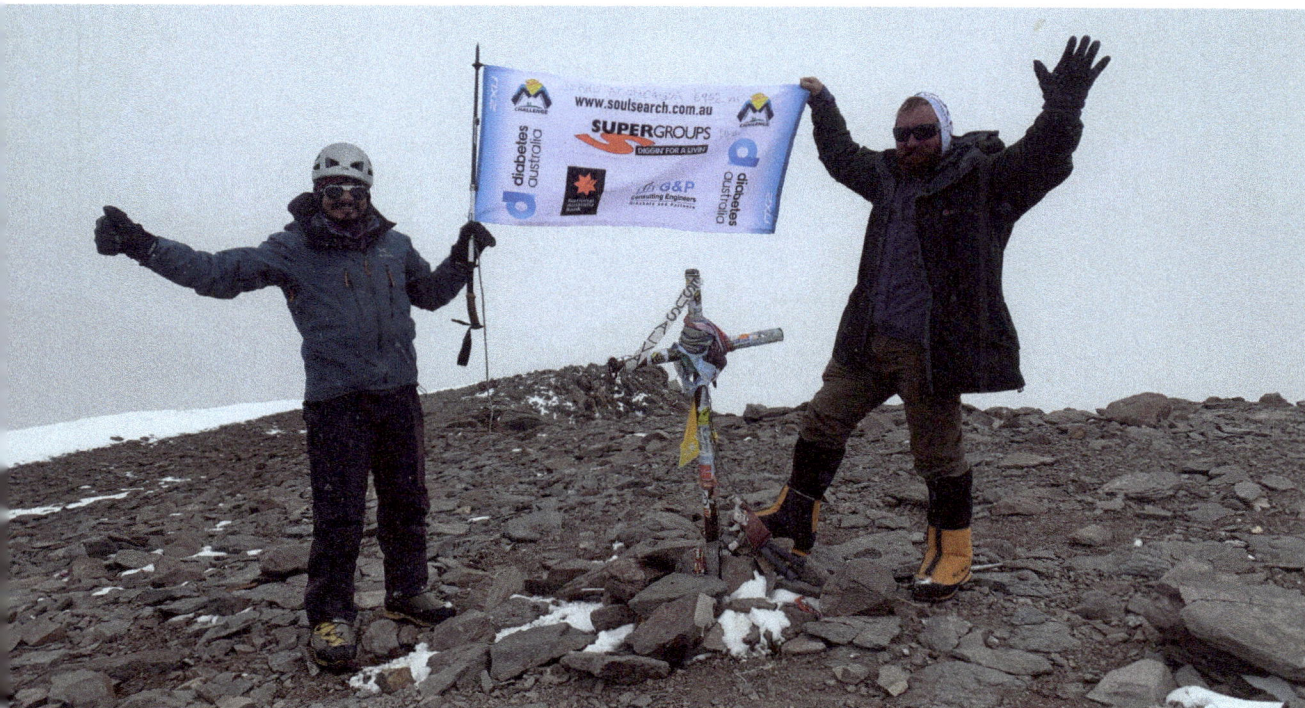

Then, suddenly, I scramble to the top of South America, Cerro Aconcagua, a mind-blowing 6,962 metres above sea level.

There's something incredibly uplifting about reaching the top of a mountain. For some reason you breathe a little easier as you have your own personal celebration after such a tough journey.

Ashley cries, vomits and laughs. Diego comforts her, then attempts a series of handstands. Unbelievable. With snow falling and the exhaustion of such a climb, he wants to stand on his head?

I'm drawn to a small, inconspicuous cross adorned with stickers, buffs and tokens of previous summits. It's clearly the symbol of this mountain's highest point.

And I have my own special task to complete—to unfold the Diabetes Australia flag, never far from my thoughts, for inclusion in my summit photo. Diego proceeds to connect the flag to my hiking pole after signing it.

'Now it's a real flag!'

While the weather deteriorates around us, we take photos and share this special moment with laughter and congratulations. Within moments the weather has turned, and we must start going down. Our crampons go back on, and we're met by rescue policemen sent to help everyone evacuate.

opposite Last goodbyes

The mountain was extremely steep to climb, so it's an almost sheer descent. Stepping, sliding, stopping; I'm thankful for the security of my crampons. La Cueva can't come fast enough. Once there, I remove the ice from my beard and try to cover up for the long traverse ahead. From La Cueva we continue, one step at a time, for hours on end, glaring into the distance for any recognisable landmarks that will herald a rest break.

Eventually we arrive at the makeshift huts, the first stop of the morning, where we can take off our crampons: snow has stopped falling and the ground has exposed loose gravel. In this exhausted state, it's not gone unnoticed that the rescue policemen have followed behind. Their presence is reassuring.

Ashley is struck with vision impairment—black dots blocking her vision, she says. With the accumulated exhaustion, she falls frequently and involuntarily. Only slowly, slowly now. We have to continue to descend.

Finally, we arrive at Camp Colera. I drop my backpack, but there is only the briefest of celebrations. I am completely exhausted. My body shuts down as I slide into my sleeping bag. Within moments I travel into a dreamless oblivion.

But we made it.

Day 16—Camp Colera to Plaza de Mulas

My body feels like it's dishing out punishment in ways I can only respond to with involuntary shuddering. Surely it can't hurt that much more if I stand? With a pounding head and

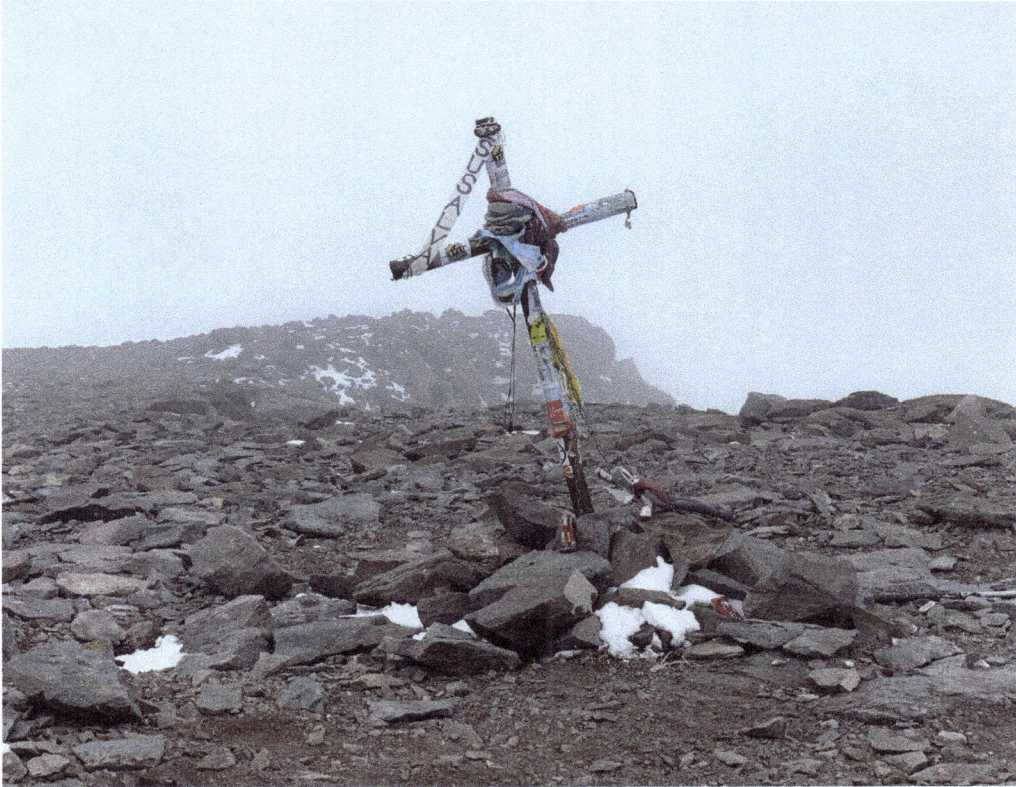

knotted stomach, I'm vaguely amazed that this is a new day. The skies are clear, the sun is out, yet it is far from warm. Once again, my world turns inward as I try to achieve just one small task at a time. Of course, we still have to pack up camp and get down.

Our exit from camp, with the burden of my backpack, is assisted by a steel guide-wire to help us navigate the steep descent over snow-covered rock formations. But any momentum that was achieved arriving at Camp 2 is lost when we collect both the balance of our personal gear and all the remaining communal gear. As the final insult, my pack is now heavier than at any previous time on our climb. I need the

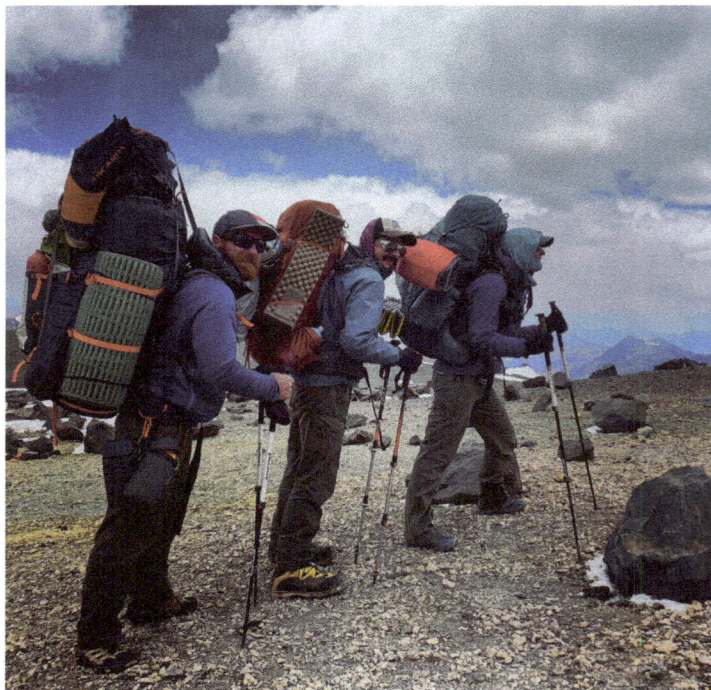

right Heavy loads down

assistance of my hiking poles just to stand, and they're now essential to stabilise my weight.

Physical pain continuously threatens to defeat me. I grimace, take a deep breath, take the next step, repeat. Though I buckle and hit the ground occasionally, now I must be strong—or so I tell myself.

It is a long, long day.

After some internal reflection back at Base Camp, eating and drinking is essential for recovery. Word has spread of our summit and, seeing our utter exhaustion, we're kindly offered some dorm beds by another company. I pull the mattress from the top bunk onto the floor. Safer to sleep down here than fall—I'm so fatigued.

Day 17—Plaza de Mulas to Horcones to Mendoza

It's only minus six degrees Celsius this morning. But the coffee is hot.

I'm ready to get out of here. Thankfully the mules will assist with our loads from here. I feel like a child shouldering a school bag, compared to yesterday's burden. Diego explains that four more days of bad conditions are forecast, but the weather is holding up for now. We descend to Horcones, the entrance to the park, relieved that the air is easier to breathe.

Climbing mountains connects you with nature, people and different cultures, and creates memories that become the stories we tell. It's about falling in love with a new environment and appreciating even more the one you left. It's about reconnecting with yourself, struggle, triumph—and realising the world is a very big place.

I DIDN'T head home after summiting Aconcagua, but I still had to travel—to America, where my family were waiting for me. We had planned an adventure together—a trip that would include every child's dream destination: Disneyland.

For most families, travelling overseas takes a lot of planning, but when you have a diabetic child that planning becomes critical. If we were not prepared to handle Fin's condition while we were away, she could face a life-threatening situation. Many travellers feel anxious about arriving at a new destination, but this was next level and the effort to prepare was immense. That effort fell largely on Heidi, as I was struggling up Mt Aconcagua in the days before our holiday.

Breaking from the family's everyday routines and travelling to a far-flung destination was a new challenge, with uncertain outcomes. We were worried, nervous, apprehensive. How would we handle any disruptions to our carefully conceived plans? What were the potential threats that could impact Fin's health? Fear of the unknown affects the way we think, feel and behave. It's no wonder Heidi became anxious and was out of her comfort zone in the days before our trip.

But Heidi has travelled extensively, and the fear of travelling with Fin's condition wasn't enough to put her off embarking on this family holiday. Any seasoned traveller knows that reducing anxiety around travel comes down to preparing for all eventualities. And that's the attitude we took to our far-flung overseas holiday as a family. Our educator at the Royal Children's Hospital, Amy, built a plan for both departing the country and returning. Expert advice on administering insulin while transitioning time zones was critical to Fin's health. But type 1 diabetes management wasn't the only thing that needed to be considered; there was also general health, available food choices at the destination and other special requirements.

And then there was the packing. Supplies of everything need to be doubled. As recommended by the Royal Children's Hospital, Finlay travels with two sets of everything, from insulin to testing strips, and we carry more than a sufficient supply of needles. Heidi packed way more than we needed for the duration of our holiday. One complete set was checked in with the luggage and one set went with Heidi in her carry-on bag, just in case the luggage went missing. An accompanying letter from the hospital had to be provided just to achieve this. The letter allowed Fin's requirements to be accommodated; requirements that include not just medical supplies, but also suitable food for the journey. But still we worried. What would happen if the authorities didn't let our special supplies through the barrage of security, customs and passport control?

There were so many scenarios to worry about—both within and outside our control.

And let's not forget the other two little kids and the teenager who were also travelling with us. They too need nurturing. How would all the kids manage on a cramped plane for such a long flight? Rightly or wrongly, additional focus tends to be on Fin. And once we arrived, how would another country accommodate a crisis? What if Fin required medical attention or advice, or lost her supplies, or had an extreme hypo? These potential problems compounded to compromise Heidi's well-being too. Even the most organised person would struggle with all the unknowns.

It was relief to arrive in America, to be reunited with my family and to see that the first leg of the journey had gone smoothly. I had ventured far and high in recent days, but the most anticipated events are often the most humble; events such as being reunited as a family. The kids are always excited to see me after I've been gone, and often the distance makes the heart grow fonder. The excitement when we were reunited this time was infectious.

Travelling to America made it easier to pivot to my next destination, and also gave me a chance to enjoy some warmth before heading to Antarctica. Heidi had always wanted to do a boat cruise down to Mexico, so that's what we did, and headed for Long Beach, California—a long way from anywhere my kids had been before, but accessible for cruising. The giggles never subsided after we boarded the *Norwegian Joy* and discovered what it was like to live in small quarters together while embracing sea life. Nobody wanted to join the kids club—we wanted to be together. The warmth of being with my family made me smile and eventually thawed my cold bones. Beachside escapes and the colourful streets of Mazatlan welcomed us. Of course there were ice-creams galore.

Still, I trained while I was on board the boat, on land, or wherever I could. Mountains demand their pound of flesh—literally. They deplete your energy and your lean muscle mass with it.

And then there was Disneyland. Heidi and I thought it would be quiet the day before Christmas at this iconic theme park. How wrong we were! Opened in 1955 by the Walt Disney Company, this enterprise is still drawing huge crowds. We

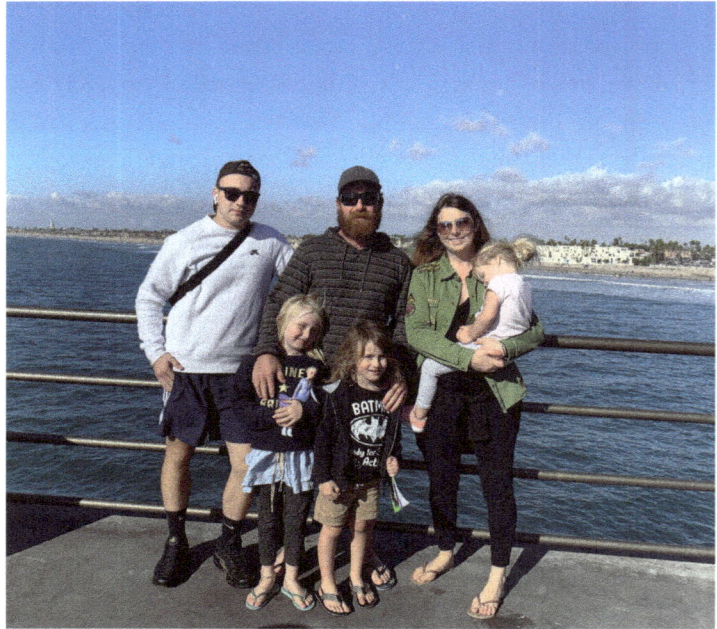

got to experience the most magical (and busiest) time of year with the full program of festivities and parades. Holiday magic brought to life all right! While Fin and Arlo were beside themselves meeting real live 'princesses', I joined Will and Kai in the queues that stretch forever for rides that last moments.

While I vowed never to return, I was the only one!

Despite being in a hotel room, Christmas Day was made all the more special by Heidi's efforts. Once the Santa business was all done, it was time for a coastal experience that only California can offer. But days building sandcastles and nights listening to street music eventually drew to a close. The sign that we posed in front of symbolically read, 'Santa Monica 66 End of the Trail'.

Teary goodbyes were eventually all that were left as we parted ways and I headed to Antarctica.

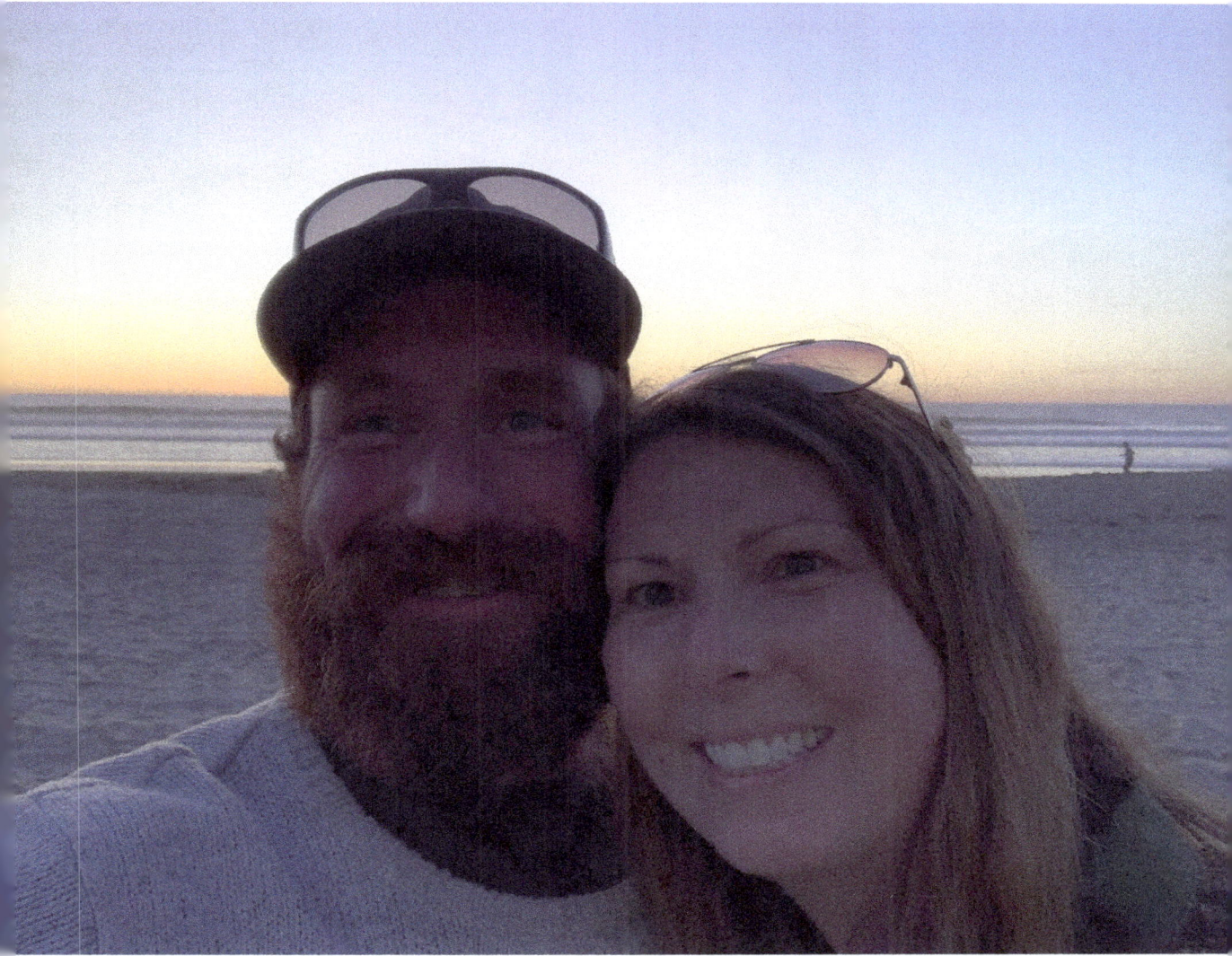

above Life's easier at
the beach—NYE 2019

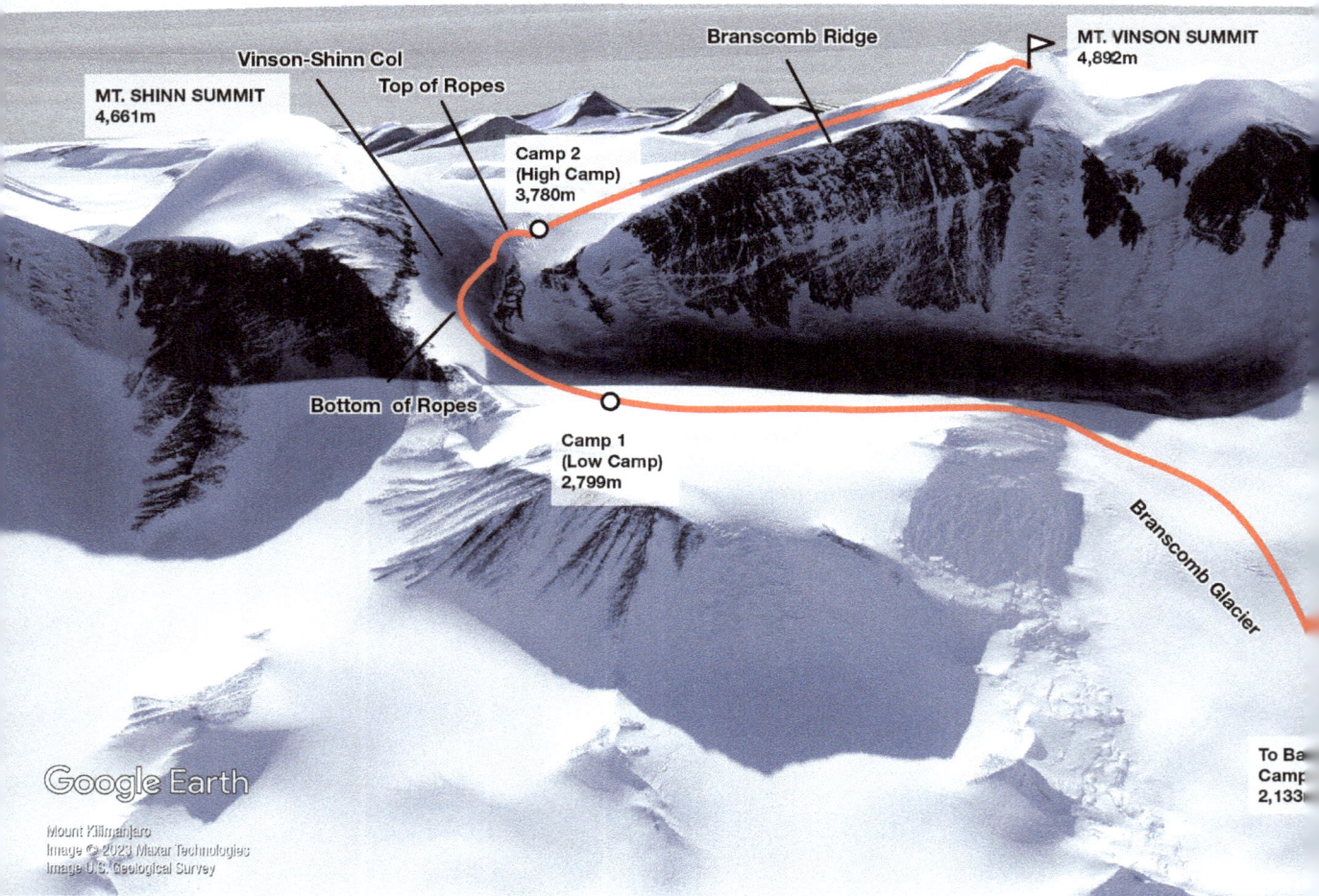

MT. SHINN SUMMIT
4,661m

Vinson-Shinn Col

Top of Ropes

Branscomb Ridge

MT. VINSON SUMMIT
4,892m

Camp 2
(High Camp)
3,780m

Bottom of Ropes

Camp 1
(Low Camp)
2,799m

Branscomb Glacier

To Ba
Camp
2,133

Google Earth

Mount Kilimanjaro
Image © 2023 Maxar Technologies
Image U.S. Geological Survey

MT VINSON

6,676km from Home

ELEVATION: 4,892m

COORDINATES:

S 78 52.548

W 85 61.715

VINSON

6 JANUARY—21 JANUARY 2020

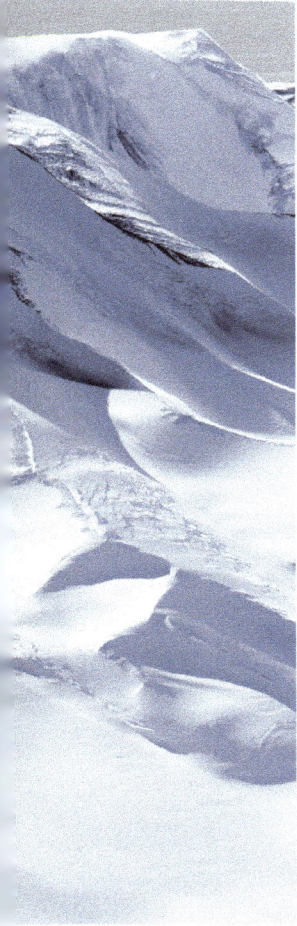

A HUGE AEROPLANE sits on the runway at Chabunco military air base in Punta Arenas, Chile, dwarfing other planes on the tarmac. It's a Russian Ilyushin-76TD, a multipurpose four-engine turbofan strategic airlifter originally designed to transport heavy machinery to remote areas of the USSR, and it's ferrying me to Antarctica and Mt Vinson, the fourth of my Seven Summits.

I've been in the city of Punta Arenas, which lies on the southern tip of Chile, for the past two days. The Patagonia region's most populous city, Punta Arenas lies on Estrecho de Magallanes, also called the Straits of Magellan, a navigable channel that links the Atlantic and Pacific oceans between the mainland tip of South America and Tierra del Fuego.

This city of around 125,000 people is just 1,419 kilometres from the coast of Antarctica, and has become a gateway to the continent. Founded in 1848, Punta Arenas is attracting growing numbers of trekkers, who are replacing the explorers, dealers and sailors of years gone by. Overcast clouds are the background to deteriorating piers and rusty ship hulls, once valuable assets now being claimed by the sea.

Walking around town, you can hardly tell that the streets were full of rioters just a week ago. The only signs of trouble are the large number of broken shop windows and mirrored surfaces smashed by rocks. As a country rife with social inequality, Chile has been witnessing its worst civil unrest in

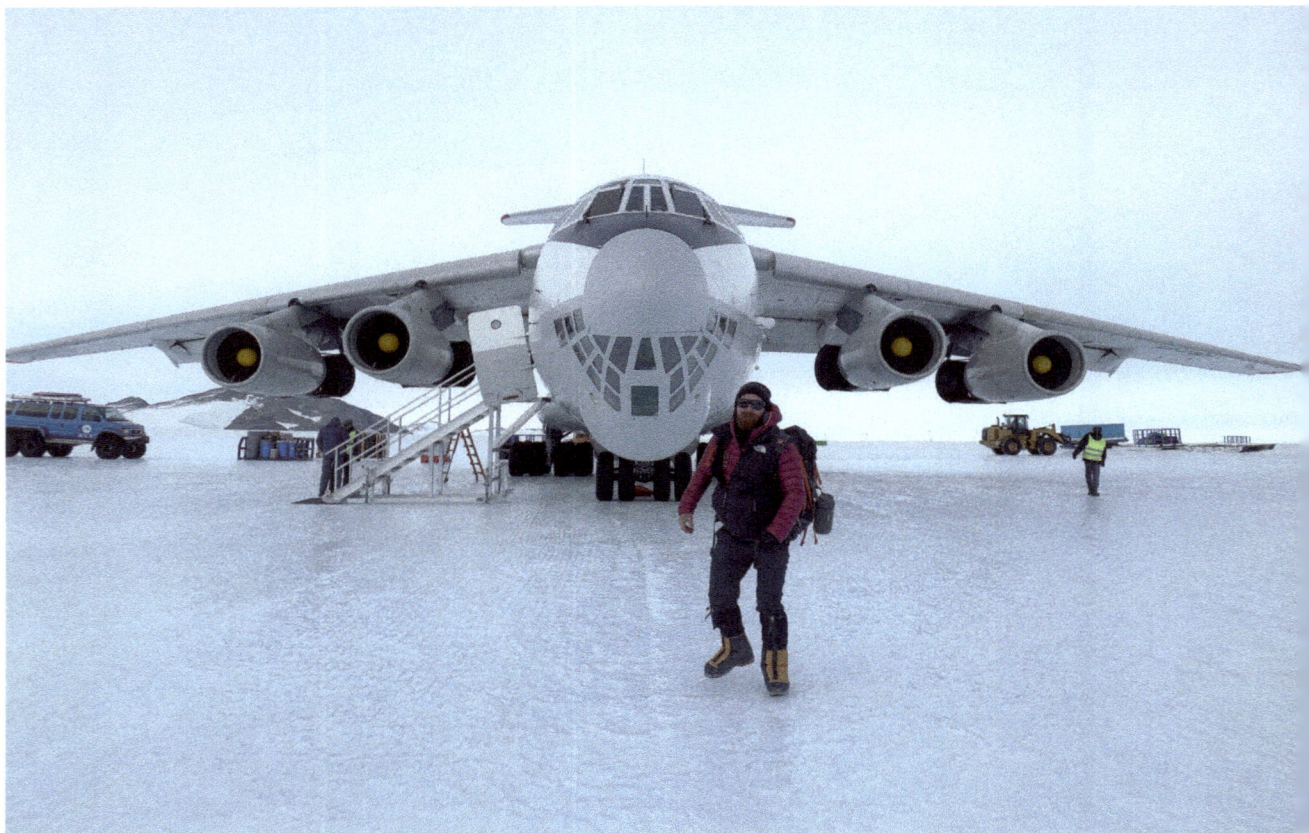

decades. There's a military presence on the streets, but locals go about their business as usual. There's no hard sell, bartering or begging as I zig-zag around this interesting town for last-minute supplies.

All is peaceful too at the Hotel Diego de Almagro, where I meet my eight fellow climbers. They include Matt, my room buddy and soon-to-be tent companion, and Josh, our guide. The passion and depth of experience of this group is evident. Half the team have summited Mt Everest, and every member has multiple big mountain expeditions under their belt.

The number of Everest veterans in this group is not surprising. Fewer people have summited Vinson than Everest, because it lies deep in the heart of the mighty Ellsworth mountain range, and until recently was very inaccessible. Organising an expedition to such a remote location was a logistical nightmare. It's only in the last few decades that guided clients have been able to climb Vinson.

Soon we're on our way. A bus ferries us to the front of the enormous Russian plane. Only ten people at a time are permitted to enter the aircraft, and no photos are allowed on the tarmac. Entering this jet is pretty special. As staff usher us to jump seats and more regular passenger seats lining the rear walls, we see huge overhead hydraulics and lifting tackle. A buzz of excitement fills the cabin. Rattling down the runway, I watch the hydraulics swing above as the plane gathers speed. The noise is incredible, and I'm glad they gave us ear plugs.

Our flight to Antarctica is expected to take almost five hours. The route crosses the Drake Passage, then follows the west side of the Antarctic Peninsula and the spine of the Ellsworth Mountains. Unlike a domestic plane, there are no passenger windows to gaze out of on our journey, which contributes to the feeling that we are embracing the unknown.

Hours later, the subdued cabin becomes a hive of activity when staff tell us it's going to get colder as we descend, and to rug up. Descent is like a high-adrenaline ride in a theme park. The plane's mighty vibrations increase as it prepares to land, and soon... touchdown. We've arrived at one of the most untouched and undisturbed places on the planet. Antarctica is truly the last frontier; a continent of rock and ice covering fourteen million square kilometres, including the South Pole.

Union Glacier, in the Southern Ellsworth Mountains, is our arrival point and where we take our first steps in Antarctica. The glacier is a large expanse of actively moving snow and ice that flows from the Polar Plateau towards the Ronne Ice Shelf. Exiting the plane, we're greeted with clear blue skies and a slippery blue-ice runway. Everyone gazes back in awe at the massive jet parked on it as we disembark. We have about twenty minutes to snap a few shots and grab a team photo.

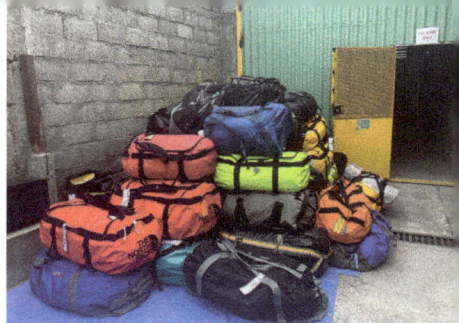

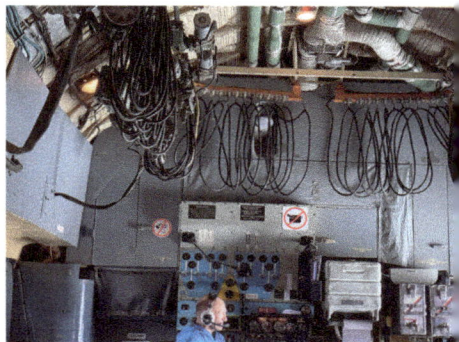

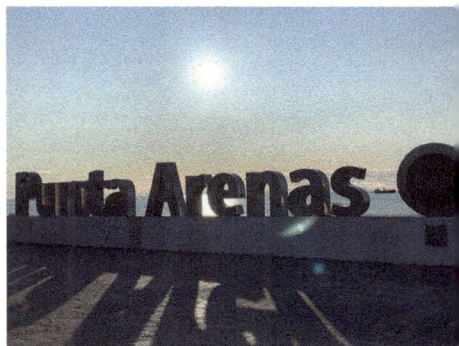

top Expedition-ready

centre Inside the main cabin of an Ilyushin 76

bottom One of the world's most southerly ports

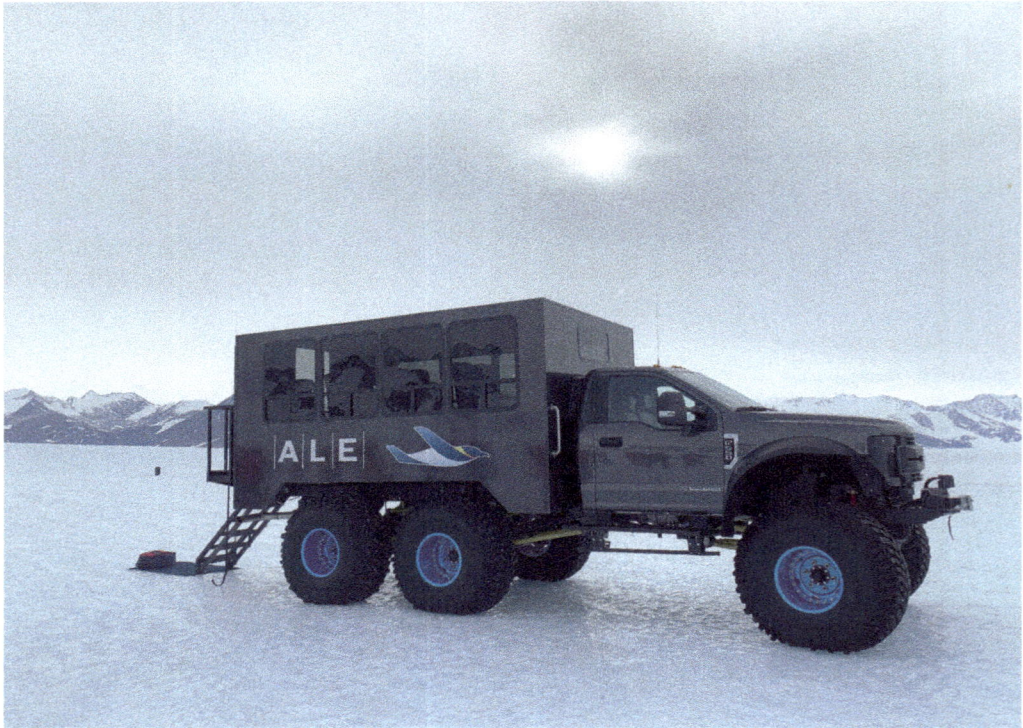

Our next ride is in an oversized Black F550 Ford truck that requires a ladder to climb into. Powering down 'Runway Road' on the eight-kilometre transfer to camp, we take in an alien landscape of rocky peaks and smooth, glistening, untouched snow. It's white-as-white for as far as the eye can see.

'If you landed on another planet, I imagine it would look something like this,' says fellow climber Darren.

Union Glacier Camp, scattered amid the snow at an altitude of 2,297 metres, has surprisingly comfortable amenities, including toilet blocks, a large heated dining tent and a library. There's even a gift shop open at select hours. It's the only camp of its kind in Antarctica, and can house up to seventy guests. Weather conditions don't permit us to continue by ski aircraft to Vinson Base Camp just yet, so for now this is home.

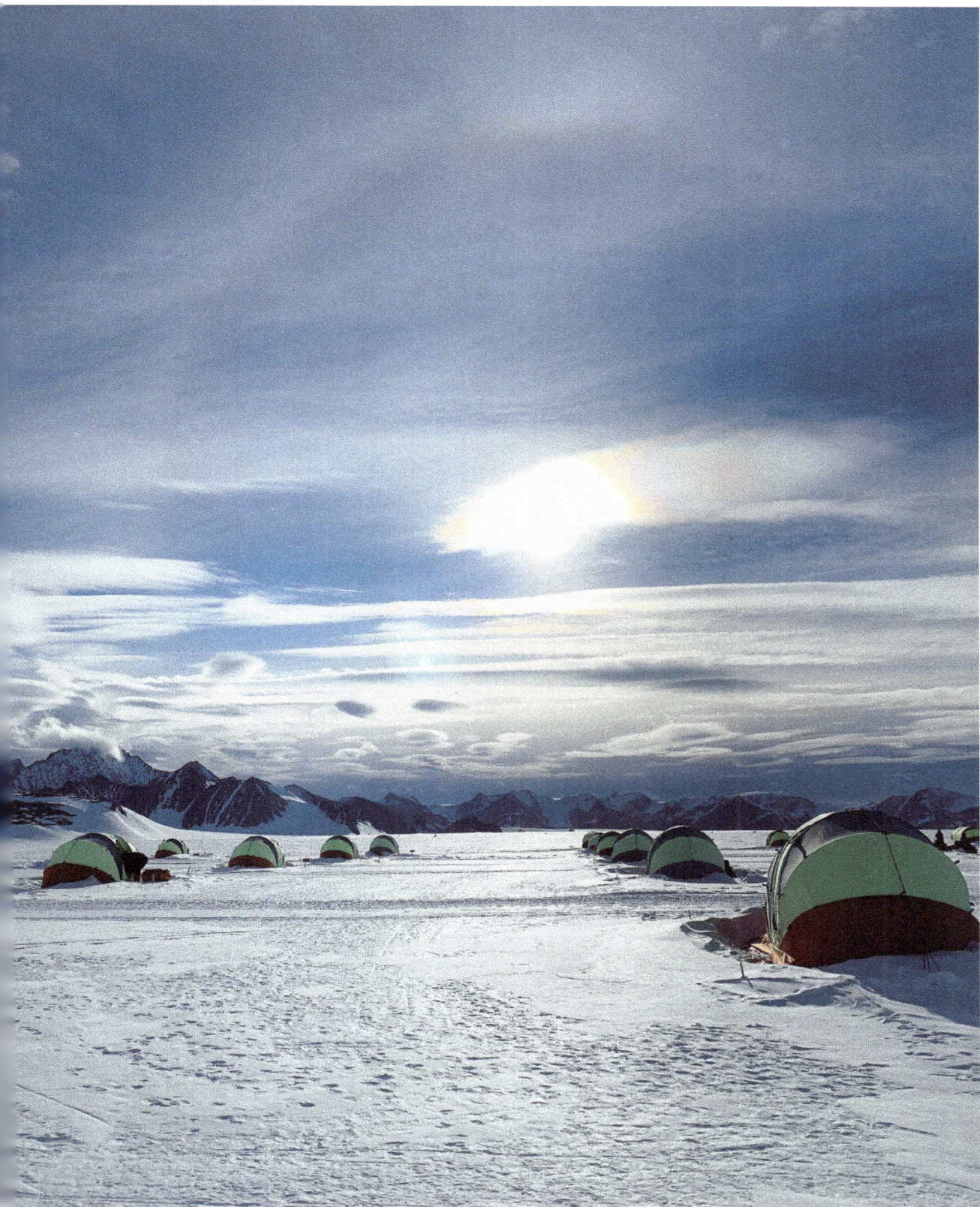

We've arrived at dinner time and I'm surprised to find, in the middle of nowhere, chefs using a fully-equipped kitchen and an extensive menu, written on whiteboards, for us to consider. A Moroccan stew, bread and red wine, followed by apple crumble, is my choice for tonight. After dinner we're reminded that while it's still light, it's already 10:30pm, so we should settle into our tents for the night.

opposite A long way from everywhere...

Clamshell mountaineering tents provide an exceptional level of comfort for our stay. Our clamshell measures five by 2.4 metres and is situated in a row of identical tents. We're close to the safety perimeter around the camp, marked by flags, that has been cleared of crevasses. Each tent has a name, and our clamshell is called 'Ponting'. With a table, two beds, padded sleeping mats and even a pillow, all that's left for us to do is roll out our sleeping bags. But with twenty-four-hour sunlight and clear skies, it's difficult to unwind. All I can do is put the eye mask on and try to relax. The day has been such a buzz and I feel extremely grateful to be here.

Day 4—Union Glacier Camp

Opening our tent door, I'm greeted with fresh snow and a different horizon from that of yesterday. Clouds hide nearby mountains and there's a fresh breeze. We're told it doesn't snow much in this area, and the Antarctic climate is generally cold, dry and windy.

We're in a holding pattern, awaiting weather updates before the short flight to Mt Vinson Base Camp, 151 kilometres away. Scrambled eggs, bacon and burritos with plunger coffee start my day; I'm again impressed by the range offered, and what's on my plate. We receive a weather brief before lunchtime and learn we're not flying today. So I meander to the gift shop, take some photos and watch the fluttering snow.

The clouds slowly lift to reveal hidden mountain tops and bring the promise of flights restarting. After ten to twenty

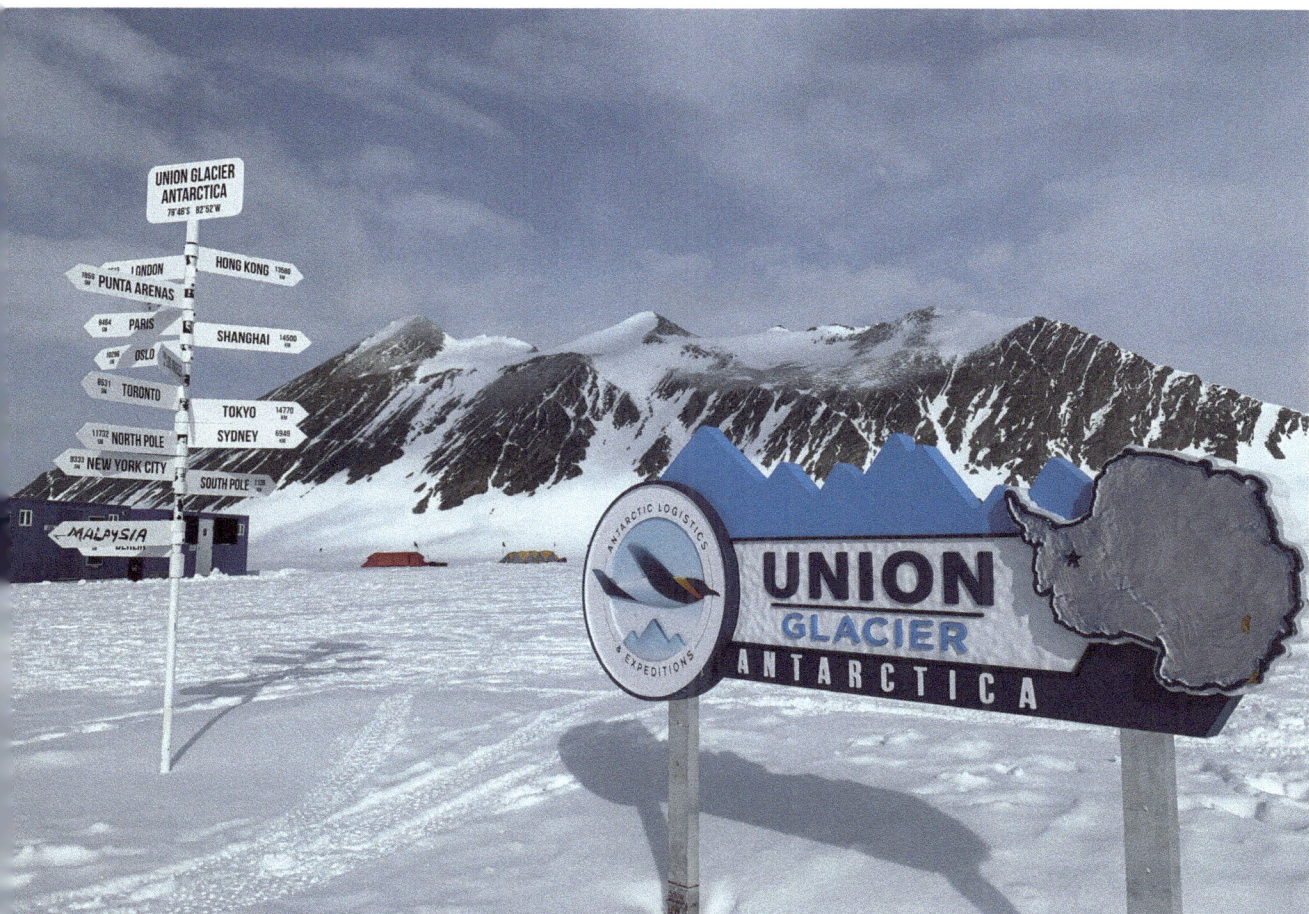

millimetres of snow, which is a lot for this region, every outdoor surface is covered in fresh white powder.

In the afternoon there's a lecture on geology and history. Afterwards it's back to the dining tent for dinner. Eating as a group is a laugh. The opening topic for tonight's conversation is toes amputated due to frostbite, complete with photos.

Adjacent to our camp is where the southernmost marathon on Earth takes place—the Antarctic Ice Marathon. With customised mountain bikes, we're able to ride on a section of the ten-kilometre flagged loop, although the weather and increasing winds prevent us venturing too far. So my tent companion and I resort to wrestling in the snow over a football, much to the shock of witnesses. Concerns about injury and appropriateness are brushed aside—we were having fun.

After expending some energy, an evening weather briefing confirms the forecast—standby.

It seems to have quickly become late, and it's time to embrace sleeping under a full sun.

Day 5—Waiting

The morning hype is all about the upcoming weather briefing. It looks to be clearing up outside, but that's no reflection of what's happening at Vinson Base Camp. A satellite phone reports a simple message: 'Still cloudy here.' Our weather briefing is presented with graphs and detailed analysis, which is beyond comprehension. In a nutshell, we're not flying yet. On the positive side, when the wind does drop and clouds clear, there are a few good days coming up.

We're cleared to walk the entire length of the flagged route we rode a small section of yesterday, which lifts morale among a few of us. It's great to really stretch the legs and venture away from the confines of camp. At the farthest point of the circuit, with mountains to both sides, a vista opens up of nothing but flat, white horizon as far as the eye can see. Each step crunches on the fresh snow underfoot. Out here there is nothing but silence.

To pass time we play football, ride mountain bikes, play cards—'Hearts', and I lose—walk some more, and study the lunch menu. And then the dinner menu. There's a shower experience to embrace. Fill one's bucket with ice, then add the hot water provided before inserting a hose next to the shower. Then with a flick of a switch, pumps are on and you're having the unique experience that is an Antarctic shower.

Weirdly, it's after midnight again, but it certainly doesn't feel like it. To unwind I've decided to read in the library. The constant sunshine has officially wreaked havoc with my body clock.

Day 6—More waiting

Waking intermittently during the night to the constant bright light, I have to squint at my watch to figure out when morning has arrived. Eventually it's time for breakfast and, more importantly, the weather update. Currently it's minus six degrees Celsius in camp, but the windchill factor is bringing it down to minus 13.5 degrees Celsius. That sounds cold, but conditions look good and positivity on the prospect of flying is high, although we're told cloud remains quite stubborn at Vinson Base Camp.

Guide Josh tells us that when it's safe for the first two Twin Otter planes to leave, we'll have two hours to pack and be ready to fly. There are six flights planned today, in three waves. Our team is wave two. Sounds great.

A game of Hearts keeps us semi-occupied as we wait for news of our imminent departure. We haven't heard any planes starting up their engines yet, but two have been loaded in preparation. We're entirely at the whim of the weather. A long lunch signals that maybe we need to find an activity for the afternoon. A few of us grab fat-tyre mountain bikes and head for the ten-kilometre loop track to exert some energy. 'If you hear planes leaving, come straight back,' Josh advises.

But back at camp, after a few games of chess and more idleness, there are still no flights. No news before we regroup in the dining tent for dinner, but lots of speculation. A breeze is picking up outside. The weather has total control over plans. Then it's confirmed—no flights tonight; departure has been called off. We've come to expect the unexpected. Our sense of adventure too goes on hold. The first wave reluctantly retrieve their loaded packs from the plane and the camp goes back into a holding pattern.

'Another game of Hearts?' someone asks. 'Yeah, I'm in,' I reply.

Conversation is light as we passively deal cards for the next game. Fellow climbers invariably ask each other why they might be here, undertaking this expedition. While scientists worldwide seek a cure, a key part of my reason for being here is to increase awareness of what living with type 1 diabetes means, not just for Finlay, but for all children who suffer from the condition. And I'm not the only one wanting to climb Mt Vinson simply 'because it's there'. The conversation is an opportunity to really listen to strangers express their purpose and perspective on everything from charities to personal missions.

opposite Touchdown

After the card game there's another engaging lecture in the library, presented by our resident historian. 'Race to the South Pole', aptly named, captures the story of the early expeditions and ultimately how the party of Norwegian explorers, under the command of Roald Amundsen, succeeded in 1911. Comparisons are made to the modern exploration that continues to take place. The resources and infrastructure that are available today just cannot be compared to the primitive conditions that the early explorers laboured under.

Leaving the lecture, we encounter increasing winds and low visibility. The latest weather briefing confirms the bad news: 'No flights tonight, it's been called off.'

Day 7—Union Glacier Camp to Base Camp to Camp 1

Light blue skies with barely a cloud! Still, crisp air!

'Today we go, 100 per cent we go,' says Matt.

Before I've finished breakfast, people scheduled on the first wave are leaving: snowmobiles fly around transferring luggage and sleds. Their efficiency catches me off guard as I pack my gear, ready to depart the clamshell tent and board our bird out of here. And we soon do.

Wow, wow… awe-inspiring landscapes abound.

To one side a mountain range, the other nothing but vast expanses of white snow blended into the horizon before a pale, light blue sky. Then the opposite. A mountain range to my right and smooth white snow as far as you can see. Shadows

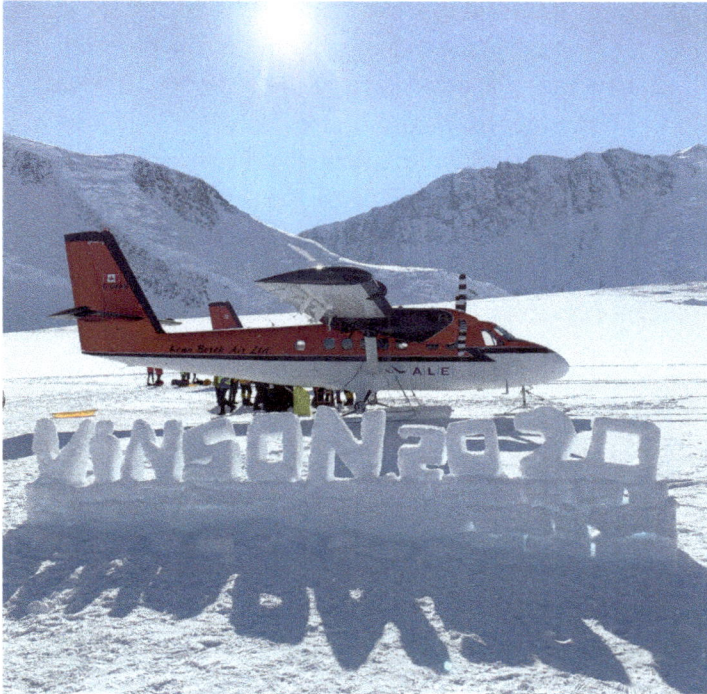

dapple dramatic mountains; sharp ridges and rocky peaks protrude from the white landscape.

We fly through a valley with mountains looming on either side. The mountain range on my right becomes higher than our altitude. It's Vinson, and so our descent begins. Base Camp, on the lower part of the Branscomb Glacier at an elevation of 2,133 metres, comes into view.

As the plane taxies, we see a small crowd: they're waiting to depart, rather than to greet us. This group couldn't summit due to high winds and have spent six days waiting for these flights to arrive to head home. The planes have a quick turnaround, and the next plane is already landing as we haul our gear onto sleds and drag them to nearby tents.

We meet our head guide, Mike, who pulls us straight in to lay out the program: due to hold-ups with the weather, we're not going to stay here. Instead, the plan is to load the sleds, pull down camp, and move to Camp 1 (2,799 metres) in one haul. This usually takes up to two days of the program, but Mike wants to take advantage of the high-pressure system that's briefly moved in, and figures we're well fed and well rested. Branscomb Shoulder Route has become the 'standard route' and is the one we will follow, he says.

It's a hive of activity—tents come down, communal carry gear is divided, sleds are set, harnesses rigged. We're divided into three groups of four rope teams, each with four members. Josh is leading our team, with Matt, Fred and myself.

It's almost 3pm when we depart and trek off into the unknown. The expanses of white snow make it difficult to discern the difference between the clouds and the horizon; they are indistinguishable from each other. Only the crunching of snow underfoot breaks the otherwise dead silence.

Breaks are short, and after days of relative inactivity, the muscles certainly know they're working. It's a toll on the hips, particularly with a full pack on my back and a loaded sled in tow.

But the hours pass quickly as I gaze upon the extraordinary landscape, a landscape like nothing I've seen before. There are no trees or bushes, that's for sure. Antarctica is essentially an ice sheet about two kilometres thick hiding a landscape of mountains, valleys and plains below. It's so cold here, it affects the global climate system. Icicles start to grow in my beard, and another layer of clothing must go on.

After a seven-hour slog we arrive at camp, at an elevation of 2,799 metres, after some 666 metres of elevation gain. Having never pulled a sled, let alone a weighted one, I know I'll need some more training as we go on.

With packs off and untied from the sleds, I've found a second wind. Which is just as well, as the next group job is to build a wall around the perimeter of the tent with ice blocks. Using two hand saws, we saw directly into the ice in a grid pattern, before popping the ice blocks out with a shovel and laying them in a brick fashion. It's a strenuous process, and

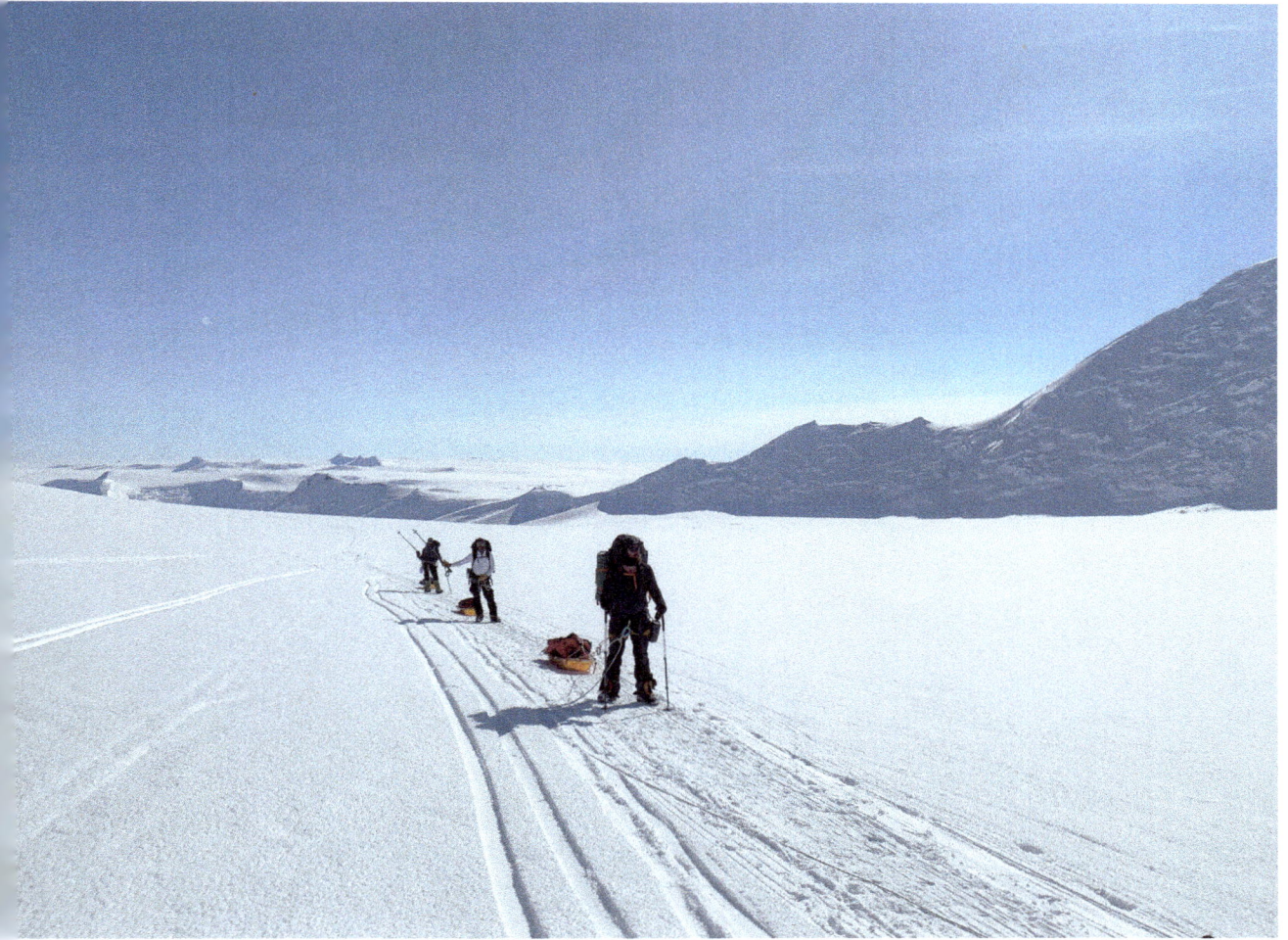

above Taking it all in

when I stop my clothes are soaked in sweat. The continuous glare of the sun has burnt my nose and any exposed skin.

Next job, pitching tents. We're sleeping three to a tent, and I'm with Matt and Fred. Meanwhile, ice is being melted and pizza is being cooked. By the time I've had a couple of small slices and received some water it's almost 2am, and I finally get my head down.

Day 8—Camp 1 to Camp 2

As the camp rattles to life, I leave the comfort of my warm sleeping bag for an Antarctic chill. An icy blast hits me when I open the tent zipper, yet bizarrely there's the sun, bright as ever. The weather forecast shows the high-pressure system will soon break down. Unless we move straight up to Camp 2 (3,780 metres), we may miss the best weather conditions of the season.

'How do we all feel about that?' asks Mike.

It's a compelling argument, requiring us to pack up this camp, and carry heavy loads up fixed lines and steep terrain. Again, normally this move is undertaken over two days, with a carry day to reduce the loads. But it's a strong group, and with Mike's recommendation that's the decision we make. It's going to be another long day, including making a new camp when we arrive at our destination.

I help pack our tent, food, and the minimal amount of clothing and snacks I think I'll survive with, but still end up with a very heavy backpack. Ice crampons go under our boots for traction, we heave on our backpacks, our rope team is tied in, and we set off from the camp we just built; a tiny sanctuary in the middle of nowhere.

It's tough walking across the moderately rising terrain. To ensure a stumble doesn't result in a long slide off the mountain we use ascenders on a fixed line to lock our position, and edge up the slope one step at a time in what is a slow process. The muscles are certainly working; the load on my back has never felt heavier. Climbing consistently at a forty-degree angle, most of the day is spent on this one steep slope. Gaining elevation does, however, give us views of surrounding peaks rising majestically in all directions.

Hours fly by as I contemplate the steps in front of me, a couple at a time, and the mind-blowing beauty of the untouched landscape behind me. I try to record videos where I can, but batteries die fast in the cold. Although I'm climbing with a group, you can feel quite isolated in the solitude of this vast, unending whiteness.

In this alien environment, unexpected thoughts can catch me unprepared. I find myself reminiscing about the good, simple moments of family life that I'm missing and that I miss. The kids' excitement in the morning as they run into our bedroom. The chaos of everyone departing the house at once for work, school and errands. Unwinding at the end of the day and hearing about what everyone got up to over a family dinner. I have none of that here, and my thoughts must fill in the blanks.

How are the kids today? This week even. Are they well? Especially Fin. Is Heidi getting any sleep? What are Fin's blood glucose levels (BGLs)? Are they okay? I wonder what my BGL would be. A healthy person generally has a range between 4.0 to 8.0 millimoles of glucose per litre of blood. But does it stay the same in the challenging environment I'm currently surviving in?

These thoughts are random, and not what usually run through my mind. The silence and the slowness of time in this ever-sunlit place have affected my mind, as has missing my family.

I've conceded that moments of homesickness will come, and then pass.

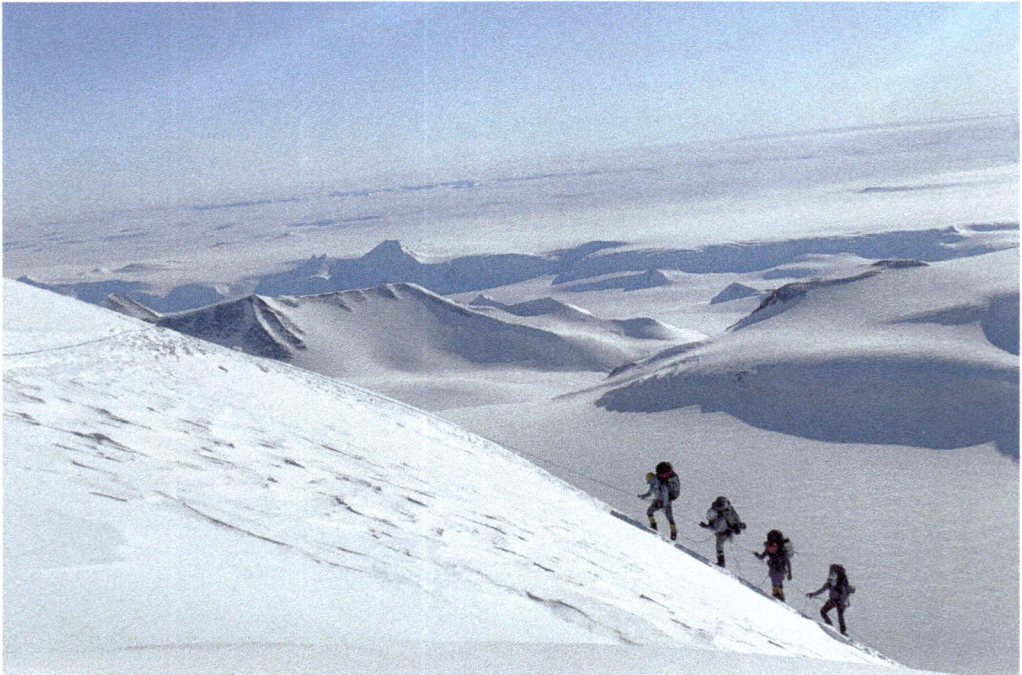

Onward we climb to the summit of this towering ridge; it's not Mt Vinson, but I certainly feel like we've climbed a mountain today. While having a rest at the top for snacks and water, Mike points to the old route, which was favoured until some climbers fell in a crevasse amid horrible conditions and a whiteout. Crevasses, often covered by just a thin layer of snow, can be hundreds of feet deep. The climbers trapped in the crevasse couldn't be rescued for four days, explains Mike, who was part of the rescue team. Exposed to the elements, frostbite cost them some fingers, though luckily not their lives. It's food for thought as we press on, with Mt Sidley now close on our left.

Finally, with one last rise to scale, we arrive at Camp 2 (3,780 metres) at 11:50pm, after an almost eight-hour effort and some 981 metres of elevation gained. While this camp has some existing ice block walls we can utilise, built-up snow needs to be levelled and shovelled out. But at least there's no sawing of ice blocks to undertake. The common tent goes up, with seats and table both dug into the ice. Then the routine continues for personal tents—level the ground, then get them up. Sounds easy enough, but adjusting to the new altitude after a day of true exertion is tough.

Finally, we crawl into our tent. My legs shake involuntarily as I lie down, too tired to find more clothes, although it's minus twenty degrees Celsius.

Day 9—Rest day

I'm keen to hear the weather update, and ultimately if we'll summit today. So I'm up early and wander around camp, but there's no-one else about. More than a few climbers are either exhausted or suffering from altitude sickness.

The next couple of days are ideal to summit, according to Mike, who has summited Mt Vinson eighteen times, and today will be a rest day. So I climb back into the tent and out of the searing sun.

Day 10—Camp 2 to Summit to Camp 2

Today's the day. Conditions are perfect, with wide blue skies, little wind, and the promise of manageable temperatures. First some breakfast, then we get away from camp at about 10am.

A couple of hours in I'm quietly struggling with nausea, and focus on breathing. My beard starts to freeze, even with two buffs on, and they too are soon frozen. It progressively gets colder the higher we scale. After forcing down some fluids and food, I start to feel better.

'If you're not drinking and eating at every stop, you're letting the team down . . .' is Mike's mantra.

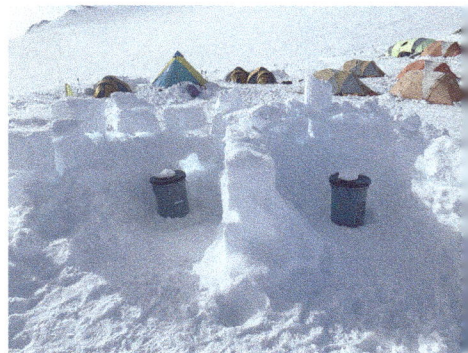

above Toilet break

opposite The serenity

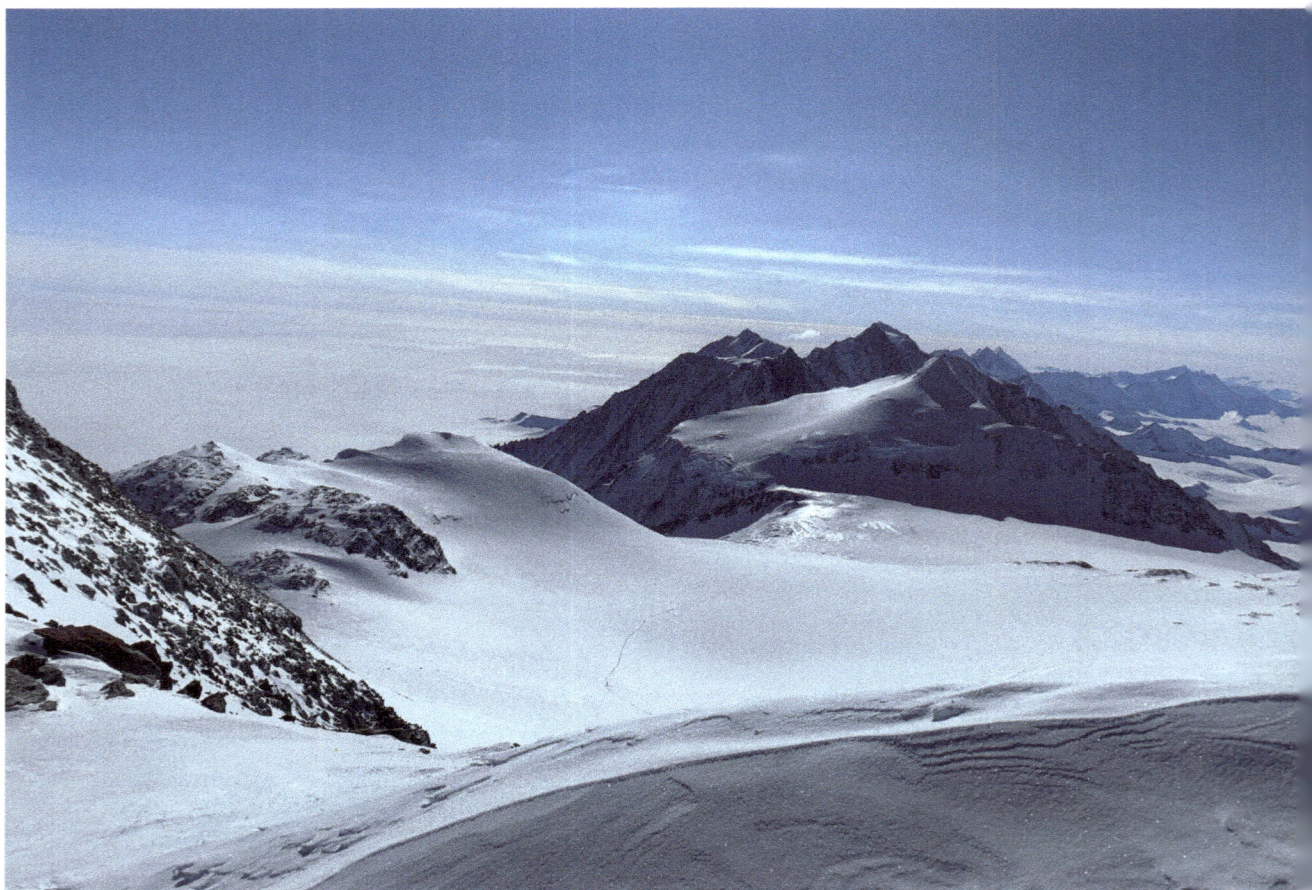

The last push to the summit includes scaling a thin path that leads ever higher, hugging exposed rock. This section twists, turns, rises and falls and continues towards the now visible summit, in total contrast to the open white plains we've crossed.

It takes an exhausting seven hours and fifteen minutes to summit Mt Vinson, at 4,892 metres.

Time stands still as we celebrate, and respect our position—we've made it to the top of the bottom of the world, and are privileged to stand on a peak that was first summited on 18 December 1966. I gaze around, simply astounded at the views. We're overlooking the Ronne Ice Shelf near the base of the Antarctic Peninsula, and a very long way from home.

After taking in the view from this ultra-prominent peak, I once again perform the most important task of the climb. The Diabetes Australia flag comes out and I plant it at the very highest point, where it flaps in the howling Antarctic wind. I need Matt to step in and grab one side of the flag so that it can be properly visible in a photo. Had I been on my own, there would have been no hope of getting a good photo and there was still a good chance the flag would fly off. Rightly or wrongly, to ensure a firm grip and avoid losing the flag, I risked frostbite and removed one glove.

At the summit of Mt Vinson we're 1,200 kilometres from the South Pole, making it the most remote of the Seven Summits. It remains the last discovered, last named, and last climbed mountain of them all. We don't celebrate for long: the weather is deteriorating. As Mike calls for our speedy exit, one last group photo is taken before we start our descent.

My face freezes and becomes painful as we cross over the ridge passage, as you would expect with a minus thirty-six degrees Celsius wind chill factor. I can feel the ice all the way up my nostrils and occasionally make an unsuccessful attempt to dislodge it. Time is of the essence as we creep back down the mountain. It's a long, difficult slog and less than exciting. When Camp 2 eventually comes into sight in the distance, it's the motivation I need to keep going towards it.

Back at camp, where our tents are protected from the worst of the wind by huge ice blocks, we're soon asleep under the midnight sun, exhausted yet satisfied. Mt Vinson has been a huge success for every climber in our group to summit.

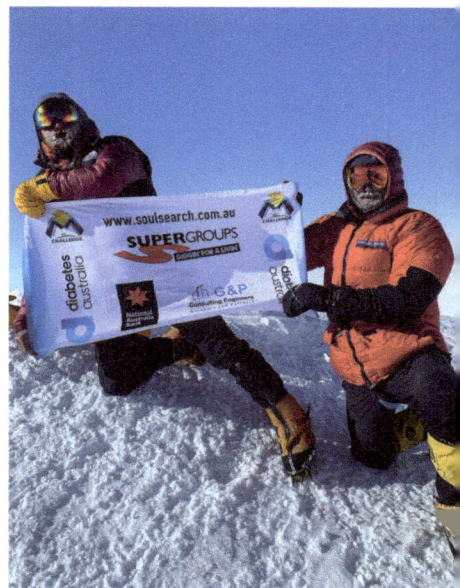

above Mt Vinson Summit

opposite Antarctica's unique environment

Day 11—Camp 2 to Camp 1 to Base Camp

Mike rouses us from a deep sleep at around midday, robbing us of much-needed rest. But he had no choice.

'We have to get out of here as quickly as we can,' he says.

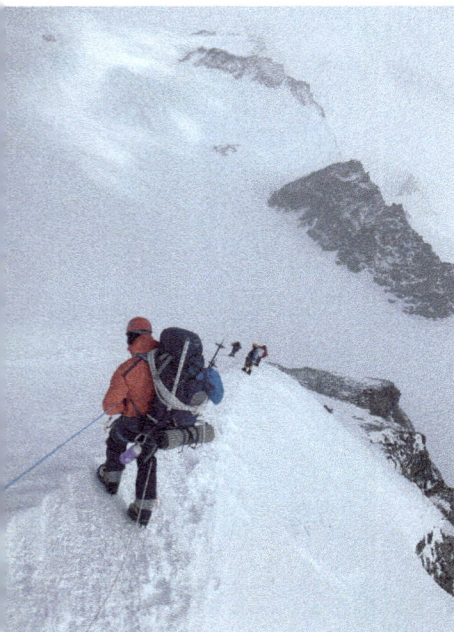

above Time to go

Our weather window has closed. Visibility is low, and it's very cold.

Loaded up and tied in to our four-man line gang, we're rope team three, led by Josh, with Matt behind me, then Fred as the 'anchor man'. As we wait, I wriggle my toes constantly. They're numb and my goggles remain frozen. Eventually we trudge off, back towards Camp 1. It's an extra effort with a full pack when you're going downhill.

Utter silence surrounds us when we stop, the type of silence you don't notice anywhere else in the world, at least not in the world I've seen. This environment and experience gives me a deep sense of calm; it's good for the soul. For me the exertion and sacrifice sets the tone to fully appreciate the planet around us. I notice new aspects of the surrounding mountains. Blocks of fallen ice. New angles that appear because sections of ice are constantly moving or breaking away.

At around 7:45pm we finally arrive back at Base Camp, drained of energy. I'm very ready to return to the comforts of Union Glacier Camp—and then Punta Arenas. But only one plane can land. Mike puts his rope team, some Canadian fellow climbers, and himself, on the plane departing for Union Glacier. He is unsure if another plane will be able to land or not, he tells us as he waves goodbye.

So we must stay at Base Camp until another plane can land. Just five of us. A plane is expected tomorrow, but if I've learnt anything in my time in the Antarctic it's that you can't predict the weather down here. Stuck in this bleak, incredibly remote place, the five of us decide to sleep in the communal tent instead of setting up individual tents. We can't help feeling short-changed in missing out on the flight.

Soft, fresh snow falls, and it's quiet, really quiet. It's still snowing as I lie awake at midnight, trying to pretend it's dark.

Day 12—Waiting

We are on continuous standby for a flight out of here. Snow slides off the tent and drips inside it like it's raining. Visibility isn't great. And it's very, very cold. Water is made by melting ice, and bacon is cooked up and served.

Josh, our remaining guide, returns from the communications tent. There is no news of any flights coming in, only uncertainty. We'll fly at some stage, he reassures us, so we start to pack. Away go sleeping bags and gear, and our bags are carted to the ice ski-way, ready to load onto the plane. We take up position sitting outside waiting for news of its arrival. After long, strenuous days climbing, keeping still and watching and waiting for a plane feels strange. It's difficult to slow down.

A couple of other groups descend from the summit and celebrate their successful campaign. Matt remains in limbo with me and our rope team, while Clayton is the new addition to those on standby. He also happens to be a pilot. We discuss the economic reality of a ten-seater plane flying full. We're advised not to pull down the main tent just yet, and the arriving party is advised to not put theirs up. We're in limbo, and the instructions feel contradictory.

Hours pass just sitting around. And we're cold, very cold. Josh comes back from the communications tent with another update, the first with any certainty: flights have been called off for today . . .

Disappointed, I trek back up to the ski-way with a sled and retrieve our bags. There's nothing to say, really, and everyone quietly starts setting up camp again. I'm then straight into my sleeping bag to try to warm up my legs.

As evening nears, the weather continues to deteriorate, and it starts to snow heavily. The weather forecast is the same for another week, says Josh, so who knows when we will get out of here.

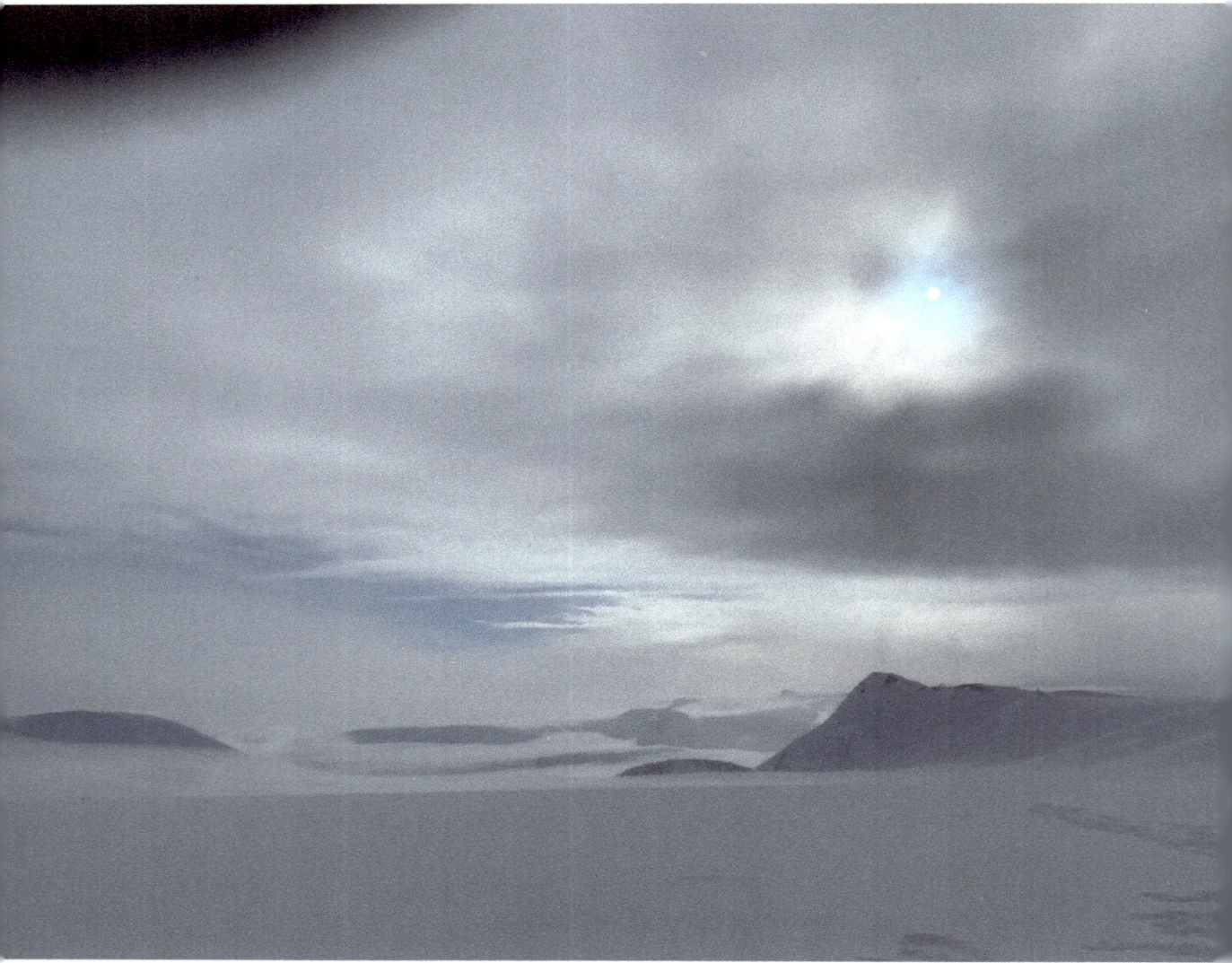

above No flying today

Our successful summit is beginning to fade from my thoughts. As the exhilaration retreats, it becomes harder to adjust to the continuing inconvenience and inertia. There's nothing to see, nothing to do. Antarctica offers a beautiful, pristine environment, but it exists somewhere past the weather that is currently right in front of our noses and preventing our return home.

Sometimes I wonder what I'd think if my kids undertook these risky adventures in far-flung corners of the world. How would I feel? What would be my concerns? When I think of my kids, Finlay always appears to be at a disadvantage compared to my other three healthy children. Well, in my thoughts anyway. There's a level of guilt there I don't yet completely understand.

Would Fin be able to cope with an adventure such as the one I'm currently undertaking? Severe hyperglycemia (high blood sugar) would quickly set in if she didn't have enough insulin or ran out altogether. That in turn would become diabetic ketoacidosis, which leads to death if untreated.

Being here in Antarctica, at the mercy of the weather, reminds me of the unpredictability of the human experience. Without insulin... well, I try not to ponder that too much. The thing about Fin's condition is that she must always be prepared. In time, I believe, that will become her superpower.

Perhaps it's my own 'take it as it comes' attitude that is rattling my thoughts. Often, I'm not as prepared as I ought to be. But that has never been a problem; in fact it gives me a sense of freedom, that I can do as I please. Not everyone is so lucky. Should I be concerned if my kids show signs of the same attitude? Finlay can't be like that. She must be prepared.

There's probably too much time to think down here as I wait in the whiteness for the weather to turn.

Nothing could be more certain than the fact that this weather is preventing my swift return home. Stopping my family from being reunited once more. There are some long hours ahead of me as I'm left in limbo with nothing to do but try to get warm in the cold that will not change.

Day 13—More waiting

Snow, snow, snow.

It's a whiteout. We're not going anywhere. We are stranded. And the news only gets worse when the weather report comes through—we might be here for a few more days.

All our food is in the cache, so a coffee and some nuts start the day. We sit around contemplating anything to pass the time. It's icy cold, visibility isn't great, and we're holed up at Base Camp. Reviewing my flight schedule back to Australia, I start to get worried. To try to avoid any negativity, I set up the iPad for a movie. The cold weather kills the remaining battery, so while it's on charge I walk around camp, and three of us have a game of Monopoly. Then it's back to the movie.

Chatter fills the silent void as another group of climbers return from Mt Vinson in high spirits after successfully summiting. I remember that feeling of elation—one that quickly died as we realised we were stranded.

Day 14—Still waiting

Another morning on the ice. I'm first up and push all the snow off the top of our tent to stop it collapsing. I go to our cache in search of coffee and some breakfast. Climbing in the snow hole, I dig out some oats, bagels, salmon and soup.

My feet are ice blocks. There's no visibility for flying. We are captive here. It's expected to snow all day, so hibernating in the tent seems the only reasonable option. There is promise of better weather tomorrow.

The wind howls in the evening: sleeping in two layers of thermals and fleece doesn't bring warmth, even in the usual comfort of the sleeping bag.

Day 15—Waiting, waiting, waiting

'Oh . . . we're living in a refrigerator,' says Matt, his teeth chattering.

The tent flaps in the wind, and fog persists. Any optimism of an early flight vanishes. The flight from Union Glacier back to Punta Arenas on the Russian jet Ilyushin-76TD is scheduled to depart today. Should we miss this flight we'll be Antarctica guests until the next flight, whenever that might be. And we're told they aren't that frequent. Still, I optimistically pack my gear and sit waiting for the now-hourly flight update.

Apparently they're really trying to get us out. I can't see it myself; winds continue to howl and it feels colder today than

below Just try and stay less cold

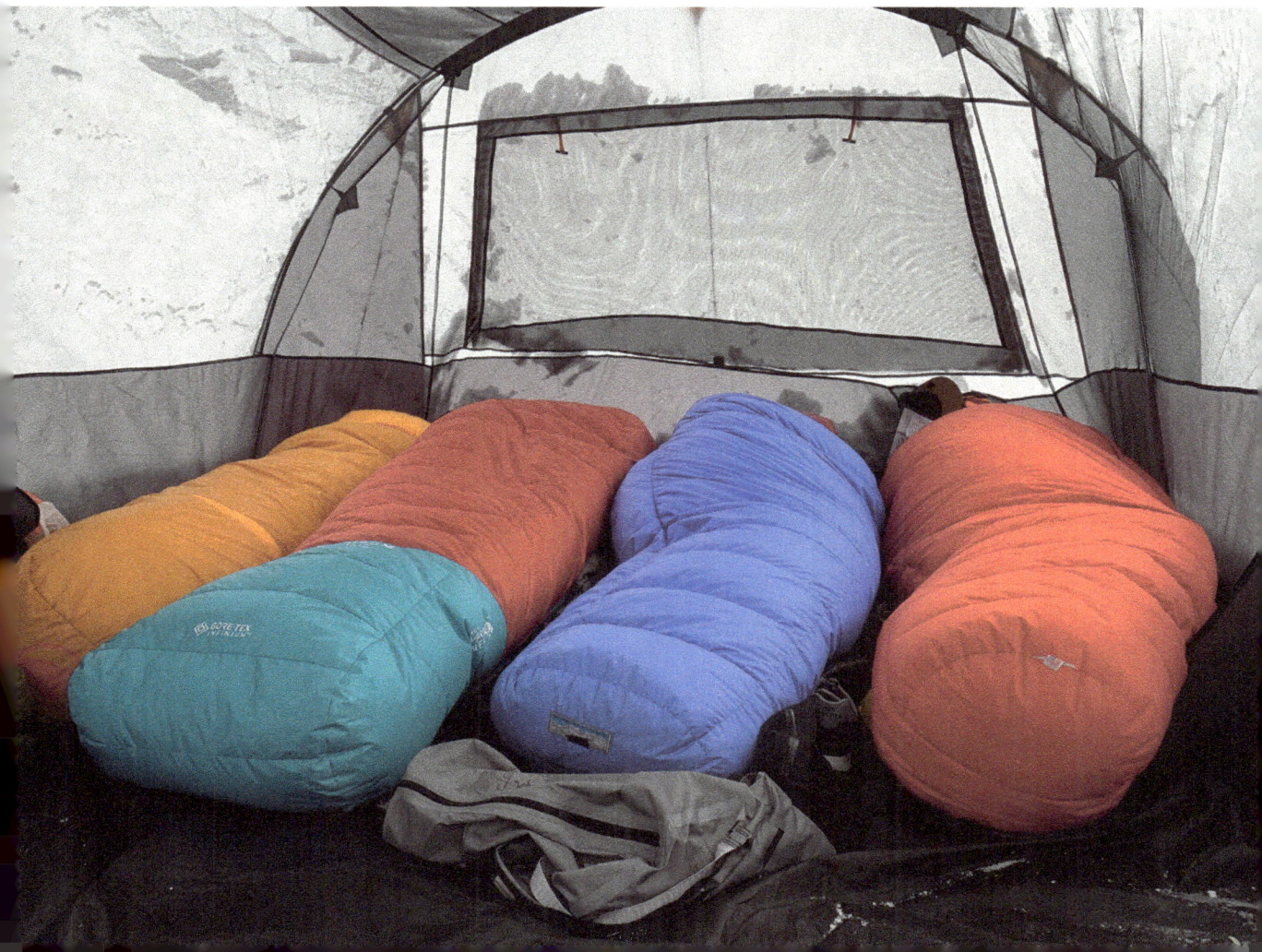

previous days—if that's possible. I've doubled my socks and checked that my toes aren't going black, as they ache with a numb chill.

Later, Josh tells us that all those who left Base Camp for Union Glacier a couple of days ago are flying back to Punta Arenas on the Russian jet today. We've now missed the flight. I'm surprised at the development and I don't feel like part of a team anymore. We're still stuck here, unable to get out of Base Camp but the others have moved on.

I have to believe there's a chance we'll get out today, or before long. Our backs will be against the wall soon, as the climbing season is coming to an end. Later, the clouds clear and we see the sun for the first time in days. Yet the planes stay grounded. So, after discovering a deck of cards, here I sit in my sleeping bag, at the table, for yet another game of Hearts.

Hopefully tomorrow will be the day for us.

Day 16—Base Camp to Union Glacier Camp

Hurrah! Clear skies and little wind has our flights confirmed for this morning.

Every face in Base Camp lights up with joy when we see those birds flying in. I'm first on the plane. Butterflies in my stomach, vibrations felt all the way down the runway, and we're out of here.

My window seat provides an unparalleled opportunity for scenic vistas, and the landscape and sky merge as one on the horizon. Gazing over the mountains, I ponder the vulnerability I've seen in myself while I was at the mercy of this incredibly harsh, yet spectacularly beautiful environment. For those who went to Antarctica before us, to open the path, I give thanks. For without them this landscape couldn't be admired from where I am, and would be forever hidden in the unknown. Having breathed the air, stood on the ice and absorbed the

opposite No words...

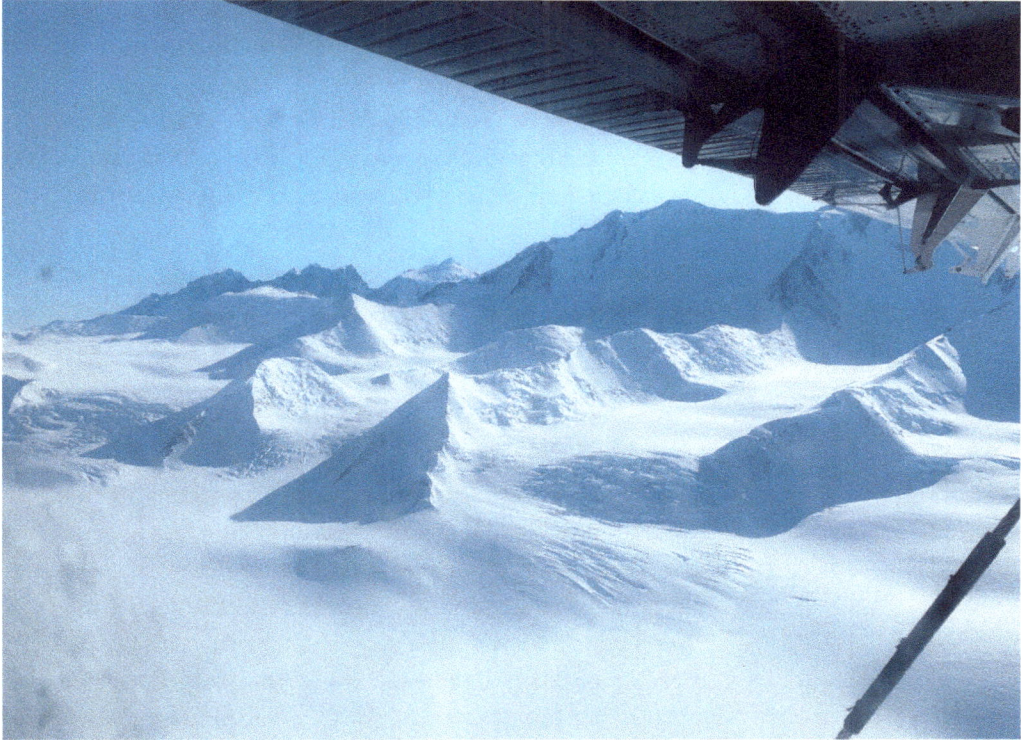

cold, my Antarctica experience has touched my soul like no other place I have visited. I would never have dreamt this experience in all its detail—ever. It's amazing that this part of the world can be accessed by and open to an individual, should you simply make the commitment to go and, of course, secure a flight. And you don't have to climb a mountain if you come here. To simply pass through can change your life.

I wanted to do more than pass through. I hope to raise donations, make a difference to the diabetes community, or at least be a good role model for my children. Great adventures are indeed possible if you dare to dream and have the courage to set out into the unknown. A cure for type 1 diabetes is unknown today, but perhaps that too is a great adventure.

Perhaps it will just take someone to believe that it is possible, gather the means to look for it, and remain determined in the face of obstacles.

Before long we're back on the Russian jet, Ilyushin-76TD, another hero that gives so many people the opportunity to visit Antarctica, and we're on our way back to Punta Arenas.

AFTER SCRAMBLING to find accommodations and enduring a series of flight changes, I eventually got back to home terra firma.

Coming home to familiar people and places, however, wasn't easy. Once the excitement of being reunited had passed, I realised that something had changed. Ironically, at home, everything seemed the same. In part, that's a credit to Heidi running a solid, reassuring routine that provides stability and security for our family. There's nothing wrong with that. But I found the sameness, on this return, strangely disturbing. Then I realised what was going on. It was me. My adventures, these mountains, diabetes—they were changing me. I no longer felt like I could fit straight back in. At least I'm good at keeping busy, which distracted me from my introspection.

In those first few days back at home, the warmth on my face of the morning's first rays caused me to wake from a deep slumber with initial confusion about where I was, like a mini amnesia. Sometimes I just wandered the streets near home, like I was discovering them for the first time. I passed the cafes and restaurants of Nelson Place and sat down to savour coffees while contemplating the urgency of locals going about their business.

There were, however, new beginnings to enjoy at home.

The kids were starting a new school year. That is a milestone, and was a big deal. They raced excitedly out the front door in the morning, tore down the street, turned the corner, crossed the road at the school crossing, waving to the familiar face of 'Vince' the crossing supervisor, and we were there.

After we led them through the iron gate and said our goodbyes, they were off, making their own way in the world. They used to be so little, and now they're becoming independent. It's evidence that time is always passing. How can I slow it down?

The Seven Summits challenge has turned out to be about more than fundraising for Diabetes Australia and increasing awareness about the disease. It's also become an existential challenge. The best way I can make sense of this crazy experience is to keep writing about it. To someone who wasn't there to experience them, my travel stories won't mean what they mean to me. I get that. Not everyone is going to be interested. I choose to share these challenges, but my words are intended for those who are genuinely interested and ask. I don't want to force my summit stories onto some poor, unsuspecting, uninterested soul.

But I do have a clear sense of direction—to the next mountain.

My lungs seem to have benefited from all the time at altitude. I run easier, and with a focus and clarity that didn't exist before.

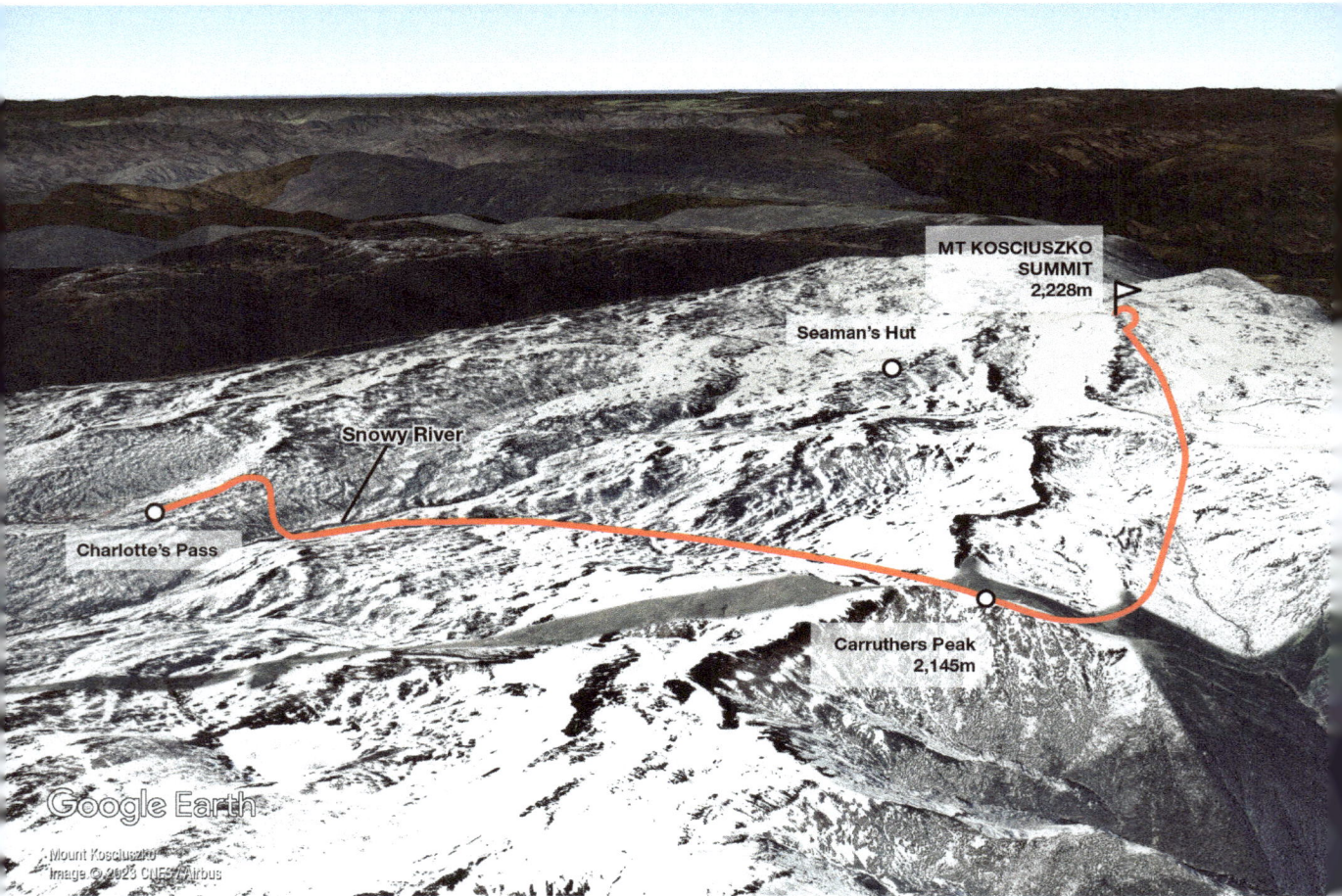

Mount Kosciuszko
Image © 2023 CNES/Airbus

**MT KOSCIUSZKO
SUMMIT
2,228m**

Seaman's Hut

Snowy River

Charlotte's Pass

**Carruthers Peak
2,145m**

Google Earth

MT KOSCIUSZKO

337km from Home

ELEVATION: 2,228m

COORDINATES:

S 36 45.604

E 148 26.379

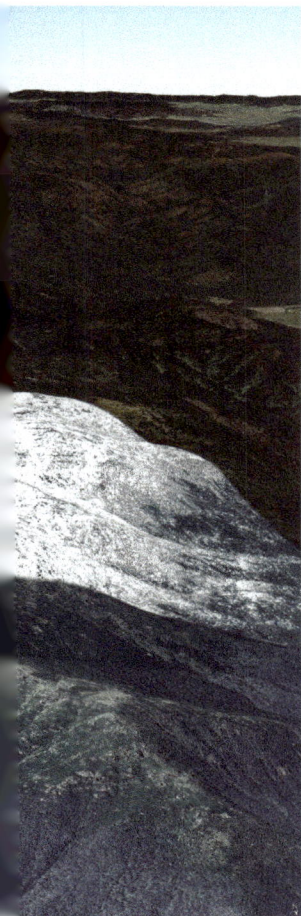

AFTER MT VINSON, the next summit on my list was the highest peak in Australia—Mt Kosciuszko. At just 2,228 metres, it's the smallest of the seven peaks. And in fact it's not a mountain you climb, so much as simply stroll to the top. No crampons, backpacks, down jackets or tents are needed. Getting to the top of 'Kozzie' simply requires a reasonable level of fitness and the ability to follow a clearly marked trail. It can be done in one day. This mountain will be far less challenging than any of the other peaks, but the decision to include it in my program wasn't automatic.

I'm not an accomplished mountaineer. Having previously described myself as 'somewhat of an adventurer', the reality is I'm an ordinary guy who tries to challenge myself and explore the world around me. I often take an idea and run with it without having all the information, and knowledge becomes an afterthought acquired through experience. My learning curve is wide, and inspiration sometimes abstract, but I train hard, aim high, and double down when the going gets tough... which also makes me a lousy gambler. And like you, before I began this adventure, I assumed that the seven highest mountains on the seven continents were easily defined. Finding out that this was not the case was part of the steep learning curve I embarked on after I set myself the challenge. The more I have travelled, the more this subjective topic has come up. So out of respect for the mountaineering community, I'll throw in my two cents and some facts, and hopefully make a constructive contribution to the conversation.

Climbing to the summit of the highest mountain on each of Earth's seven continents is an accomplishment coveted by mountaineers worldwide. The concept was first proposed by Richard Bass, an American businessman and mountaineer, in the early 1980s. Bass had a degree in geology from Yale University, and with a fellow climber called Frank Wells (future president of The Walt Disney Company), he drew up a list of the Seven Summits as follows:

opposite Mt Kosciuszko

- Kilimanjaro (5,895m), Tanzania
- Elbrus (5,642m), Russia
- Aconcagua (6,962m), Argentina
- Vinson Massif (4,892m), Antarctica
- Kosciuszko (2,228m), Australia
- Denali (6,194m), United States
- Everest (8,848m), Nepal

Dick Bass and Frank Wells duly reached the summit of six of the mountains on this list, with the exception of Mt Everest where they were rebuffed on their first attempt. After a second failed attempt, Bass finally reached the peak of Everest, without Wells, on his third attempt on 30 April 1985 and became the first man to summit the highest mountain on each of the seven continents.

Or did he?

Enter famed Italian mountaineer Reinhold Messner. In 1978, Messner and Peter Habeler reached the summit of Everest without supplemental oxygen. In 1980, without Habeler, Messner repeated the feat from the Tibetan side in what was also Everest's first solo summit. This extraordinary mountaineer suggested a different definition of the Seven Summits, eponymously called the Messner list. In this version of the summits, a mountain in West Papua on the island of New Guinea, Carstensz Pyramid (also known as Puncak

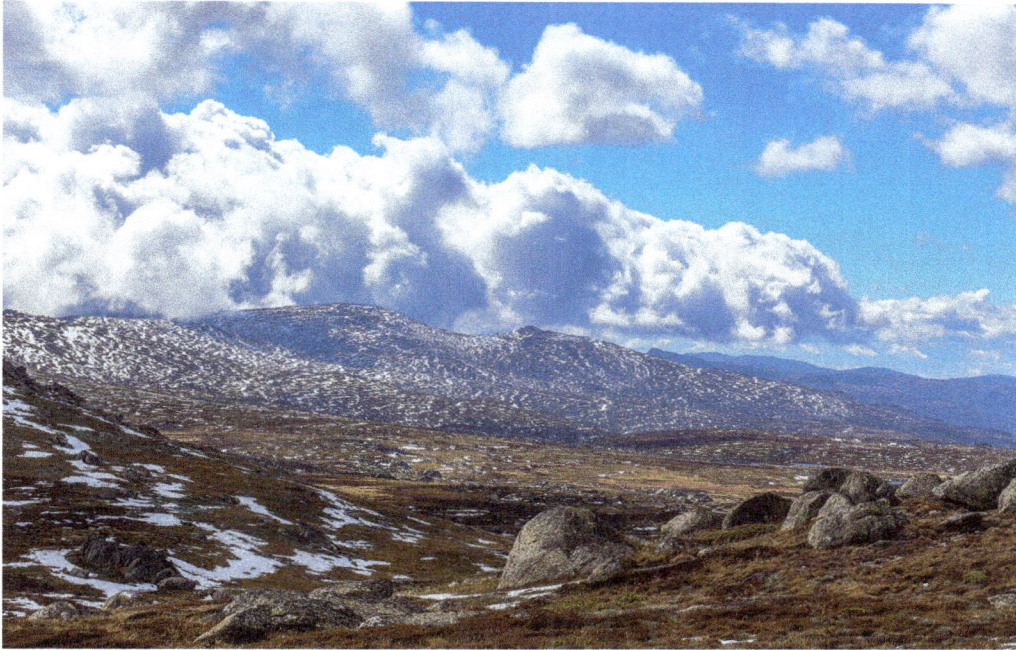

Jaya), replaces Mt Kosciuszko. In May 1986, Patrick Morrow, a Canadian climber, was the first to climb the Seven Summits as defined by the Messner list. Messner himself completed the list in December of the same year when he summited Mt Vinson.

But the question remains: why would you replace Mt Kosciuszko on the Australian continent with a mountain that sits on an island?

Because it turns out that continents are subjective.

The *Oxford Dictionary* defines a continent as:

any of the world's main continuous expanses of land (Europe, Asia, Africa, North and South America, Australia, Antarctica).

But while the *Oxford Dictionary* is sure about what a continent is, other authorities are not. Different geographers and scientists have long debated how many continents there are on planet Earth, because the geography isn't clear. Some claim six, some seven and, more recently, some have claimed eight.

North America and South America are treated as separate continents in the seven-continent model, but they may also be viewed as a single continent known as America or the Americas. Some say that Europe and Asia should be a single continent, as they aren't separated by an ocean. Experts argue that Europe and Asia are separate because mountains run between them, but there are debates about exactly where the continental line should be drawn. In 2017, a group of geologists claimed we should recognise an eighth continent. Earth's 'hidden' continent, they argue, is a mostly submerged land mass beneath New Zealand and New Caledonia—an elevated part of the ocean floor, about two-thirds the size of Australia, called Zealandia.

And what about Australia? Australia is clearly defined as a continent by many, but some authorities have argued that it's just a really big island. In fact, the concept of Australia as a continent really didn't exist before the 1950s. As plate tectonics have become better understood, the definition of the Australian continent has expanded to include several neighbouring islands, including New Guinea. The reason for this is that New Guinea is separated from mainland Australia by a barely submerged continental shelf. Critically for our discussion, when you define the Australian continent as including the island of New Guinea, Carstensz Pyramid in West Papua becomes its highest mountain.

The main point of difference between Bass and Messner was whether the definition of a continent should include the continental shelf. But it's unlikely that Reinhold Messner and Patrick Morrow felt that Carstensz Pyramid should be included as one of the Seven Summits because they were passionate about a particular definition of the Australian continent. It's more likely that they favoured Carstensz Pyramid over poor old Kozzie because it's an actual 'climb' and has the character of an expedition, rather than a simple hike. As we've learned, you can simply walk or run to the top of Kosciuszko.

Legend has it that Bass and Morrow were competing to be the first to complete the Seven Summits. Ironically, Morrow created a more difficult task for himself by replacing Kosciuszko with Carstensz Pyramid, and Bass was the first to triumph. Also interesting to note is that Morrow and Messner both later went to the top of Kosciuszko, where the whole idea of 'covering your bases' may have come from.

Perhaps the whole debate and controversy wouldn't exist if Morrow and Messner, an influential climber of his day, weren't so highly respected. Due to their favoured definition of continents, division was created among the climbing community. In 2005, the Seven Summits list was revised by the American Alpine Club to include both Carstensz Pyramid and Mt Kosciuszko as valid choices for the highest peak in Oceania. This created two legitimate versions of the Seven Summits list, although opinions still vary and the subject continues to be debated. One thing's for sure, however—all the men in this story deserve distinction for their contributions, and undeniably created a path for the future of the Seven Summits, which many more have followed.

I believe it was up to me to define my Seven Summits, and equally you're entitled to your own opinion. I've been to Indonesia several times and can't use travel and cultural experience as the sole reason to scale Carstensz Pyramid, which is no doubt a worthy achievement. But does being a worthwhile climb make it one of the Seven Summits? A lot of thought went into the concept of continents as a 'social construct'. In the end, cultural diversity led my rationalisation and ultimate decision not to include Carstensz Pyramid in

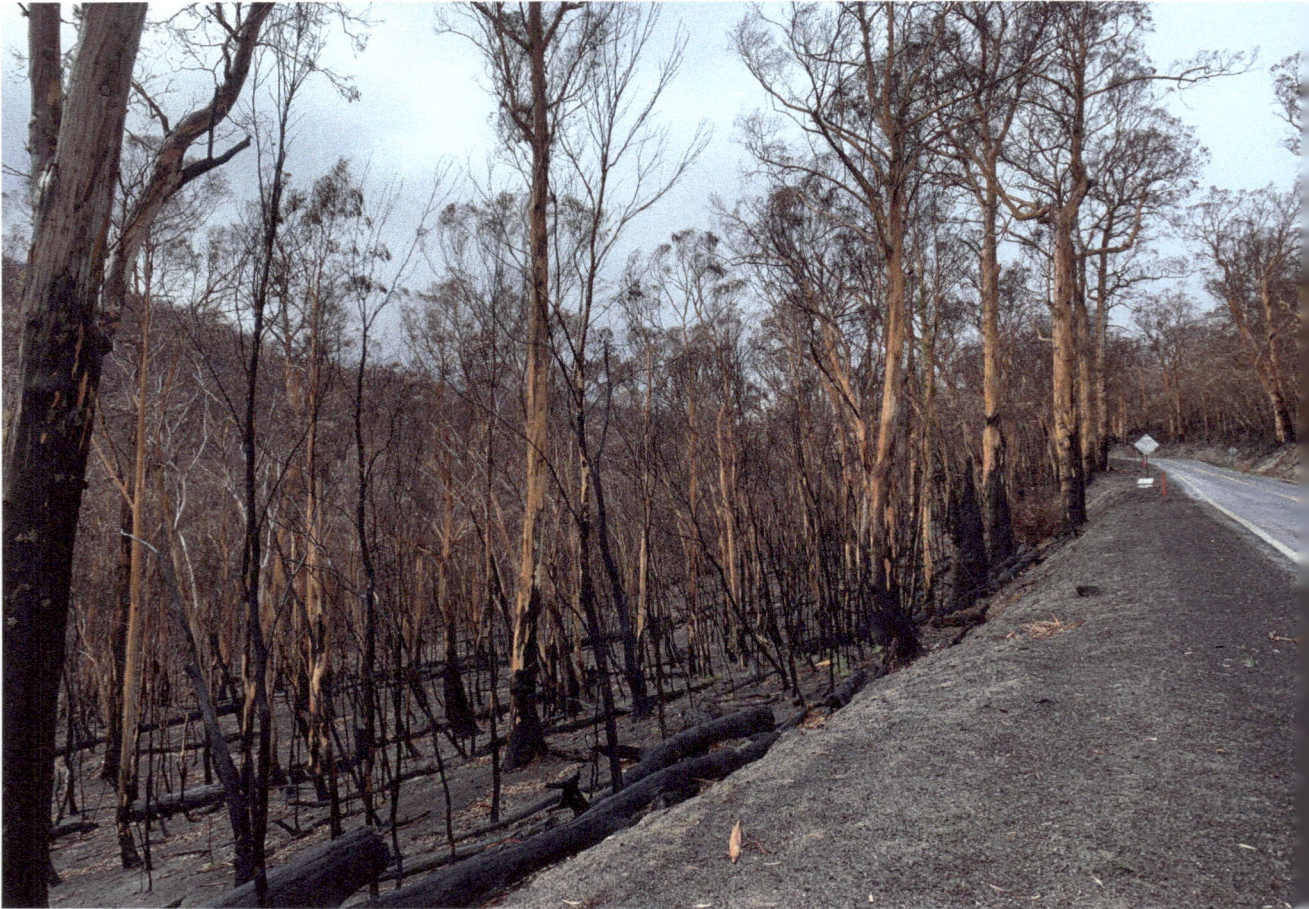

my Seven Summits challenge. For me, seven summits meant seven mountains. And it didn't really matter which ones. The beauty is that we're free to make up our own minds.

Bass argued that Mt Kosciuszko should be included instead of Carstensz Pyramid because it is easier to climb and accessible to a wider range of people. His rationalisation was the opposite of Messner's. But if you think that Kosciuszko is an easy climb, try achieving the summit via a fifty-kilometre ultramarathon—as I did. That will challenge you, should you choose to make it your seventh summit!

A marathon and a mountain

From Melbourne it's 329 kilometres northeast to Kosciuszko National Park in New South Wales, which covers 690,000 hectares. Within the park is Mt Kosciuszko, Australia's highest mountain at 2,228 metres above sea level. As we've discussed, the summit of Mt Kosciuszko isn't technically difficult to achieve, or a difficult route from a mountaineer's perspective. But it remains undeniably the highest point in Australia, and as such accomplished climbers come here from around the world to climb it.

On the drive to Mt Kosciuszko we pass blackened signs and silent, empty forests—once verdant landscapes that have been charred by the bushfires that devastated the state's southeast region in December 2019. While the main road into the park is now open, many other roads remain closed because of the fires that razed parts of the Snowy Mountains on both the New South Wales and Victorian sides of the Australian Alps. To travel through fire-ravaged countryside, see the beauty still within the Snowy Mountains, and cross her incredibly beautiful rivers is a great privilege. As an Australian, I am determined to give all my efforts to summit our highest mountain.

We're travelling to the park for the Australian Alpine Ascent, a fifty-kilometre ultramarathon that takes competitors to the summit of Mt Kosciuszko from the village of Charlotte Pass, a wintertime ski resort. Given this is the easiest of the Seven Summits, it seems fitting to climb this mountain while at the same time completing my first ultramarathon.

Until 1977, it was possible to drive within metres of Mt Kosciuszko's summit. These days it's preserved for environmental conservation and recreational use, and instead thousands of people hike to the top each year. During the winter months a pristine white blanket of snow falls on the Kosciuszko National Park and its four popular ski resorts: Perisher, Thredbo, Selwyn Snow Resort and Charlotte Pass, the closest village to Mt Kosciuszko.

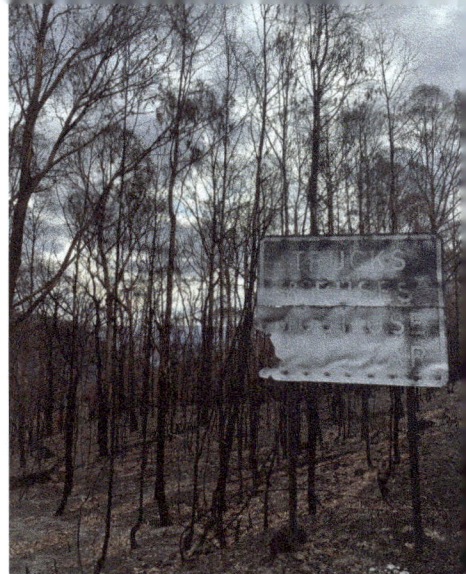

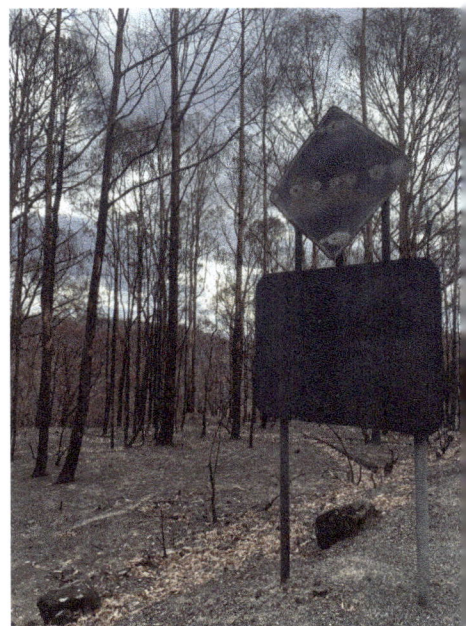

above The signs tell the story

opposite After the bushfires

When the snow melts in spring and pristine waters flow into mountain streams, the winter wonderland changes into a vast network of alpine trails snaking amid magnificent alpine scenery. The scenery can't be described as magnificent on the day of the Australian Alpine Ascent, however. Much-needed rain pours across the mountains, which are shrouded in fog. The marathon's 700 participants pack into a Charlotte Pass resort dining room along with officials. The overflow take up positions in the halls, on the stairs, and even fill the reception area. Waiting outside really isn't an option; nobody wants to get wet.

Although it's mid-summer, the forecast doesn't look great and the rain radar looks worse. The weather can be unpredictable in Australia's alpine region—just weeks ago the area was blanketed in bushfire smoke. Most runners are wearing rain jackets, which makes me doubt my minimalist approach of shorts and running tee. But while it's really fresh waiting to start, I anticipate warming up quickly.

Just before start time everyone shuffles down to the starting line to hear the quick race brief, and within a few minutes we're off, with a thick fog hovering and rain splattering down upon us.

Straight out of Charlotte Pass, it's all uphill. Then we're onto an old paved route that heads sharply downhill towards the usually glorious Snowy River in the valley below. It's a change of pace and relief for some tight muscles.

With all the sharp bouncing down the descent, I realise I've had a gear malfunction. The dry bag holding my jacket has bounced out of my pocket. Then it dawns on me that my Diabetes Australia flag was tucked securely, or so I thought, behind my dry bag. When I check I realise the flag is gone and is somewhere back up the hill. This is the first time I've ever dropped my flag, let alone lost it altogether.

With a deep, deep sigh, I turn around. I don't even know if I'll find the flag.

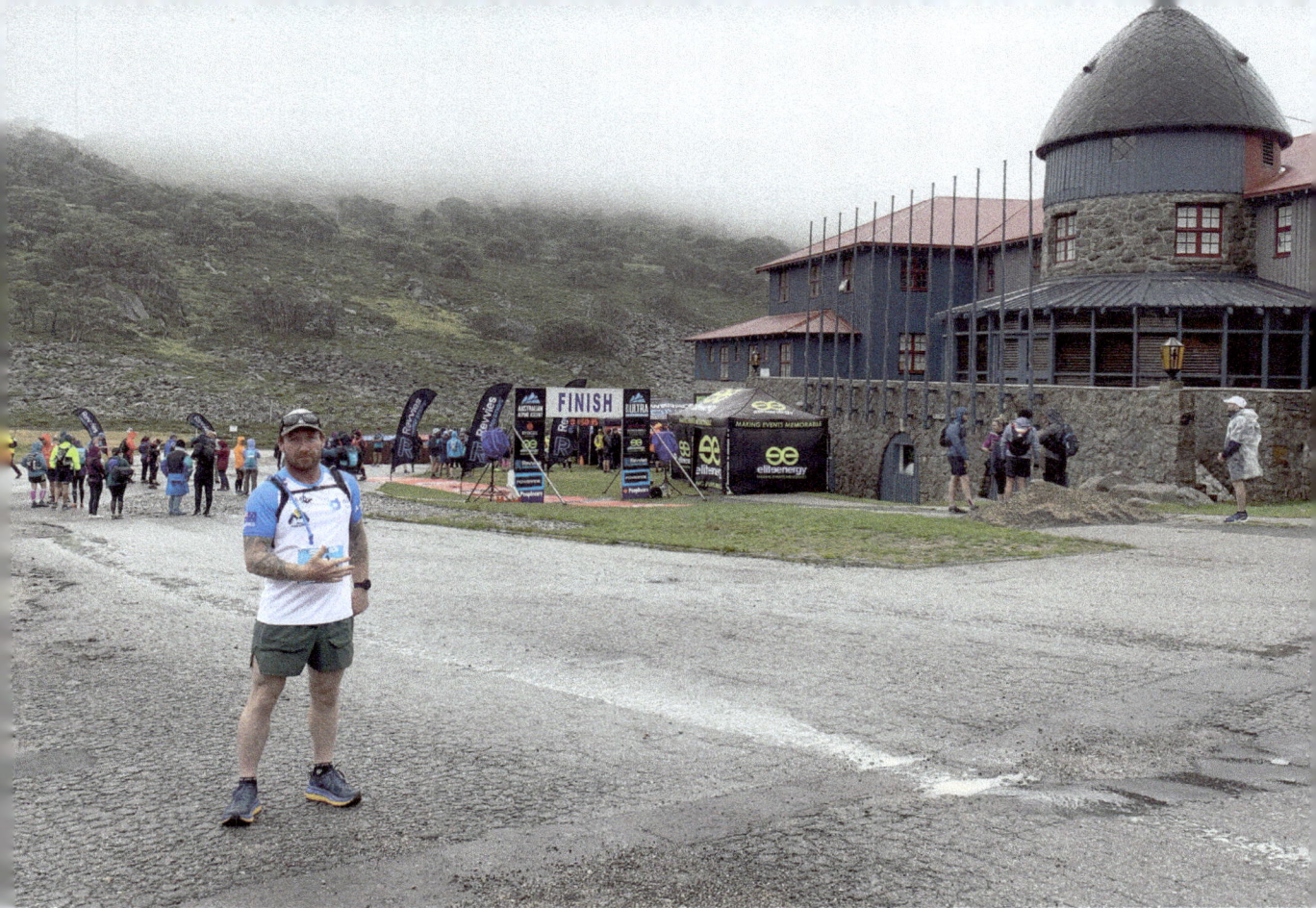

Unaffected by any personal disasters, hundreds of runners are moving forward as intended. It's obvious that I'm travelling against the tide as I run back uphill, my eyes darting around and scanning the gravel track and roadside scrub for any signs of my lost belongings.

I hazard a guess that I've backtracked a couple of hundred metres, but I may as well be at the starting line. Standing in everyone's way certainly gets more than a few strange reactions. Nowhere in the starting brief did they say, 'Take caution while descending down the first steep section, for there's a man running the wrong way in the middle of the narrow path and heading straight for you.'

There's the flag on the trail! Lucky save, unlucky additional effort. Picking up the flag, I feel like I've won a prize and proceed to stuff it back in my pocket. I'm not taking any more chances with it, and quickly back downhill I go, now seamlessly fitting back into the event.

After rock-hopping across the Snowy River, grateful the water level is low enough to allow crossing without getting my feet wet, I look up and notice it's all back uphill from here. I realise this event is a combination of running and climbing, and requires a Fartlek technique. 'Fartlek' is a Swedish term that means 'speed play' and involves varying your pace throughout the run, alternating between fast segments and slow jogs.

Wild winds greet us the higher we scale the mountain, and blasts of rain cool the heat I've developed from the exertion. Underfoot are any number and shape of rocks to leap across, and care has to be taken so as not to twist an ankle.

Upfront I see a metal boardwalk that crosses part of the terrain, protecting fragile alpine plant and animal species. I'm finally striking a rhythm and settling in speed when I notice a runner crouched on the boardwalk against the now-howling wind. This section is seriously exposed to the elements, with gales strong enough to stop runners in their tracks. Leaning hard into the wind, I manage to stay upright as I charge along it: a slip here hurts. As I discover later, many participants ended up with an injury from slipping on this metal pathway, dubbed 'The Cheese Grater'.

Still higher we climb, as the trail follows the undulations of the mountain. Although it's raining, and the middle of summer, I spot a solid pack of ice preserved in the shade. The steady climb continues before finally I reach the junction to the Summit Track. Here the wind blows hard and the rain has pin-sharp force. Oh, and it's still all uphill. It's uplifting to meet the first of the runners, who are now descending the mountain, and hear their words of encouragement.

opposite With thanks to that stranger

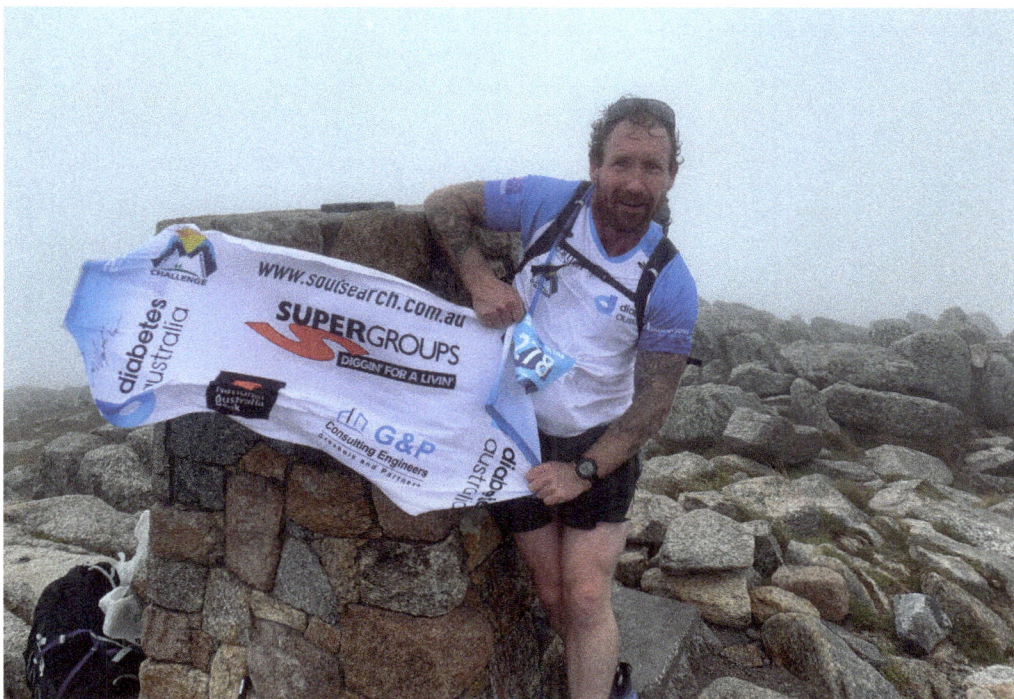

One step at a time—I'm stepping very quickly, rather than running, because the wind pushes me backwards—and then I round the last upward left-hand corner. Here a race official, bravely bearing the worst of the wild weather for us to take part in the Australian Alpine Ascent, is dutifully recording bib numbers.

The runner in front of me continues up the mountain, and I follow him just a few more metres to the stone monument at the summit. This stranger kindly takes a moment out of his race to take a photo for me and the cause. The Diabetes Australia flag, last unfurled on Mt Vinson, Antarctica a few weeks ago, is again hoisted among violent wind gusts.

Summit No. 5 is complete.

But the ultramarathon is far from over. No time is wasted to enjoy what would in clear weather be breathtaking vistas across the Australian Alps. It's back to racing. I'm fortunate to have summited when I did—moments after I started to descend, organisers closed the final stretch to the summit due to severe winds.

My muscles appreciate going downhill, and it's finally possible to make real progress. A continuous downhill run for the best part of the next hour isn't the only welcome change in the conditions. Equally welcome is the easing of the tempestuous weather the further I descend.

opposite Trying to smile

All too quickly I'm back where the race began—at the start line. 'You going again?' asks an official. I take a moment to catch my breath as I contemplate his words, which don't seem to make sense. Then their meaning registers. The distance I signed up for is two laps of this course. I'd almost forgotten. Arriving here signals only the end of the first lap.

It takes me a further moment to respond. 'Yep!' I affirm. At the thought of the next lap, I can only shake my head—I haven't paid my pound of flesh to the Snowy Mountains yet.

Turning around, I'm greeted with the same gruelling hill to climb up—again. It's exactly how I remembered it from the first lap, only more difficult. Up, down, up, up, up. The rain pours, and water fills my running shoes. I momentarily contemplate walking to prevent the discomfort of running in my sloshing shoes, then stride forward. The longer I'm on this course, potentially the more damage I'll do to my already fatigued legs. So I run where I can, walk the steps, and concentrate intensely on foot placement on the rocks.

Pushing my stamina, I pass a few participants, but among the wind and dense fog I'm often running with no-one else in sight. I have no goal to catch up with other runners, no expectation to press harder; with the successful summit behind me, I'm just intent on finishing now.

The wind is just as brutal as I approach The Cheese Grater for the second time. I cross it cautiously, then try gaining speed again. Arriving at the junction to the Summit Track,

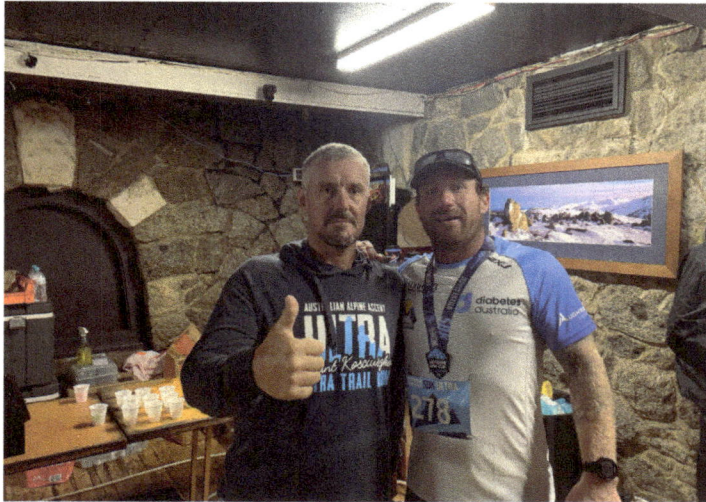

officials are taking bib numbers again and this time adding a little encouragement. 'Well done. It's all downhill from here...'

My second descent is a similar experience to descending other mountains. With energy spent, it's the individual's responsibility to manage under sufferance. So I back off just a little. Then, entering the final two kilometres, I find extra energy from somewhere, pick up the pace and welcome the finish line.

In the final steps, a high five from my mate Jim brings a smile. He toughed out the marathon's twenty-five-kilometre route and fell on the metal causeway, grazing his face and legs. Yet here he is, cheering me on over the finish line. It's the essence of mateship, courage and determination on 'Kozzie'— Australia's highest mountain.

If climbing is about visiting each of the seven continents and experiencing different mountains and different cultures, here I've witnessed grit and determination amid an environment of raw beauty and regeneration.

My result? Thirteenth place overall in 05:32:10.

Training, training, training

I completed my run to the top of Kozzie on 8 February 2020. A few days earlier, on 25 January, the first case of Covid-19 was detected in Australia, in a man who had flown to Melbourne from China. It was a time of uncertainty and apprehension, but few could have predicted the profound effect Covid would have across the globe. When I first set out to complete my Seven Summits challenge, I certainly didn't think that travelling to each continent would be a problem. But just a few weeks later, on 19 March, Australia closed its borders to the rest of the world indefinitely. I had wondered how I would get to the summit of Everest; now I wasn't sure I would even be able to get to Nepal.

But I had to remain hopeful. Surely the borders would reopen as the pandemic slowed down. And with the measures being put in place around the world, this would happen soon. Hopefully. In any case, I had to look on the bright side. At least this unplanned hiatus in my challenge would give me a chance to improve and intensify my training regimen.

In climbing five mountains I had experienced new and undiscovered levels of pain and perseverance. But there was an elephant in the room—Mt Everest. By now I knew enough to appreciate that these mountains demand respect and, in order to achieve success, I needed to be ready. I needed to be in optimal physical and mental condition for an attempt at my sixth summit and the world's highest mountain.

I've only heard of one other Australian training for and completing the Seven Summits in recent history. Steve Plain, in May of 2018, not only reached the summit of the highest mountain on every continent, he completed the feat faster than anyone in history. Mountaineers who have crossed his path tell me he trained as a triathlete and was a really strong climber. That's a good enough recommendation for me. If a triathlon can provide a solid base of endurance, and optimal full-body strength, surely I should try it?

opposite, left

Learning to ride

opposite, right

Learning to swim

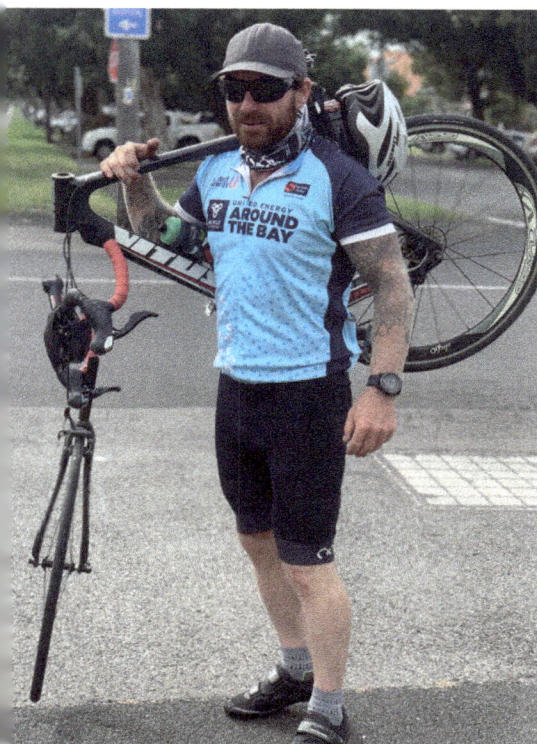

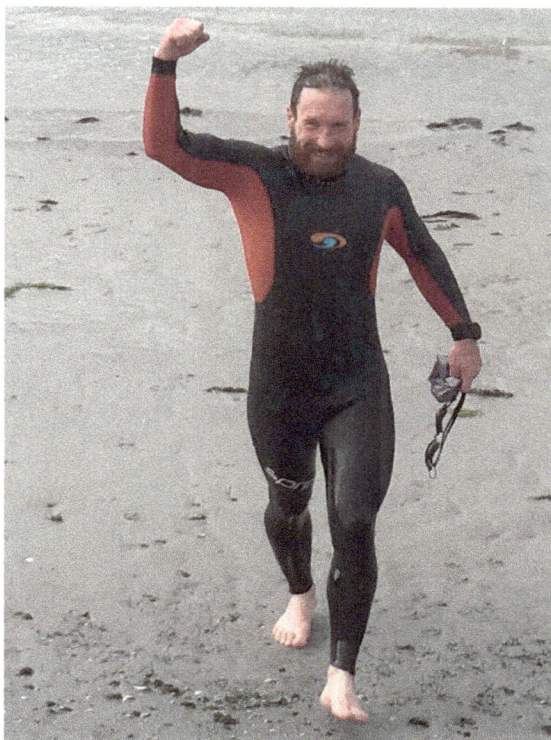

I signed up for an Ironman 70.3 and headed to the bookstore. In the book *Triathlon Training for Dummies*, the 'Half-Iron' description opens with, 'Calling this race half-anything doesn't do it justice.' And closes with '... don't start here. This is not a first-triathlon kind of event, regardless of your fitness level and experience.' The Ironman 70.3 challenge requires swimming 1.9 kilometres, cycling ninety kilometres, and running twenty-one kilometres. Swimming in the ocean was foreign to me. In fact, to be honest I couldn't really swim. Nor had I ever ridden a road bike or 'clipped in'. But hey, since I'd bought the book, I thought I may as well give it a go. After all, I can run. Well, trot along at a decent clip for a middle-aged, stocky sort of bloke. And despite the book's dire warnings, it sounded like good training for Everest. If I could survive the experience ...

I also hoped training for and competing in a triathlon would give me the structure I needed to save myself from the

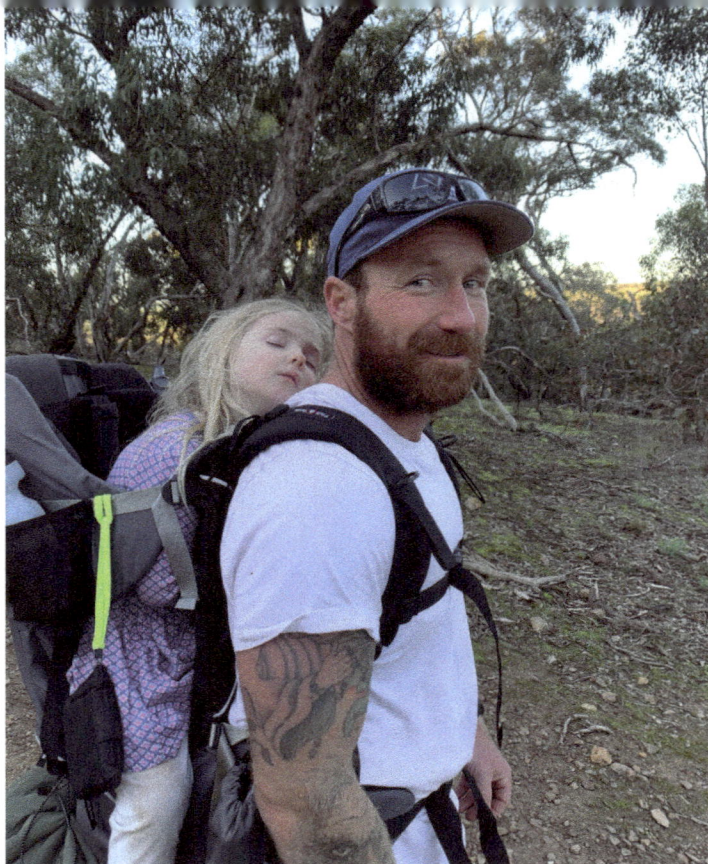

right Taking my daughter
Arlo training

opposite Our family

dysfunctional training routine that I had cobbled together based on running, weights, more running, and carrying heavy backpacks around. I even bought a specialised child-carrying backpack to load my children into. Will would come home and plead with me to stop carrying the kids around the streets, as everyone notices his eccentric father. I also tried to learn how to swim via self-education while attending my children's swimming lessons—with little success. Heidi watched in disbelief as the children's swimming teacher encouraged me to 'Reach for the edge.' I continued to thrash about, undeterred.

None of this was easy. But I can do suffering, and so I suffered.

To find time for training between family and work commitments, I got up between 4am and 5am most days. I practised, applied myself at capacity, and focused with the intention of

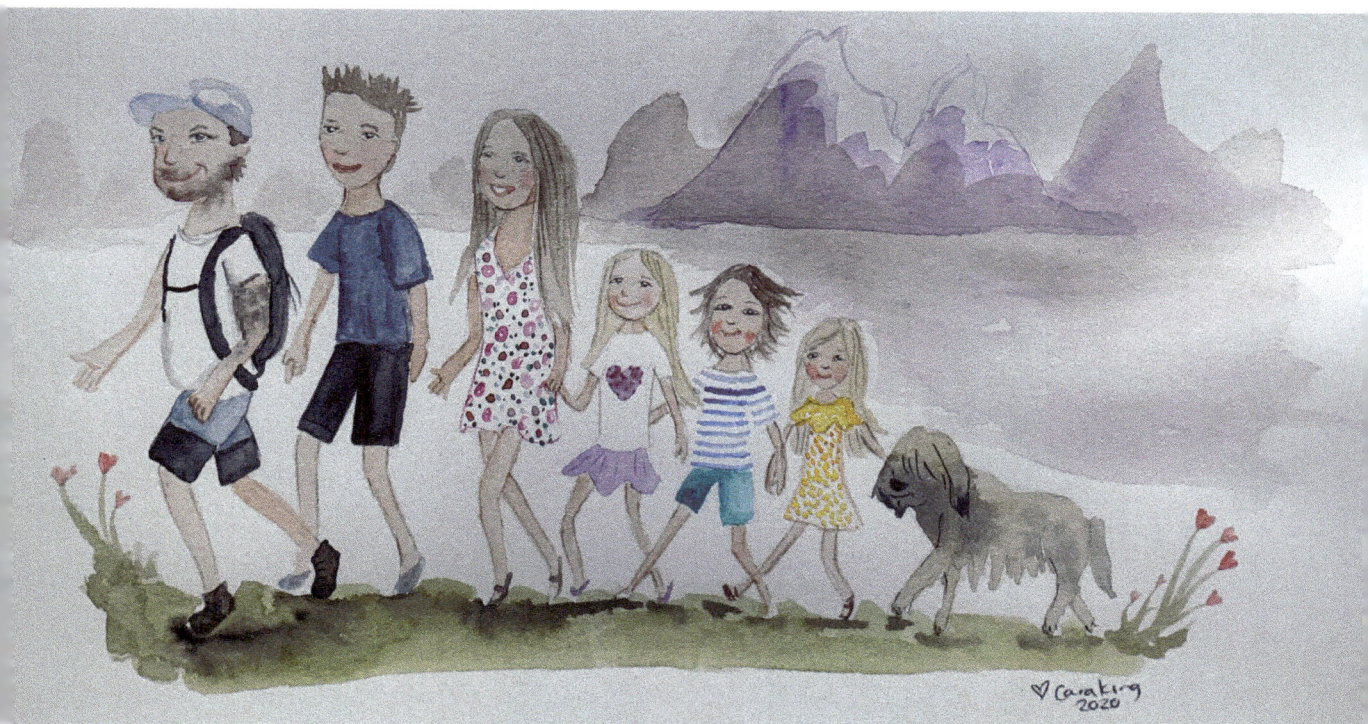

improving. I trained up to twenty hours every week, with an average of ten to fifteen hours. Every day was a training day. If I had a day off, some form of recovery was required ... stretching, sauna, massage, physio. I was aiming to optimise my own performance.

Then, just as taper week was in sight before my first Ironman 70.3, the Victorian Government announced a snap five-day lockdown, the state's third lockdown since the Covid-19 pandemic arrived on our shores. The Ironman 70.3 was postponed. A new date was set. The race would take place the day before I was due to fly out for the biggest climb of the Seven Summits—Mt Everest.

I was determined to prove that book wrong. Surely there is always an exception.

Training and working, working and training... Although at times fatigued, I was ready.

THE DAY before I was due to fly to Nepal to tackle Mt Everest, I somehow managed to complete my first Ironman. Five-and-a-half hours after the gun went off, I took the final right-hand turn down to the red carpet. It all happened so quickly—one minute you're done with the swim and the cycling, you start running, then there are cheers, a photographer, and the voiceover guy calls your time, '... with the best beard of the day award, David Morgan clocks in at 05:27:42.' Next minute, you're done.

I was glad I had shifted my focus to participate in local events such as the Ironman 70.3. In the autumn of 2021 I was in good health. I was physically the best I'd been in the last two years of the Seven Summits challenge, and also enjoying good mental and emotional health, which supports my motivation. Adding to the atmosphere of optimism was the fact that Covid vaccines were starting to roll out around the world. I was amazed at how quickly a vaccine had been developed. This is what happens when you throw money at a cause. It made me think of Fin and her diabetes, and I was more determined than ever to raise money and contribute to that elusive cure. There finally seemed to be a path towards 'Covid normal'. And I know I'm an optimist, but in March of 2021 the dark days of the pandemic seemed to have retreated and everything was coming together so that we could all move forward.

At least, that's what I thought as I packed my bag for Mt Everest.

PART 2

EVEREST

'the Head in the Great Blue Sky'

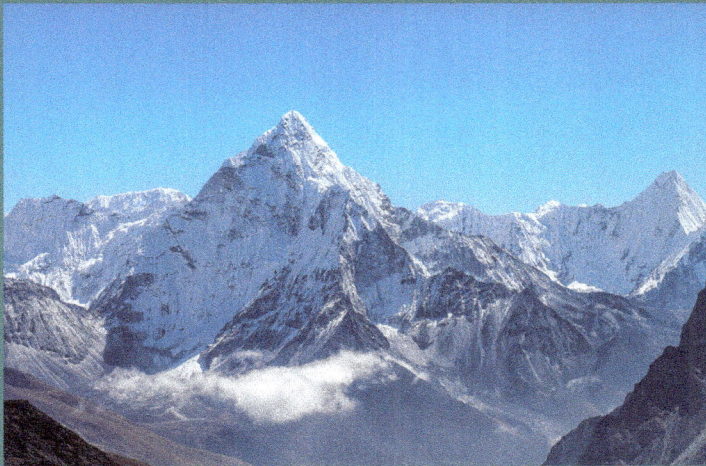

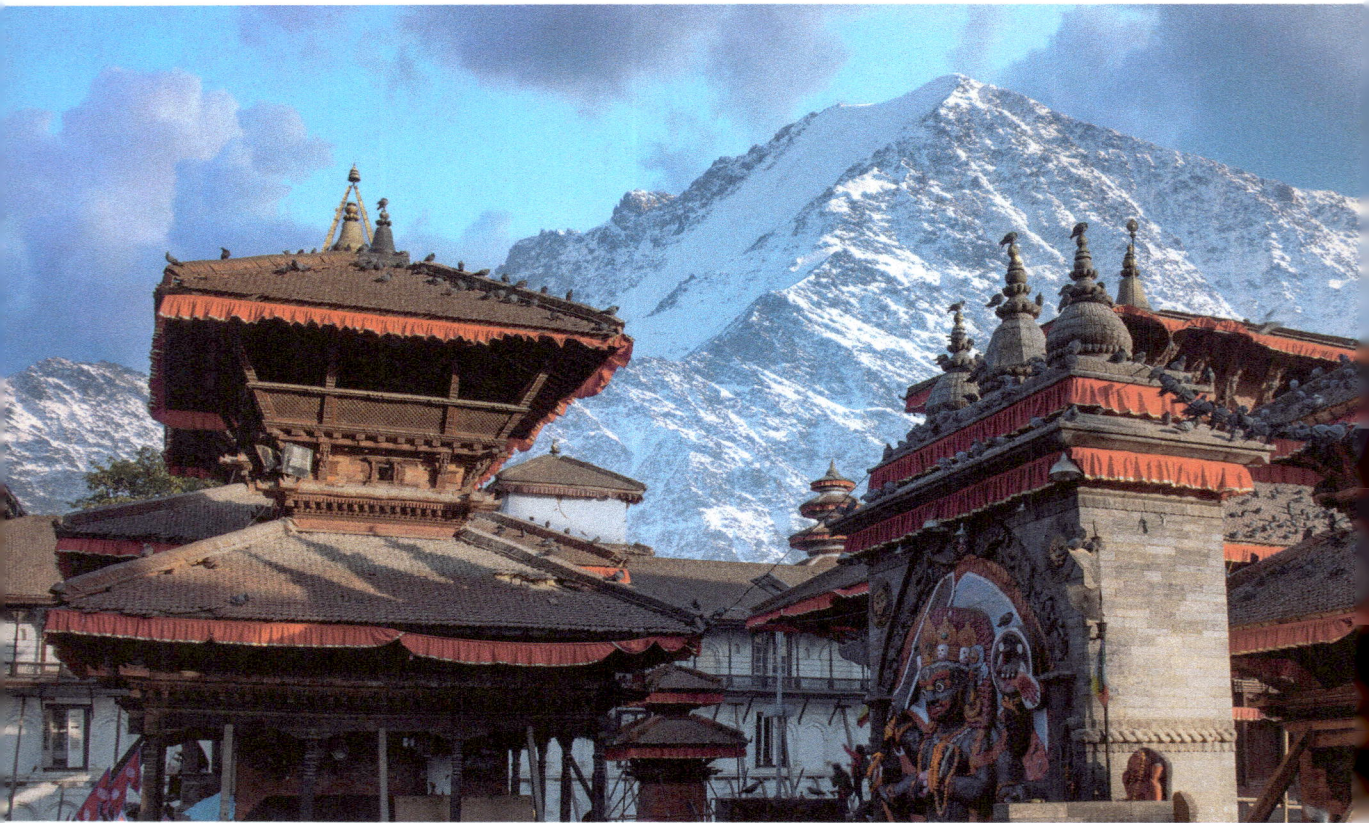

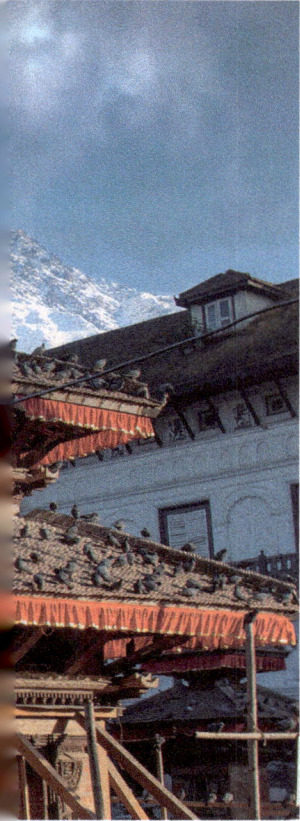

MELBOURNE TO KATHMANDU

6

TRAVELLING WITH EXEMPTION[1]
30 MARCH 2021

I have considered your request and determined that your application to travel is authorised on the following grounds:

Travelling overseas for a compelling reason for at least three months.

Your departure from Australia is subject to standard border clearance processes—an exemption to travel restrictions does not exempt you from these requirements. You do not need to re-apply for permission to depart if your flight details or departing port change. A record of this outcome is available in border systems, in order to facilitate your departure.

AUSTRALIAN DEPARTMENT OF HOME AFFAIRS

IT'S VERY DARK as we approach Melbourne Airport, highlighting how few cars are on the roads in an area that, pre-Covid-19, was usually crowded day and night. Tonight there are no lines of cars, no people in sight, just a lone security guard at the front of the terminal. A single taxi drops a passenger behind us. There's no-one else.

---

1   The curious reader might like to know that when departing Australia and applying for my travel exemption, I adhered to all criteria the Australian Government requested to continue my Seven Summits journey, and would not have left if I had been refused departure.

I check my paperwork once more. Yes, Terminal 2 is where I say goodbye. Goodbye to my family and familiar routines. Goodbye to all I love. I think of the special occasions I'll miss. But I won't miss the work. There's no more of that, no more training, no more of the chaotic life I've somehow adapted to. In moments like these I'm confused about my choices. I enjoy the hugs, but these moments affirm what we'll miss. What I'll miss.

My young daughter starts to cry, breaking the silence of the night. I heave my forty kilos of gear onto a trolley as a distraction, and start walking along the empty pavement towards Terminal 2. Covid restrictions mean my family can't come into the terminal and say goodbye at the gate, as we would normally do. Turning, I wave one last time and hope they see.

Deep breath, put on mask, enter the terminal.

Nothing. No hustle and bustle, no crowds, no life. There are just a few staff here and there as I wander around looking for the check-in desk. I'm early. Few signs are lit, and the terminal resembles a vacant warehouse more than the gateway to the sophisticated, international city that is Melbourne. I take a photo with not a single soul in sight. The hopeful feeling I'd had earlier, that there was a road out of Covid, disappears. There's nothing 'normal' about this scene.

I check the screens—there are seven flights in total, and a mere two desks are open for international travel. My flight is next, with check-in opening at 8:30pm, almost three-and-a-half hours before departure. There's one gentleman before me as I take my place in an otherwise empty queue. A woman joins the line. It's an airport I'm unfamiliar with; an airport that is quiet, too quiet. There are more staff than travellers.

The check-in process begins. Straight to the counter I go. It all starts normally enough.

'Passport please,' asks a woman. I pull out a pile of paperwork. 'You have an exemption, yes?'

I can't help but ask, 'Does anybody arrive and say no?' Some exemptions can expire, I learn. Okay.

'Nepal visa?' I have pre-approval. 'Is that all you have?' I'm getting worried.

I supply another online visa form from Nepal. A Nepalese portal, Covid-19 Crisis Management Centre, provided another approval via barcode just this afternoon, and only after I'd contacted customer support and made five attempts at lodgement. Yes, need that barcode too.

'Are you aware that you must quarantine for five days on arrival?' the woman asks.

She then takes all my documents and proceeds to another desk, with my phone, to enhance the barcodes. It's a concerning process. I look behind me. Not a single person in the line. I've never seen this before. The woman calls ahead to check my Australian exemption before finally weighing my bags. The entire check-in process takes around half an hour. This is caution with a capital 'C'.

With a wave of relief, I see two boarding passes churn from the machine.

Boarding passes in hand, I take a seat nearby to return some overdue phone calls. There's nobody else here, so I don't even feel the urge to whisper.

Then it's progression through customs, which is usually a slow process in a packed customs hall. Instead, today a sole staff member waves me through after checking my boarding pass. I walk straight up to the only body scanner that's open, present my carry-on luggage for scanning, and walk through. Then an automatic passport-reader does its thing while I'm photographed. I walk straight through this checkpoint too, and on the other side I find some actual people. There are lots of customs officials and a few travellers forming a single line. No-one is in a hurry.

We wait. Then a friendly gentleman begins his job: 'Where are you off to today?' 'What's the purpose of your travel?' Unlike pre-Covid times, this isn't some brisk interaction. Instead, the customs officer spends a lot of time with each person, fully understanding their travel plans. The gentleman in front of me is taken for further questioning in a nearby room. I think my story is straightforward, but after a full conversation with customs officials, and seeing the man being led away, I can't help but feel a little intimidated.

Just two of us stroll through the duty free store, where about ten staff stand at their counters. 'Gee, it's quiet in here,' I offer.

'Yes, we really need a sale if you can help,' is the cheerful reply.

In this part of the terminal the toilets are closed off, all shops except the duty free store are closed, and the lounges are empty.

By the time I reach gate 11 there are only twenty minutes left until boarding. The whole casual feel of the abnormal Covid airport is surreal. I usually appreciate busy airports: chaos, nervous energy, people boarding, disembarking, in transit.

With no sense of urgency, the boarding gate opens. Nobody lines up. People just stroll over and progress straight through, down the passage and onto the big bird. Flight crew, wearing masks and gowns, individually take us to our seats. One row per passenger—now that's social distancing. I feel slightly awkward placing my bag wherever I like; there's so much space.

As the aeroplane thunders down the runway, I feel a weird, slightly familiar sensation. It's several confused minutes before I realise what it is . . . excitement. I'm in the air, experiencing 'Covid normal travel', and heading to a part of the world that I have not previously visited. It's also a country that is dealing with the Covid crisis in a way that is surely different from Australia's strict approach. It feels like travel is new again, and something not to be taken for granted.

Butter chicken and rice sounds good to me. Washed down with a chilled red wine. A flight attendant presents the bottle as if I'm in a five-star restaurant. It's nice wine, so naturally as I'm enjoying this delicious meal, I ask for another.

'Of course, sir.'

Dessert is also top quality. 'May I have another?' I ask.

'Of course, sir, please enjoy two.'

This is starting to feel more like business class than economy. Maybe it's the red wine, but I do feel extremely fortunate to have this opportunity to travel, to explore, to participate as a global citizen.

I walk the aisles, just to stretch, but curiosity has me counting the people on this A350, which usually carries up to 350 passengers. Entire sections of the plane are empty: I'll take a guess there are twenty-one souls in cattle class. Time for a movie while I stretch out, relax, and grab an extra blanket before some badly needed shut eye.

I'VE WOKEN because there's some turbulence. We're cruising at 40,000 feet. Hours have passed; I'm a long way from home now.

Aah ... I add some cream to hot coffee. Another coffee and it's breakfast time. The turbulence has subsided, and the first-class economy service continues ... as if I can turn down another helping of apple pancakes.

I'm sitting here typing and reflecting on the last few days. Time has passed quickly, the otherwise long and tedious thirteen-and-a-half-hour haul is almost over and the A350 is now descending. The on-board hospitality will be what I remember most from this flight to Qatar.

Disembarking from the near-empty flight is a breeze. Yet, walking into the familiar surrounds of Doha's Hamad Airport, I'm surprised to see how busy it is. People are milling around, transfer screens are filled with details of upcoming flights, lounges are full, and people are being driven around in carts as usual. This is very different from the vibe I experienced in Melbourne. In total contrast to my flight from Melbourne, the Boeing 787 Dreamliner I now board for the four-hour, twenty-minute flight to Kathmandu is packed to the rafters. This is more like the travel of old.

I take up a middle seat. Two gentlemen soon flank me on both sides, meaning social distancing is out. There's no refined customer service here. I'm locked into back-to-back movies to ride this journey out.

Smoke has filled Kathmandu's skies due to ongoing bush-fires, prohibiting any visibility on descent. Although my face mask has now been a constant fixture for more than twenty-four hours, best I keep it on for both Covid and respiratory reasons.

The wheels drop with a thud, the runway appears, and we land in Kathmandu, the capital and largest city of Nepal. This city of one million residents stands at around 1,400 metres above sea level in central Nepal, and is the gateway to the Nepalese Himalayas.

When the plane pulls to a halt everyone jumps up at once, clamouring for space, grabbing bags, all bunched together. I almost laugh at the captain's voiceover: 'Please maintain social distancing when exiting the plane.'

But Covid is not a laughing matter. Every cough among the crowds brings unease, suspicion, fear—a reaction that didn't exist pre-Covid. I manoeuvre my trolley through the crowds and find the exit.

Outside, the roads are full of cars and scooters, and the sidewalks are busy with people. The city is a functioning, fast-paced metropolis. There are traffic jams, pollution, smoke. The infrastructure looks dated, and the exposed electricals I see along the streets gives an insight into the developing nature of Kathmandu.

Nepal is one of Asia's poorest countries and has a population of around twenty-nine million. Its public health system is weak, several generations of families often share crowded accommodation, and there is a vast migrant workforce returning from India.

To date there have been 277,640 cases of Covid and 3,031 deaths. The country's vaccination campaign against Covid-19

opposite Yak & Yeti, Kathmandu

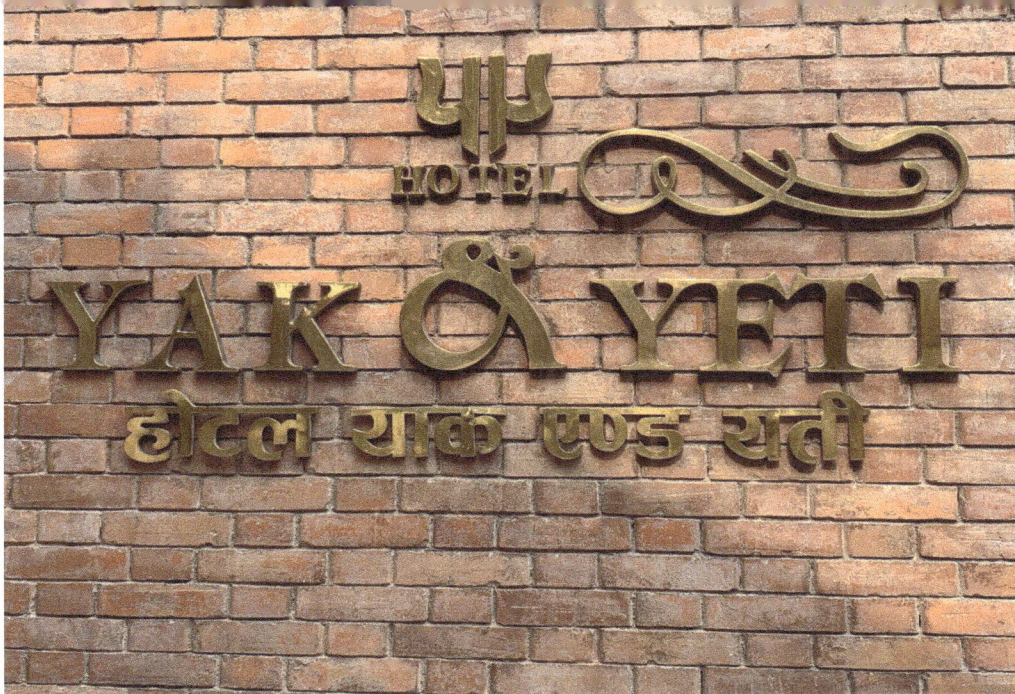

began on 27 January 2020. So far more than 1.7 million people have been inoculated, according to Nepal's Ministry of Health and Population.

'Many people have had the vaccine now,' says my driver. 'I don't know if vaccines help, but we are lucky to have a low death rate.' I only wish there was a vaccine for diabetes. Fin would have to endure perhaps just a single needle in her lifetime, rather than several a day.

We navigate streets crammed with people, sweep along Durbar Marg—a long, broad avenue that leads to the Royal Palace—and swing into the spacious, manicured grounds of the Hotel Yak & Yeti, a five-star oasis in the heart of Kathmandu. First impressions are good.

Here I am—arrived . . .

I WAKE early the next morning, but for the first time in a while I've had a full eight hours' sleep. No jet lag, but I'm hungry and it's time to explore the hotel, formerly a Rana palace built in 1890 by Bir Shumsher for his youngest wife, Top Kumari Devi.

The whole splendid place has been a hotel since 1977. I find fellow climbers lingering in the vast, open communal spaces surrounded by views of the Yak & Yeti's manicured grounds. There's a pond, gardeners tending to the lawns, and an array of beautiful flowers and trees.

Mike from CTSS, our expedition organiser, emerges, and it's nice to say hello and exchange a few stories. Covid-19 testing is to start at 9am, and the diverse group of climbers have plenty of questions to move through before that. I learn I'll be leaving in the third wave with Mike to fly to Lukla Airport on 5 April.

Between now and then there's plenty of downtime. On journeys like this, we're often waiting for weather reports, for guides, or for logistics coordinators to tell us what's happening next. Today's highlight is about to begin. In the Yak & Yeti Hotel's vast foyer, two medics have set up their Covid testing wares in full view of all guests. No consulting room, no privacy, just an audience. Fortunately, the poke up the nostrils is over fairly quickly. But the spectacle isn't—onlookers are quite welcome to share a laugh and some chit chat while witnessing the discomfort of others.

Mike introduces me to Tendi, our CTSS Sirdar (lead Sherpa), a legendary climber who has summited Everest thirteen times. Despite only one year of formal education, he is said to speak ten languages—most of them fluently. Tendi is generous with his time, and he knows the answer to almost every question he is asked. He's extremely happy we're all here, he says, and that this is a special time for him and the team he leads.

'Couple hundred porters, couple hundred yaks have also moved our gear to Base Camp, all of them very happy you're all here finally. They are all very happy to be working. And all the Sherpa too.'

Tendi tells me that my lead guide is Big Tendi, one of the most tenured guides in Nepal, and also the current technical director for the Nepal Mountain Guides Association. A veteran mountain guide, Big Tendi has guided seventeen climbers to the top of Everest in three separate expeditions, and has more than thirty years of climbing experience. Any concerns about having a capable Sherpa guide disappear in an instant.

Big Tendi usually does the private International Federation of Mountain Guides Association's (IFMGA) Sherpa Guided Climb, which is essentially guiding with a single climber, but I'm fortunate to have his oversight as lead guide on my IFMGA Sherpa Team Climb. This means a maximum one in four Sherpa guide to client ratio, with the benefit of autonomy above Camp 2 on the summit rotation to summit with a personal Sherpa.

To pass the time, I wander around the grounds of the hotel. I watch ducks glide across a pond, admire the architecture, and loiter in the foyer. Due to Covid-19 restrictions we are not meant to leave the grounds, but this isn't monitored. Somebody tells me the Nepalese government has changed the Covid quarantine requirements—again—down from five days to none. But who knows? Such whispers simply add to a feeling of uncertainty.

After another day of loitering around the beautiful setting of the hotel, which is hardly representative of most people's quarantine experience, I realise I'm going to struggle if I don't get out soon. 'Hey mate, are we expecting Covid test results back today?' I ask Mike.

'I think the deal is if we haven't heard back from them that it's positive, then we're good. I think you passed.'

I have to trust that face masks, social distancing and hand sanitiser all work in preventing Covid, because I feel the need to be engaged outside these walls. It's time to venture past the self-imposed barriers of confinement. A short stroll from the hotel and I'm back in the real world—dozens of bikes buzz past, and the streets are chocked with cars. It's organised chaos. Police direct the busiest intersections under the watchful eye of a few armed military personnel.

I get some money changed. 300 US dollars for 34,500 Nepalese rupee.

On the way back to the hotel I see Steve, one of my break-fast buddies, heading out of the hotel grounds. He's been here before and knows his way around, so I do an about-face and join him. As nice as a five-star hotel is, a city can only be experienced through its streets and people. Travelling is not just about getting to the destination, but also everything you see along the way.

Off we trot back into the land of the living, with Steve showing me his favourite haunts, including a pizza shop, a restaurant, and a bookshop well stocked with English volumes. We pass construction sites that are quite simply dangerous—occupational health and safety just isn't a thing here—and explore some interesting streets off the car- and bike-choked main thoroughfare. Mandala Street, paved, quiet and clean, reminds me of Italy. Back amid the chaos of the main street, I'm offered everything from drugs and spas to girls. Walking back to the hotel we see a guy carrying a wardrobe on his head. Moving house maybe? I can't describe how it's possible, but there it is. Oh, and we spot a goat being carried on a scooter through the traffic. Unusual sights, and not something you can experience from the hotel. Final purchase: a block of chocolate as a treat.

Back at the Yak & Yeti, I get a call from Ryan, who is soon to be my room buddy and possibly a tent buddy for a lot longer. He arrived from the USA a couple of hours ago, and I've asked him to join me for dinner. Ryan is a breath of fresh air—goal-orientated, ambitious and adventurous. In this case the goal is the summit of Mt Everest, and it has brought together two people from opposite sides of the planet who have much in common. Ryan's a Delta pilot, I'm a builder, and yet we're both runners and travellers with similar climbing experience. Ryan plays chess, runs ultramarathons, and is married with two stepchildren. He also enjoys an alcoholic beverage or three. We should get along fine.

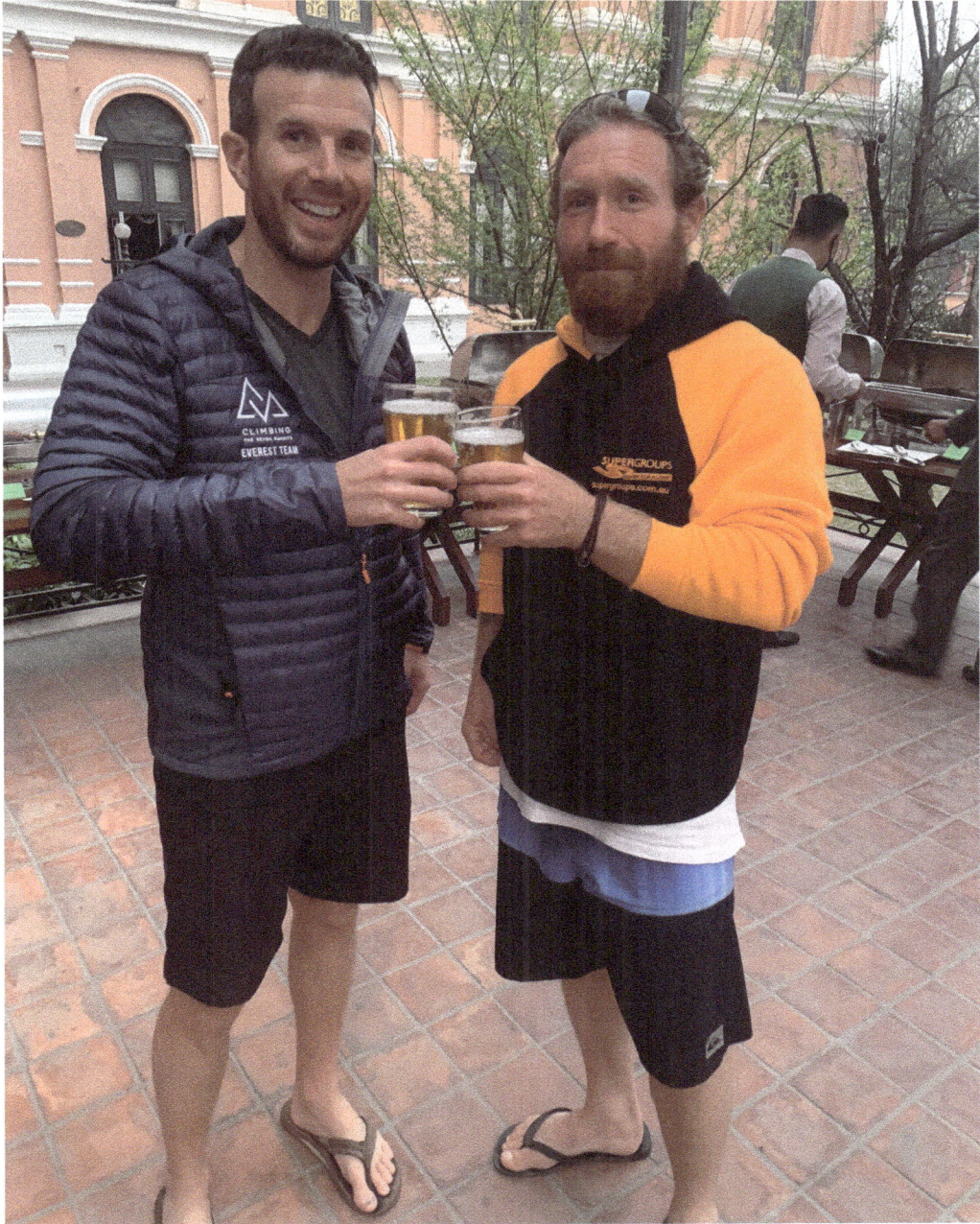

I CAN'T think of much to do today, so I drink coffee and sit in the morning sun. Nobody's around, adding to the peace.

I wander into the hotel foyer where I meet Tendi, who introduces me to Big Tendi. Ryan's here too. It's great to start coming together with the people whose company I'll keep on this adventure, at least initially. Mario from Croatia has arrived, minus some of the critical gear to climb the world's highest mountain. Ryan and I join him and Big Tendi on a trip downtown to a mountaineering store to stock up.

Big Tendi wants to see our gear, so I pull it all out for his inspection. 'Where's your spare light?' he asks. 'These gloves, not good enough. Lithium batteries for summit only, these no good.'

I thought I had it covered, but obviously a few adjustments are in order. I'm not arguing with such a respected veteran.

April, our remaining team member, has flown in and we all move together for a meal.

THERE'S A team meeting at 10am the next day. Mike addresses the group. 'Sherpa are incredible people, I think you'll really enjoy being immersed in their culture and the Khumbu Valley,' he says.

Khumbu is a region of northwest Nepal on the Nepalese side of Mt Everest, where the elevation ranges from 3,300 metres to 8,848 metres at the summit of Everest. It's one of Nepal's most popular tourist destinations. Mike says the weather is unpredictable throughout the Khumbu, so we pack for every outcome.

We're introduced to the people flying into Lukla. The weather looks good to fly tomorrow, Mike says, with the helicopter as a contingency option. Last-minute brief details are explained, and there's a short Q&A, which hopefully indicates everyone is ready. I certainly am. All that's left for me to do is to venture out for a couple of last-minute adjustments to my kit, including, importantly, the correct gloves—'If you want to keep your fingers,' Big Tendi advises.

One of the Sherpa guides offers to take me shopping. On his moped. In no time we're weaving through traffic, beeping constantly and stopping frequently as we pass a chaos of construction sites, police and military personnel, local traders, people crowding the pavements. It's a great way to see the city in its rawness and authenticity.

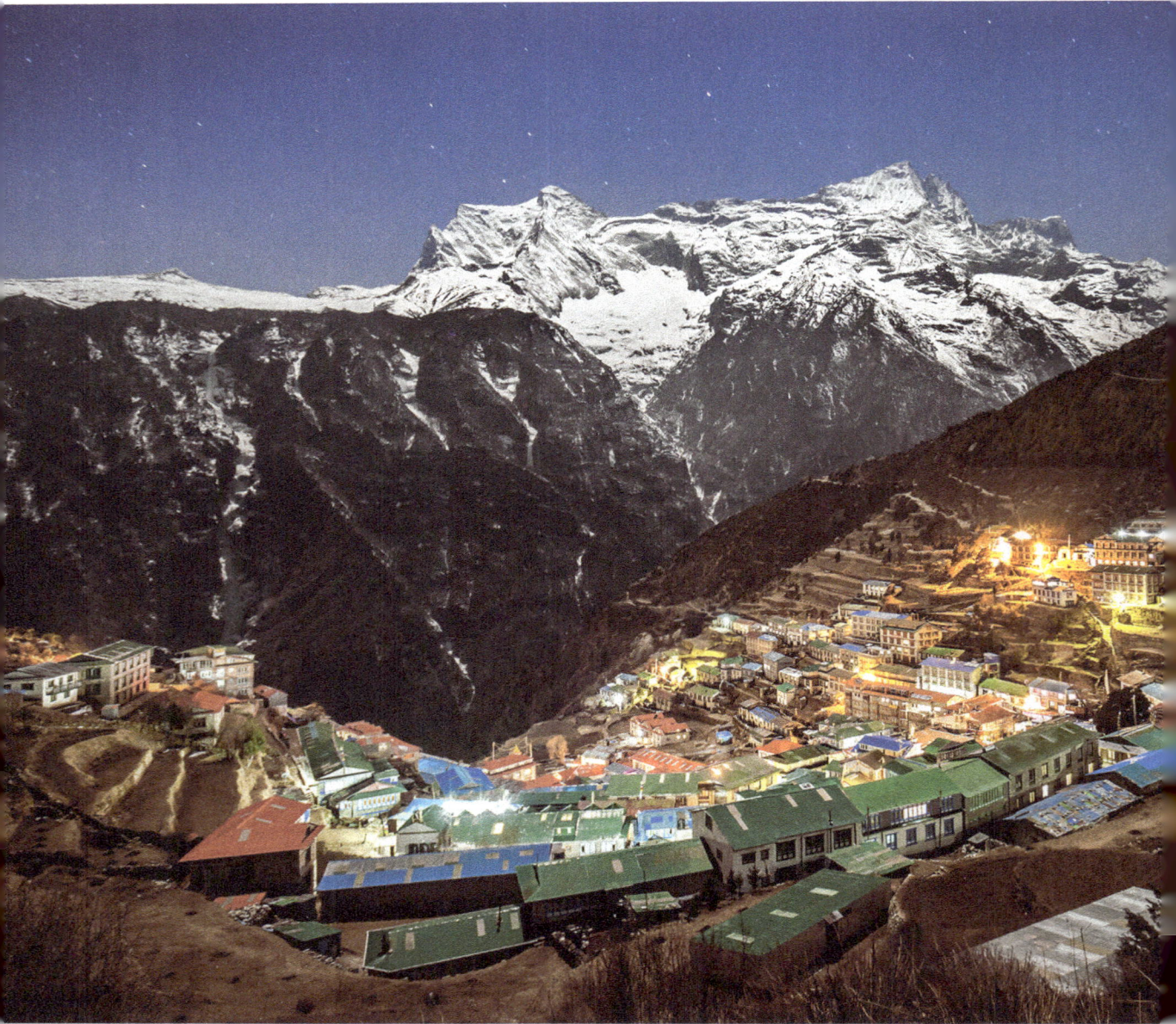

KATHMANDU TO EVEREST BASE CAMP

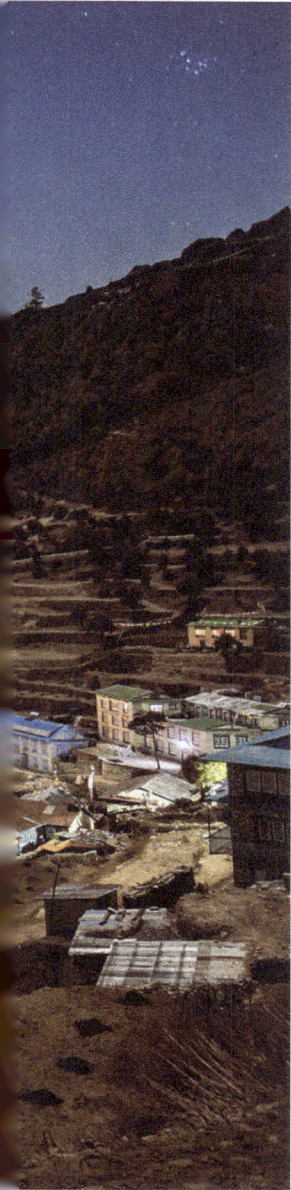

7

VEREST IS a mountain unlike any other. In stark contrast to my fifth mountain, which took a matter of hours to summit, I expect Everest to demand months of my life.

The time it takes to climb Mt Everest depends on a number of factors, such as the route taken, weather conditions, the climber's experience and physical condition, and the availability of support services. Typically, the average length of an Everest expedition is two to three months, with most climbers spending several weeks acclimatising to the altitude before attempting to summit.

Acclimatisation essentially means waiting for your body to increase its number of oxygen-carrying red blood cells. Extra red blood cells are essential in high-altitude environments where the air is 'thinner'—that is, contains less oxygen. Monitoring oxygen saturation levels using a pulse oximeter can help determine whether the body is adapting to the new altitude or whether there is a risk of altitude sickness, which can be a potentially life-threatening condition. Checking our 'pulse ox' will be a daily ritual.

Everest Base Camp is the starting point for climbers attempting to summit Everest via the South Col route in Nepal, and is located at an altitude of 5,364 metres in the Khumbu region. But when I say 'starting point', just getting here is a trek in itself. The journey typically takes eleven to fourteen days, depending on the itinerary and pace of the trekker.

There are fourteen of us on this expedition, and on the way to Everest Base Camp we will share the same teahouses, regardless of whether we're private or Sherpa climbers. Along the way we will pass through traditional Sherpa villages and past Buddhist monasteries. We will witness stunning landscapes, including the Khumbu Icefall, a treacherous section of the climb to the summit of Everest.

Everest Base Camp is a popular trekking destination for non-climbers as well, offering stunning views of the surrounding Himalayan peaks and an opportunity to experience the unique Sherpa culture of the region.

The actual climb to the summit can take anywhere from ten to twenty hours, depending on the climber's pace and the conditions. But for now, I have to focus on the first half of my adventure—getting to Base Camp. Kathmandu has been fascinating, but I'm pumped and ready to head for the mountains.

opposite Lukla Airport— the most dangerous airport in the world?

PULSE OX: 89%

Kathmandu to Lukla to Phakding

It doesn't matter that I've had a terrible night's sleep; we're finally underway. A buzz of excitement fills the Yak & Yeti foyer, and after a quick bite to eat we board buses for the five-kilometre journey to the airport.

'Ten-minute wait on coffee,' a barista advises in his otherwise empty shop at the airport. In a most awful turn of events, we're now boarding the plane minus coffee. And with that our thirty-minute flight to Lukla in a L410 UVP-E20 aircraft commences, courtesy of Summit Air.

Tenzing-Hillary Airport was built in 1964 through the efforts of Sir Edmund Hillary's fundraising, and is perched 9,383 feet above sea level in the tiny Himalayan settlement of Lukla. It is also regarded as the world's most dangerous airport. This is because the short, 1,729-foot runway, perched on little more than a shelf, is surrounded on all sides by steep,

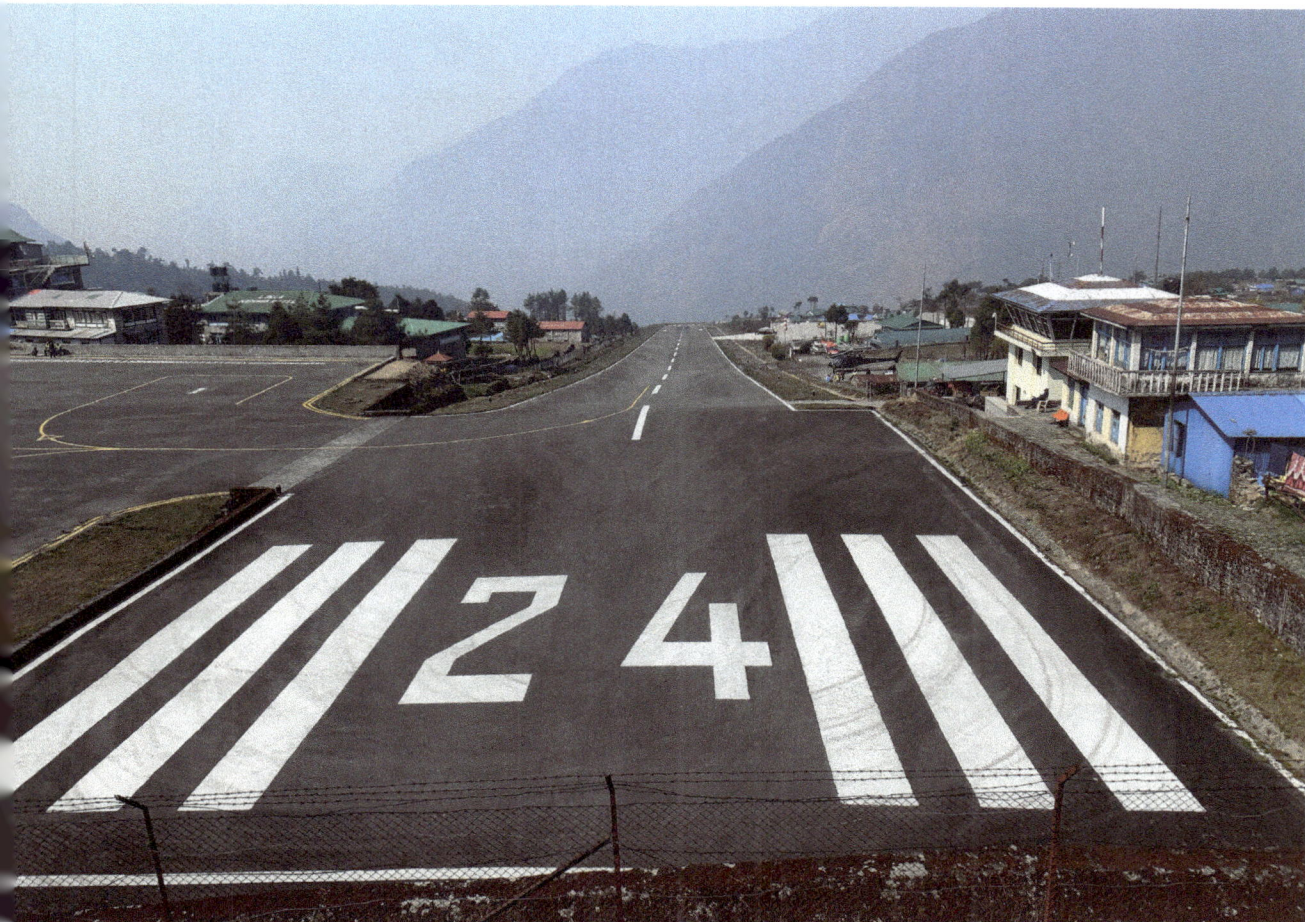

mountainous terrain. At one end there's a wall and at the other a steep drop into the valley below. But Lukla is the only airport you can fly to for the start of the Base Camp trek. Landing here can be dramatic, but thankfully today we touch down efficiently enough. In fact, I felt safe throughout the flight, and in just an hour-and-a-half we've been transported from the smoke and pollution of Kathmandu to the crisp mountain air of the Himalayas, altitude 2,830 metres. It feels surreal to finally be here.

Kami Rita, the current world record holder with twenty-four Everest summits under his belt, arrives at our teahouse.

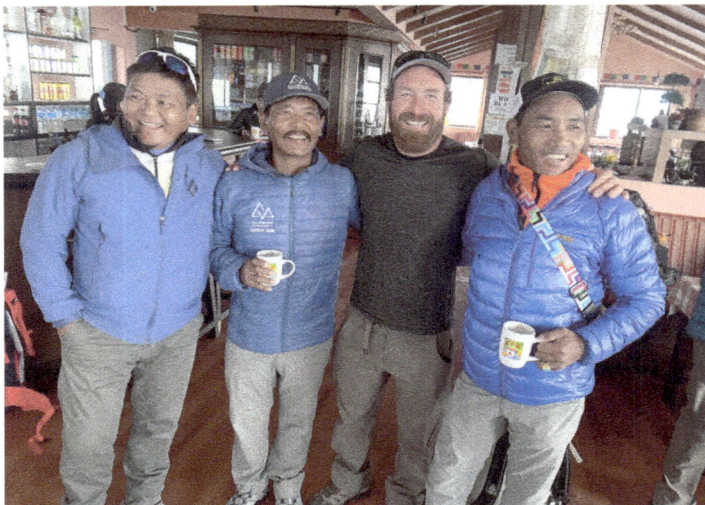

right Legends of Everest

This legendary mountaineer was born in Thame in the Solukhumbu district, which is the same district where Tenzing Norgay, who guided Edmund Hillary to the summit of Everest in 1953, was born. Kami Rita's celebrity status is evident and meeting him is an inspiration. Hopefully, he will achieve his twenty-fifth summit this year.[1]

Everyone gathers, Mike shares a few words, and our adventure begins. Our small team strolls to Pasang Lhamu Gate for a photo opportunity.

Big Tendi tells us of his plans for our summit success. Many golden nuggets of advice are woven into his stories, such as switching your active hand on the rope. Sounds simple, but repetitive use of only one hand when you have to lift it above the heart results in poor circulation in that hand. In turn, your fingers can be more susceptible to frostbite. Not a problem for Big Tendi though. 'I don't really get cold until it's minus thirty degrees Celsius, I have warm blood,' says the guide who has summitted Everest nineteen times.

---

1   Kami Rita went on to scale Mt Everest for the twenty-fifth time on 7 May 2021.

It's also great to get to know the man behind the legend. Big Tendi, forty-five, is a family man with a fifteen-year-old daughter and four-year-old son. After mostly guiding private clients in recent years, we're certainly privileged to have him allocated as our lead guide, which was made possible by a client's last-minute cancellation. Last time Big Tendi did a group gig it was 2012, and he led thirteen people to the summit.

The start of our trail is mostly large stones and well-compacted earth, with care still required for foot placement. There's nobody at our rest stop, Wind Horse Lodge and Restaurant, because of Covid-19 restrictions. Normally the track would be busy, with streets lined with people, yaks and donkeys, Ryan tells us. It's nice for us that it's so quiet, but devastating for locals trying to make a living.

After our rest stop we cross a cool suspension bridge that spans a deep gorge. A second bridge to our left has fast-flowing rapids and transparent, light blue waters that you just want to jump into. Yaks and donkeys occasionally pass us on the trail. But where are all the people? We seem strangely alone, and aside from a few locals here and there we have the mountains to ourselves.

After a morning's trek we arrive at Phakding, a small village that lies in the Dudh Kosi River valley, 6.75 kilometres north of Lutka. The altitude here in Phakding is 2,642 metres, and when I take a deep breath I can feel that the air is starting to thin. From now on, my body will work a little harder to get the oxygen it needs. So far the climb has been easy. But it's lunchtime and I'm starving.

Tonight we're staying at Sherpa Guide Lodge and Restaurant. It's a lovely, cosy place with a welcoming ambience and manicured gardens. It'll just be our group, due to Covid mitigation strategies. With infrastructure all the way to Base Camp and a quiet climbing season, this is a good start to the limited number of quality establishments on offer in this region. Cheese momo, vegetable momo and a pizza with the lot are my selections for lunch. The food is delicious, there's

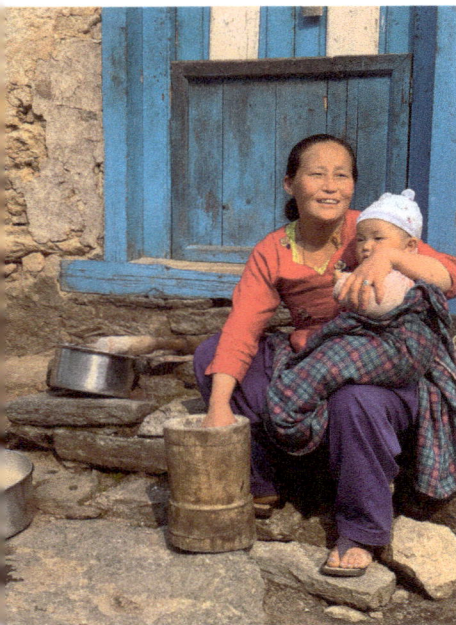

above Pounding grain

opposite Typical suspension bridge

lemon tea in abundance, and the rooms are excellent and come complete with ensuites. I'm not sure how long this perfect run will continue, but everything is working out so far.

After a lazy lunch, I wander off to explore the village. I try interacting with a woman and her small child who are pounding grain on the step of their house. A donkey pushes past, another eats the roof of a nearby shelter. While local kids seem inquisitive about our presence, they continue to run and play.

A few of us hike back to one of the suspension bridges we crossed earlier. There are prayer flags of all colours flapping towards the centre of the bridge. They're a constant feature along the trek, and when they're all gathered in places like this they look spectacular. Mani—prayer wheels—are also common in the villages of this region, some of more significance than others because of their plaques. One reads: 'Please turn this mani to purify your soul: Lama Dorji.' I've learned today that you always walk around prayer rocks clockwise and always spin mani clockwise while chanting the ancient Buddhist mantra 'Om mani padme hum'. In English, this rhythmic chant translates to 'Praise to the jewel in the lotus'.

There are flowers blooming early because it's been a warm season, but other than a few porters and the occasional local, only our small group gets to admire the beautiful scenery. It's very quiet. A loud chopper hovering over our hotel soon shatters the silence. Our luggage, which hadn't made it onto the plane, has arrived. Our bags are dropped from on high and bounce straight onto the front lawn. Peace returns when the helicopter turns around and disappears into the distance.

It's been a day full of new sights, sounds, smells and adventure. I can't wait to do it all again tomorrow.

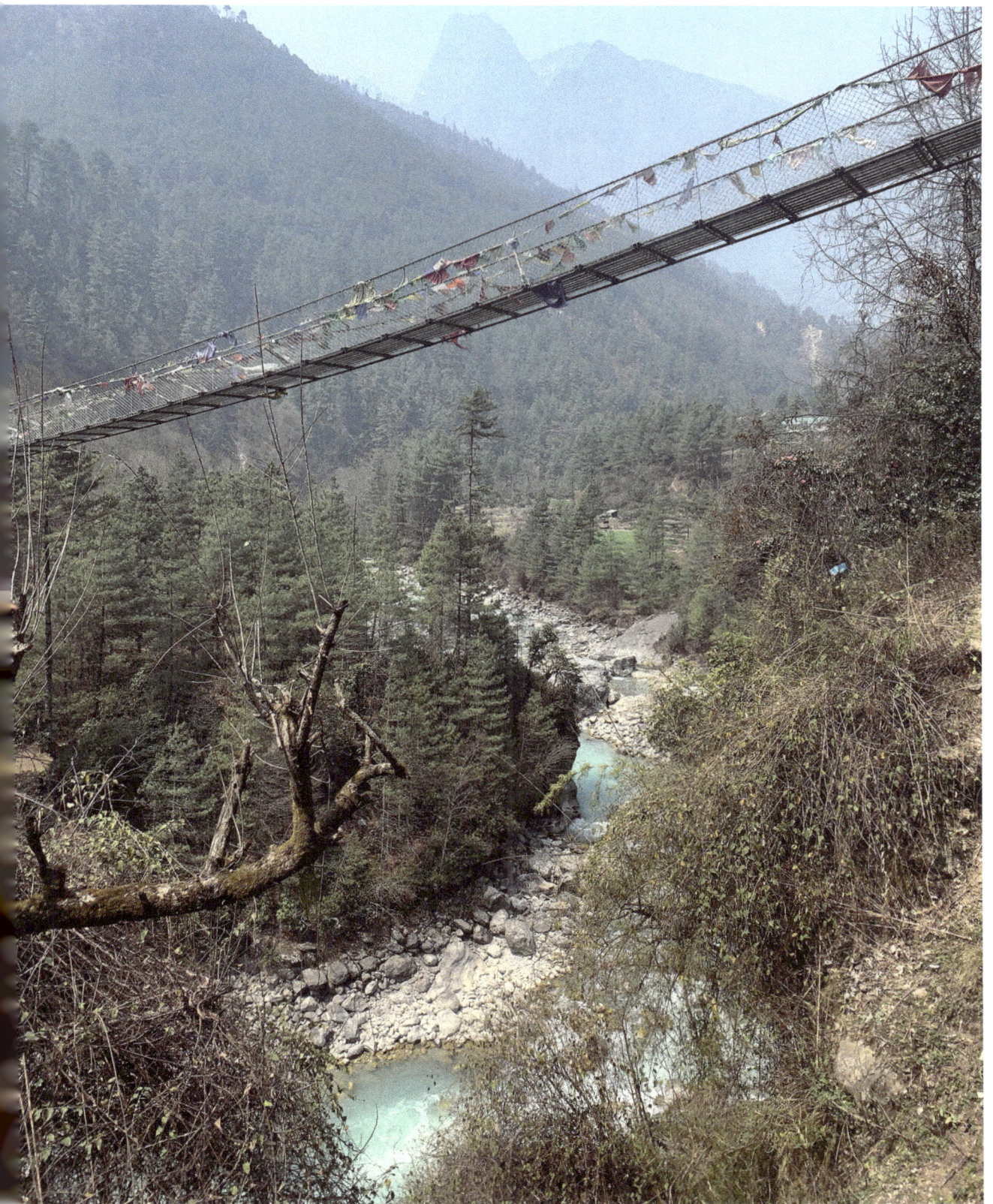

Phakding to Namche Bazaar

750m of elevation gained

DISTANCE: 11.32km

TIME: 05:30 hrs
(total time with break)

ASCENT: 1,084m

DESCENT: 262m

ALTITUDE: 3,392m

PULSE OX: 95%

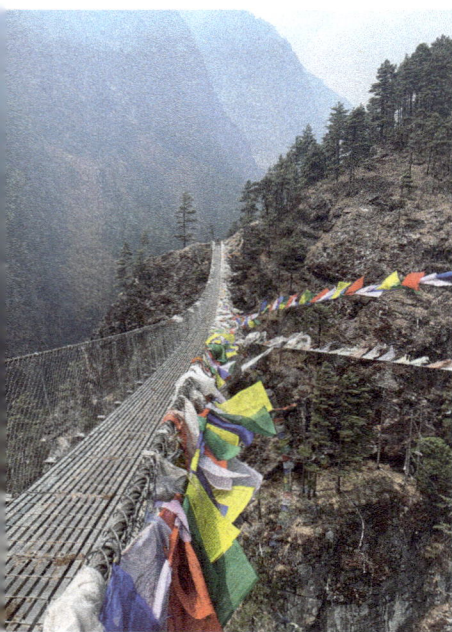

above Prayer flags
fluttering

It's a crisp new morning with a light haze through the valley and we hit the trail following a breakfast of apple porridge. The trail is undulating as we track the Dudh Kosi River and traverse it several times via suspension bridges. It's all slowly, slowly to warm up and get some elevation gain behind us.

Men are digging trenches and constructing walls to the side of the trail to cater to trekkers. Tourism here is a multi-billion dollar affair, so it's great to see some money going back into the communities. I can see women tending to the cooking and washing laundry. Little kids amuse themselves in the streets, never too far from the huts we pass.

We cross a small bridge that has a beautifully peaceful ambience. There's nobody else here. A brisk wind blows through across the valley, causing prayer flags to flutter. There are two waterfalls in the distance cascading from higher above. It's so enchanting I linger a little longer after our group passes through.

A security checkpoint informs me we're in Sagarmatha National Park, a UNESCO World Heritage site covering 124,400 hectares of dramatic mountains, deep valleys and glaciers that is home to several rare species, including snow leopard and panda. Sagarmatha National Park also has more than twenty villages and a population of over 6,000 Sherpa, whose ancestors have inhabited the region for the last four centuries.

As we enter the park, a few military personnel count our numbers and check paperwork. The sheer rock walls here have been used for climbing practice, and Big Tendi points out two rock anchors he has embedded. All the lower sections are carved with prayers painted white. The craftsmanship is incredible, considering the time it would have taken to carve lettering into these solid, towering rock formations.

More donkeys and yaks seem to be on the track than yesterday, but we're mostly the only group underway. There's a

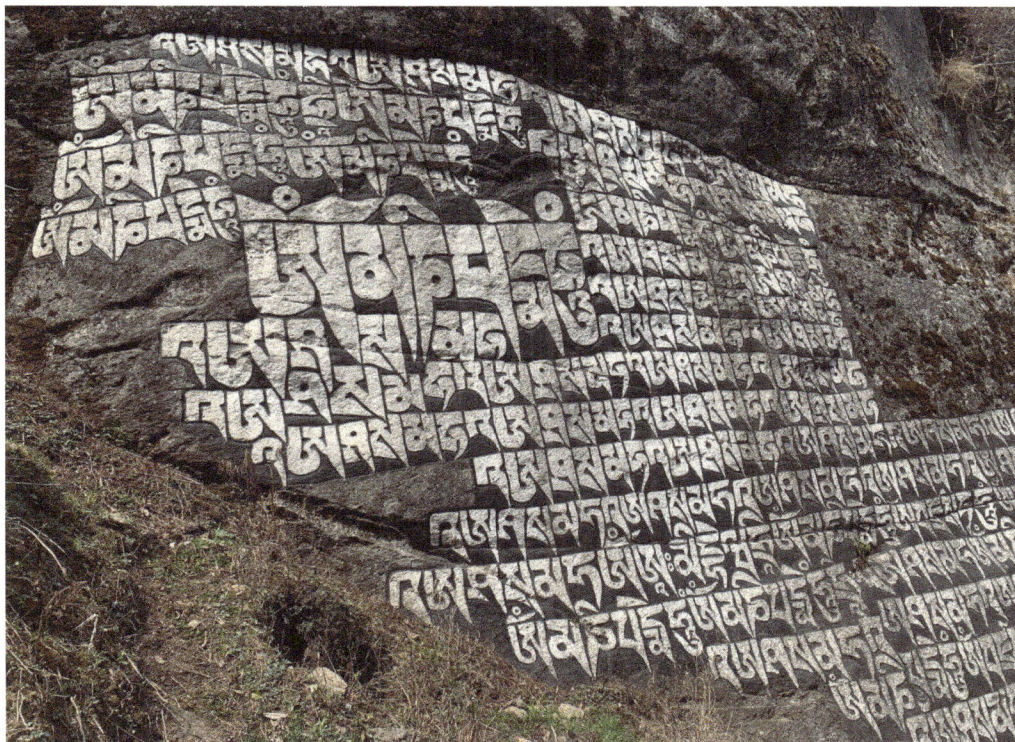

above Just some of the many carved prayers

small group of Scottish trekkers, and I'm not sure what the French guys were up to as they push past in a hurry—day trekkers, I suspect.

I never tire of enjoying the awesome suspension bridges that cross the raging rivers below, surrounded by incredible vistas of towering mountains. But horsing around, I've dropped my sunglasses. They've landed on the banks of the river, so of course I'll have to retrieve them. Just jogging down the embankment has my lungs pumping. The effort takes my breath away, but I persist, grab the glasses and attempt running up the embankment, now gasping. Yes, the altitude has arrived.

There's a spectacular double bridge in the distance. Big Tendi tells me that 600 years ago his family crossed here to

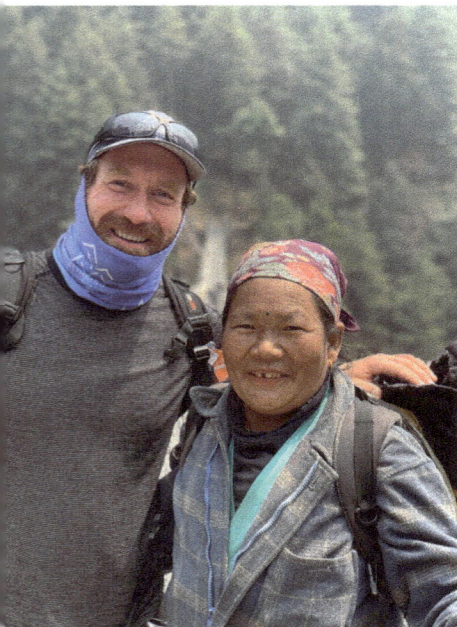

above Joining in the fun

opposite Namche Bazaar

take up lands. Lucky… otherwise he'd still be in Tibet. The winding trail to the bridge has picture-perfect panoramas at every turn. The river rushing below has morphed into raging rapids; the wind is blowing enough to keep me cool and allow the prayer flags to flap and create their own spectacle. It's simply breathtaking.

Stepping onto one of the higher suspension bridges, we pass an elderly couple. Big Tendi stops and shakes their hands. He tells me the man, a former monk, is a 100-year-old Sherpa who has been voluntarily building the track with stones—manually—for the past thirty years. His name is Pasang Sherpa, and even at his venerable age he and his wife continue building the track. Trekkers give small donations, which Pasang Sherpa and his wife live off and use to pay others to assist them in this massive undertaking. I'll be sure to contribute too.

Pasang Sherpa's wife crosses the bridge, dancing as she realises I'm filming. I ask if I can take a photo too, and show her when it's taken. She is all smiles. I hope this wonderful couple see out all their days in this place, which must be so very special to them both.

It's up Namche Hill from here. The trail is steep in sections, but has the shade of the forest and is less exposed. There are lots of switchbacks and we rest once. With a last push, the trees give way to reveal Namche Bazaar, at 3,500 metres.

The unofficial Sherpa capital, Namche Bazaar is a historic trading hub famous for its yak cheese and butter, and is literally built into the side of a hill. I'm surprised at the size of the town, which is home to 1,600 hardy souls. There are multi-storey buildings and streets lined with shops. Large statues are everywhere, and paintings adorn ceilings and structures.

Staying here is critical for acclimatisation before trekking to higher altitudes, I'm told. Hotel Namche, said to be one of the town's upstanding establishments, is our digs for tonight. I believe we have 'super deluxe' rooms.

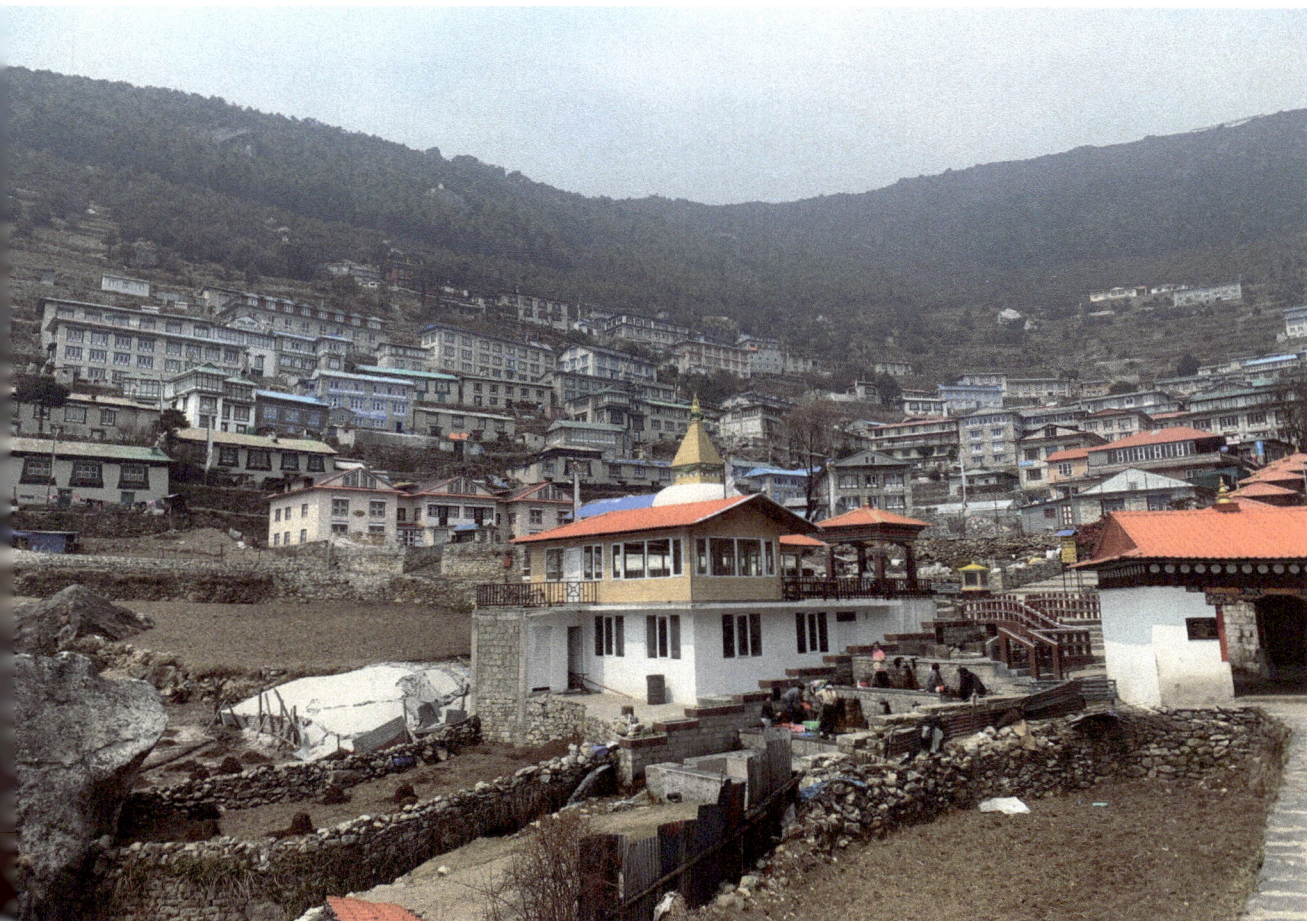

LUNCH IS a big occasion, and I've certainly got an appetite after the 11.32 kilometre hike. The 'Sherpa' beer behind the bar is all out of date, and our guides tell us not to drink it. Unfortunately, the repercussions of Covid lockdowns reach even these remote settings. Fresh German beers are purchased next door, and our hosts miss out on the beer money. At the table it's cheers all round for our small but social group. Laughs, stories and highlights are shared, and the German beer is refreshingly cold.

The weather seems to have cooled down. Strolling about Namche Bazaar's shops, I realise there's only a handful of other tourists here. There are more monks than visitors about town, which has German bakeries, many cafes and even an Irish pub. The pub is named, inventively, The Irish Pub, and is said to be the most remote Irish pub in the world.

Ryan and I are scoping out a coffee. There's no-one at all at the first café, not even staff. No-one at Himalayan Java Coffee around the corner either, but a lone staff member turns on the lights and is happy for our patronage. Ryan's been here before and is shocked by the contrast. 'These joints would normally be pumping,' he says. The cappuccino and chocolate slice are certainly first rate. There's even free wi-fi.

We pass a multi-storey building site with its steel structure being assembled. Three men cling to a column up high as welders work in the open below. No scaffolding or safety here.

Later we enjoy dinner in a private room off the hotel's restaurant filled with colourful flags, photos and memorabilia. The atmosphere is set by Ron, one of our trekkers, strumming the guitar. I notice he's playing Men at Work's 'Down Under' for me. Mike can play a decent riff too.

I've eaten a lot. Even managed a glass of Aussie shiraz. All the way up here, that bottle has not only travelled, but survived a long journey from Australia. Naturally, it makes me think of home, and I wish my family could have the opportunity to see these amazing sights and have these life-changing experiences I'm having. Then I remember how challenging travel can be when you have a diabetic child. I wonder if Fin will ever be able to have an adventure like this. Could she manage her condition in a remote corner of a developing country?

THE NEXT day we're off for a hike and to take in some acclimatisation.

Just out of Namche Bazaar, following a steep climb of steps, there's a viewing point that takes in the town, which sits in a horseshoe-shaped bowl amid the Himalayan mountains. The sun is up, and the trek up here has warmed me up despite a

opposite Namche Bazaar bowl

DISTANCE: 7.5km
TIME: 04:07 hrs
ASCENT: 527m
DESCENT: 539m
PULSE OX: 95%

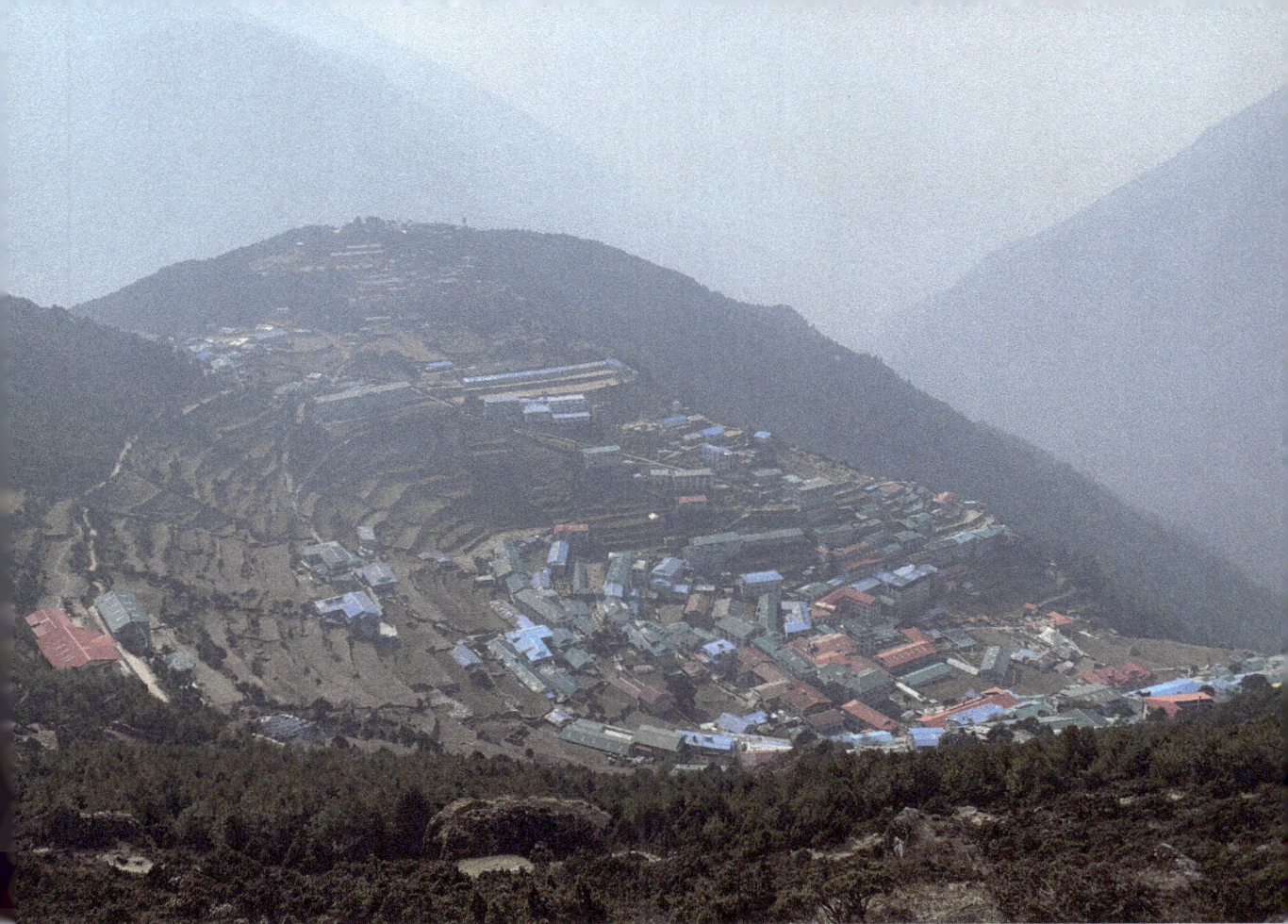

slight chill in the air. There's a stubborn haze, which Big Tendi says melts the snow on the mountains much faster as the haze carries particles of dust. His hope is for a large dumping of snow to restore the balance.

Our hike takes us further, to Kunde, one of the larger Sherpa villages. Entrances to the village are lined with memes and stone-engraved plaques. The village has its share of monuments too. Before the advent of paper, all writing was done on these stone plaques. Now they're lined up, stacked in neat rows, still intact. I haven't seen any trekkers or fellow climbers in transit today. Though the season is open, it appears in a very limited capacity. Kunde is altogether quiet. A few people are out sowing crops; someone is washing clothes.

There's a hospital here, built in 1966 by Sir Edmund Hillary and the friends and volunteers he persuaded to help him. Kunde Hospital services up to 8,000 local people, plus the thousands of trekkers who pass through the region during the climbing seasons.

A doctor on duty has offered us an inside view. Two general practitioners and other medical professionals provide healthcare for the people of the Khumbu region for 100 rupees—essentially free. Babies are delivered here, and they've started their own Covid-19 immunisation program. The tourists pay for consultations, with all proceeds going back into the hospital. The doctor here gives a generous insight into the work he generally undertakes, with the most common problems including respiratory issues, gastric problems and diabetes. On my enquiry, the doctor advises he has only ever had one case of type 1 diabetes, and that patient had to go to Kathmandu for treatment.

Covid-19 vaccines have made it here for the essential workers so critical to the area. One shot has been administered to high-risk people aged over fifty-five, which is promising. The doctor himself admits being infected in December 2020.

'Seventy-five per cent of people up here have been infected,' he tells me.

What?! This is a complete shock, given the information I received in Australia. I believed Covid-19 hadn't reached the remote Khumbu region, that once we made it through Kathmandu we'd be safer. I wonder about the long-term impacts for the region.

After thanking the doctor, and donating to the hospital, I press Big Tendi on this point. He tells me he spent three months sleeping with another guy in a tent who had tested positive three times with Covid, yet he didn't become infected. For this reason he doesn't think he'll get vaccinated, he says.

The amount of information available about coronavirus is dizzying. It's hard to keep track of what's current, what's known, what's myth, and what actual guidance one should follow. Visiting the hospital has been something of a reality check. Somehow, amid the beautiful scenery of the Himalayas, and distracted by new and exotic sights and sounds, I'd forgotten about this deadly virus. Now I'm reminded of how serious this pandemic is.

We hike to Khumjung village, directly adjacent to Kunde on the valley at the foot of Khumbu Yul-Lha, the sacred mountain of the Sherpa, where Edmund Hillary built a school in 1961. The legendary mountaineer built and ran forty-two schools, hospitals and medical clinics in the Mt Everest region. Khumjung school—the first that Hillary built—became known as 'the schoolhouse in the clouds'.

Namche Bazaar to Debuche

It's still and clear this morning. Light rain overnight has cleared the haze, for now. The skies are blue, and there are great views of Kongde Ri mountain from the Hotel Namche dining room.

We trek north from Namche Bazaar and pass the Tenzing Norgay Memorial stupa monument, which is our first drink stop. Continuing on, some giants of the Himalayas slowly reveal themselves. I reach the first view-point for Ama Dablam (6,856 metres), a mountain that intrigues me more and more as I continue to hear stories of it. There's Lhotse (8,516 metres) in the far distance, Taboche (6,367 metres), and on our right the sun is hitting the ice-covered slopes of Kangtega (6,685 metres) and glistening in a way that no photo does justice to. With a little help from our guide, Anup, who was my moped driver in Kathmandu, the South Summit of Mt Everest can be identified above the South Col.

DISTANCE: 10.46km

TIME: 04:53 hrs

AVERAGE SPEED: 2.2kph

ASCENT: 850m

DESCENT: 546m

ALTITUDE: 3,740m

GAIN: 348m

It's a little busier on the route today. Small guided hiking groups, one larger group of climbers and plenty of locals are out on the track. In the small villages we pass, kids and mums smile and wave, only too happy to have their photos taken.

It's the porters that I'm most impressed by. They carry loads between fifteen and thirty kilos, with a fixed price for their labour. Some opt to carry two loads—up to sixty kilos—for double pay. Just as I'm admiring these strong guys hauling such big loads, I see one carrying what can only be described as a monster load. I ask Anup to ask the man how much weight he's lugging. The answer is three loads, weighing a total of eighty kilos! Just incredible. I watch the porter heave the load onto his back using a strap on his forehead, with his arms left to balance the incredible weight.

One group of four porters run down the track past us, while we labour up in the opposite direction. Jovial and laughing, they've already delivered their loads for the day and are heading back to Namche Bazaar to get in line for tomorrow's loads.

Although it's a continuous incline for the rest of today's leg, the scenery around is inspiring. The further we trek, the bigger and more distinctive the mountains become. I can now see Camp 2.7 on Ama Dablam, and where the old Camp 3 was. It's a magical mountain that holds your attention and imagination. The snow upon her is the whitest of white, with the sun accentuating its balconies.

If the porters haven't been impressive enough, a new type of porter is labouring under loads of a different type—construction materials. Long, thick timber beams, more precisely. At first I see a porter carrying two beams strapped together. I just shake my head at the size of the load. A little further, a rest stop appears where three Sherpa are taking a break. A break from their loads of four long, large timber beams strapped together. I ask Anup to ask them the weight of those loads. 'Between ninety and ninety-five kilograms,' he replies.

The first real example of the dangers of Mt Everest also passes us by. A young local holds a man's hand, guiding him down the mountain. The man being led stumbles and stares at the ground. It's mountain sickness—the effects of altitude—Arup tell us.

Our next stop, after a long, continuous climb, is Tengboche Monastery, also known as Dawa Choling Gompa, which suddenly appears from nowhere. This huge structure, an important Buddhist monastery, was built in 1923, destroyed by an earthquake in 1934, subsequently rebuilt, destroyed again by fire in 1989, and rebuilt again. A large colourful arch frames the stairs that lead up to the impressive building. I learn that Tenzing Norgay was born in the area, in the village of Thani, and was once sent to Tengboche Monastery to become a monk.

Tomorrow we'll revisit for a blessing ceremony, but for now we're just passing through. It's only a short walk downhill to the village of Tengboche, our base for the next two nights. Just off the track, we see the first hard, compacted ice.

The lodge is new, the hosts are very happy to welcome us, and the rooms exceed our expectations. I'm carb-loading ... well, that's what I tell myself as I move through a big bowl of pasta, a plate of chips and a Mars bar pie. I am shooting for that extra cushioning after all. Sated and comfortable, I pay homage to the mountaineers who paved the way for the average person to follow in their footsteps. I can't represent my country in a world first, but I can follow my individual journey and bring awareness to a deserving cause—Diabetes Australia.

Tonight we sit around a warm fire with hot drinks and high spirits. We listen to music, play a dice game, Farkle, and laugh as I come from behind to win.

One trekking companion has missed dinner with a migraine. A few more have retired early with headaches. Despite the comforts, the body must work to adapt to the changes in altitude.

DISTANCE: 4.07km

TIME: 02:05

AVERAGE SPEED: 1.9kph

ASCENT: 460m

DESCENT: 453m

ALTITUDE: 4,230m

IT'S DEFINITELY colder this morning. Outside, a thin frost covers the grass and ice builds beneath the corrugated roof runoff. Yet the sky is blue and clear again, promising warmth, and from the grounds I take in views of Mt Everest and the equally commanding Ama Dablam on the horizon.

Our outing today is to the Tengboche Monastery for a 'puja'—a blessing—by the monks for our expedition. I've never been to a ceremony like this: the chanting, the prayers, the serious approach and careful organisation. It's a formal affair, and there's no talking, filming or photos.

One monk coughs and splutters continuously. A couple of years ago we would have dismissed this as an old man with a cold. In today's environment I'm not alone in concerns he may have Covid-19. Worse still, as we circle around the outside of the monastery, pass the giant Buddha and head back to the central area, this same monk places a string of 'sungdee' around our necks, which is to remain until we're successful in our journey or until it falls off.

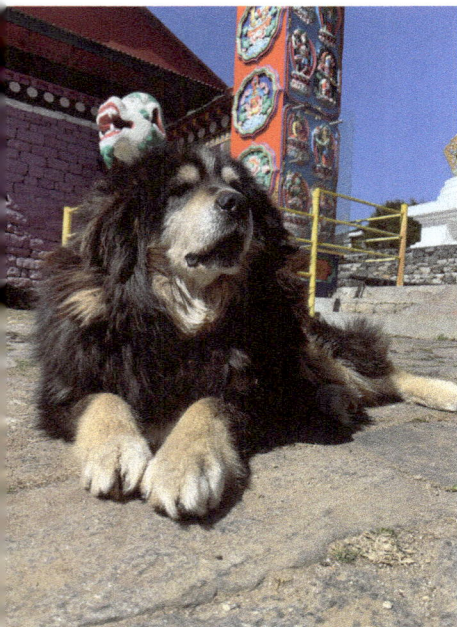

The ceremony continues, and we are then presented with a 'kata'—prayer scarf—'to ward off evil spirits and to protect along the long journey, and upon the mountain.' I appreciate the monks' devotion, and pay respects in turn, although a monk's lifestyle doesn't resonate a lot with me.

Newly blessed, we set off from Tengboche Monastery.

Debuche to Pheriche

DISTANCE: 9.34km

TIME: 03:55 hrs

AVERAGE SPEED: 2.4kph

ASCENT: 660m

DESCENT: 152m

ALTITUDE: 4,230m

GAIN: 490m

It's a 5am start, planned to capture a time delay on my GoPro of the new dawn hitting the mountains. It's dark and cold, and the valley is blanketed with thick grey clouds. It's still though ... too still, in fact. The clouds don't budge. Not ideal.

Ryan joins me, and we stand and chat in the dark. Will these clouds ever move? My fingers are getting cold, although I'm wearing gloves. It takes an hour, but slowly the clouds break up and small patches of blue sky emerge. We nearly

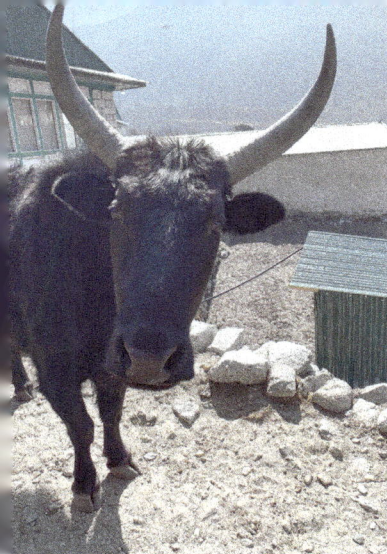
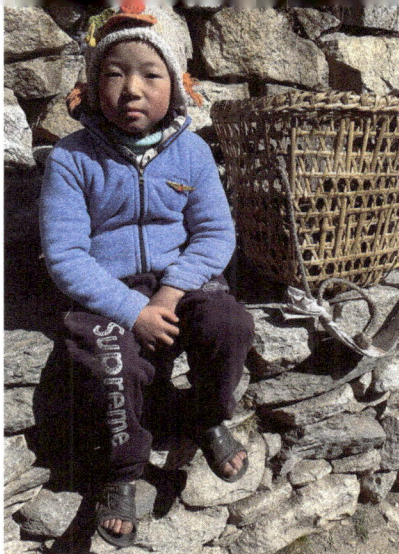
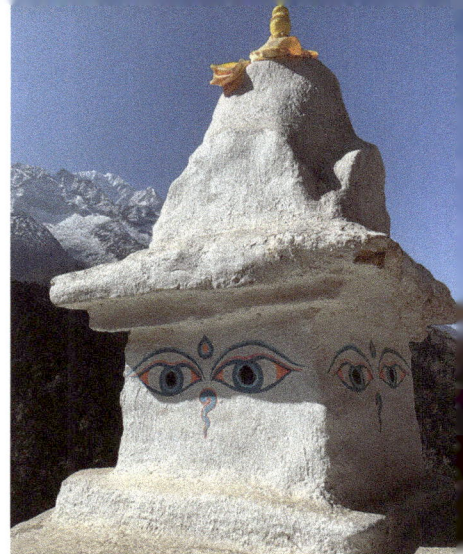

call it and go inside. But we're rewarded by staying; the grey clouds disperse and daylight starts to emerge, bathing the mountains in incredible light. I'm just in time to see the full sunrise from the hotel dining room after getting my bag out for the porters and changing for the day's hike.

Nirmal 'Nims' Purja is also staying at our accommodation, leading another team. A holder of multiple mountaineering world records, he's quite the celebrity around here. Prior to taking on a career in mountaineering, Purja served with the British Armed Forces as a Nepalese Gurkha. In 2019, he climbed all fourteen of Earth's 8,000-ers (mountain peaks above 8,000 metres) in a record time of six months and six days, beating the previous record of just under eight years.

The track is getting a little busier today, or, more accurately, we don't just have it to ourselves. It's an undulating walk mostly following the river. There are plenty of yaks out today, so I'm always on the lookout for a 'yak attack' on the narrow track. More than a few people have had their trip cut short by an aggressive yak, and I'm told one person died.

We stop for drinks at one of our Sherpa's teahouses en route. It's a cosy place, with tables and colourful cushions on bench seats set around the perimeter. The owner has climbed Everest numerous times and has certificates and memorabilia

left I was just watching the helicopter

centre Saying 'hello'

right Always something new

opposite Hanging out at Tengboche Monastery

adorning the walls. He even competed in the Mt Everest marathon many years ago.

It's not a long or difficult walk today: there's nothing to complain about as I gaze at the many angles of the mountains and how they change when we approach them. But at 4,000 metres the air is getting thinner, the lungs are really working, the heart is pounding. Soon enough Pheriche is in front of us, and another day's hike is done. I always feel we can go further, climb higher, but that's not how acclimatisation works. 'Slowly, slowly' is the mantra to progress.

The Pheriche Aid-post, established by the Himalayan Rescue Association in 1973, hosts lectures on 'mountain sickness and other hazards in the Nepal Himalaya', which strive to reduce casualties in the mountains. HRA also runs the seasonal Everest ER medical clinic at Base Camp. Although it's a light-hearted presentation, the topics of acute mountain sickness and acclimatisation are very real. Nepal can be deadly. The country has the widest altitude range of any country on Earth, ranging from 200 metres in the Terai to 8,848 metres at the summit of Everest. 'Don't go too high too fast' is the cornerstone of acclimatisation.

I ask the doctor if he is concerned about Covid-19 spreading through Base Camp. 'I'm really concerned actually,' she replies.

'What are the chances, do you think?'

'It will be really lucky if it doesn't spread through Base Camp.'

Not the comforting commentary I was hoping for. After being infected, you can return a positive Covid PCR test for two to three months. If I catch the virus, I could be stuck in Nepal for months. I'm starting to think that it's only a matter of time before I hear about a Covid situation at Base Camp. But I'm in the Himalayas now, so I just have to keep on rolling.

On a brighter note, the Hotel Edelweiss Pheriche is another great place to stay. The main lounge feels more like a local bar, and oozes with character. The rooms are basic, and cold, but that's okay—it's minus one degree Celsius outside. I chill out (pardon the pun) at the hotel for the afternoon with hot drinks, good food, good company and a few games to pass the time.

Later Tenji Sherpa is introduced to everyone, and will be joining us from here on. Tenji is an incredible athlete with extensive time on the big mountains. He'll be assisting Big Tendi in our small team campaign to the summit.

IT'S EARLY, minus five degrees Celsius outside and the only person up is the hotel owner, who is starting a fire in the common area. I've jumped on the wi-fi and get a chance to call home. There's nothing like starting the day talking to the family, hearing about what's happening at home—the old normal. Home is nothing like the Himalayas. It's a suburban setting we all retreat to at the end of our daily routines. A place to relax after daily challenges. But more than that—the reason I'm on this crazy adventure in the first place is the people who share our home. It's not easy balancing this undertaking, this intention, with home life. I'm enthralled by the Himalayas, but at the same time I ache with homesickness when I talk to my family. Regardless, I try to stay positive and manage our limited interactions genuinely.

Heidi has taken the kids to Grazeland—'A playground for foodies'—to eat a variety of desserts. Fin's eating Spanish donuts, one of their favourites, with everyone. In many ways, my family has endured similar sacrifices to mine to let me complete these summits—my absence, my worries—but our diets might be the exception!

Today is an acclimatisation hike. As we exit Pheriche, there's basically a vertical hill to scale. Not everyone is coming, and that's okay, as some climbers need the rest day. It's a dusty, single-file, worn-in track; nothing too impressive. What is impressive is the different sides of Ama Dablam in view. As we hike towards it I can see more detail in the mountain, and it's amazing.

DISTANCE: 4.76km

TIME: 03:15 hrs

AVERAGE SPEED: 1.5kph

ASCENT: 630m

DESCENT: 663m

ALTITUDE: 4,845m

PULSE OX: 93%

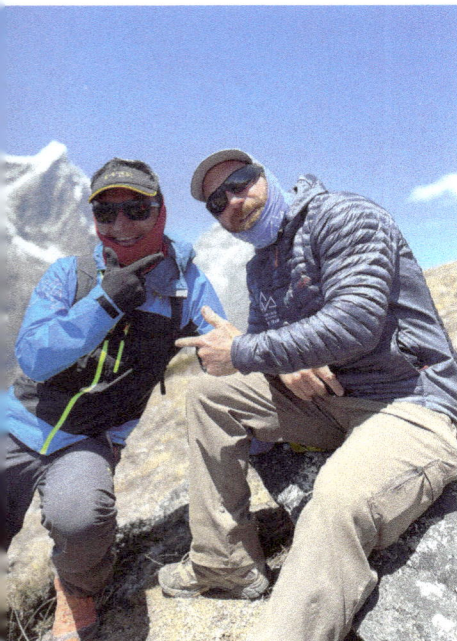

above Tenji Sherpa

opposite Summit's just over there...

We're accompanied by Tenji Sherpa, now part of our Everest team. It's a good opportunity to get to know this awesome guy. Tenji has an extensive climbing resume that lists six Everest summits, including once with no oxygen. He has guided and climbed throughout the Himalayas, Europe and the USA and, like Big Tendi, is an IFMGA internationally certified guide.

Once we reach our objective height, I take some photos, drink all my fluids and relax for our fifteen minutes. Big Tendi is onto me straightaway. 'Get your jacket on, man. If you want to summit with me, you need it,' he says. 'It's not like Australia here, the cold will get in your chest and you'll get the cough.'

I like his direct advice. I'm not cold, but with a single base layer on, I appreciate that the wind is up here. With Big Tendi's finger pointed at me, I happily don my jacket.

After a group photo it's time to roll out. The descent is always quick, and we're soon back at the Hotel Edelweiss. Here, an angry yak jumps out of its enclosure. Quick with the camera, I capture the moment. Not something you see every day and I'm wary to stay out of its way. I didn't come all this way for a yak attack.

After some warm drinks and food, the highlight of the day has arrived—a hot shower. Gee, it's good, just standing there, clean, refreshed and ready for a change of clothes. It's the little things that matter.

Pheriche to Lobuche Base Camp

DISTANCE: 5.47km

TIME: 03:30 hrs

AVERAGE SPEED: 1.5kph

ASCENT: 556m

DESCENT: 32m

ALTITUDE: 4,805m

PULSE OX: 86%

With the duffle re-packed once again, it's time to make tracks. No more hotels, teahouses, menus or beds. No real toilets or showers. No common room fire on those cold nights. We're off to Lobuche Base Camp. Tenji Sherpa, who tells me he is twenty-nine, is leading our trek today.

Lobuche is no small hill, or single-day hike. As her snow-capped peak and looming presence come into view, I take the

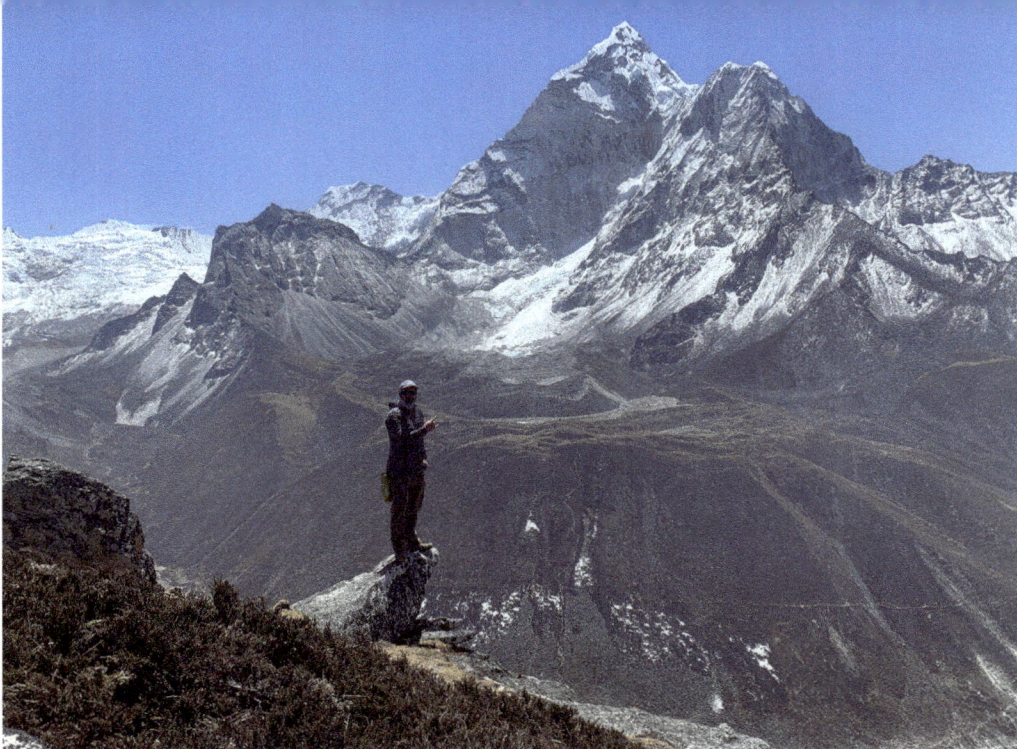

opportunity to snap a few photos and admire the landscape. Presently Lobuche Summit grows closer through grey clouds and fog circles. Fast-flowing creeks have ice on their banks, and some are completely iced to the surface. The morning sun is usually enough to warm me up, but not today. I think I'll be digging out more down jackets later.

Eventually Base Camp comes into view. The CTSS site has a 'Big Tent'—an eight-metre circle with an igloo entrance. We arrive at camp and there are a few brief introductions, as the CTSS crew are already here. Ryan, CTSS owner Mike and I wait for the rest of the group to catch up. After a short orientation to camp from Mike, it's straight to the Big Tent for lunch.

I'm impressed. The tent is lined and has a tarp floor and two rows of tables. There's a cook at hand who serves hot drinks to warm us up. Noodle soup is then served, followed by a basic main meal. It's relaxing kicking back on the comfy seats in the warm tent and out of the elements.

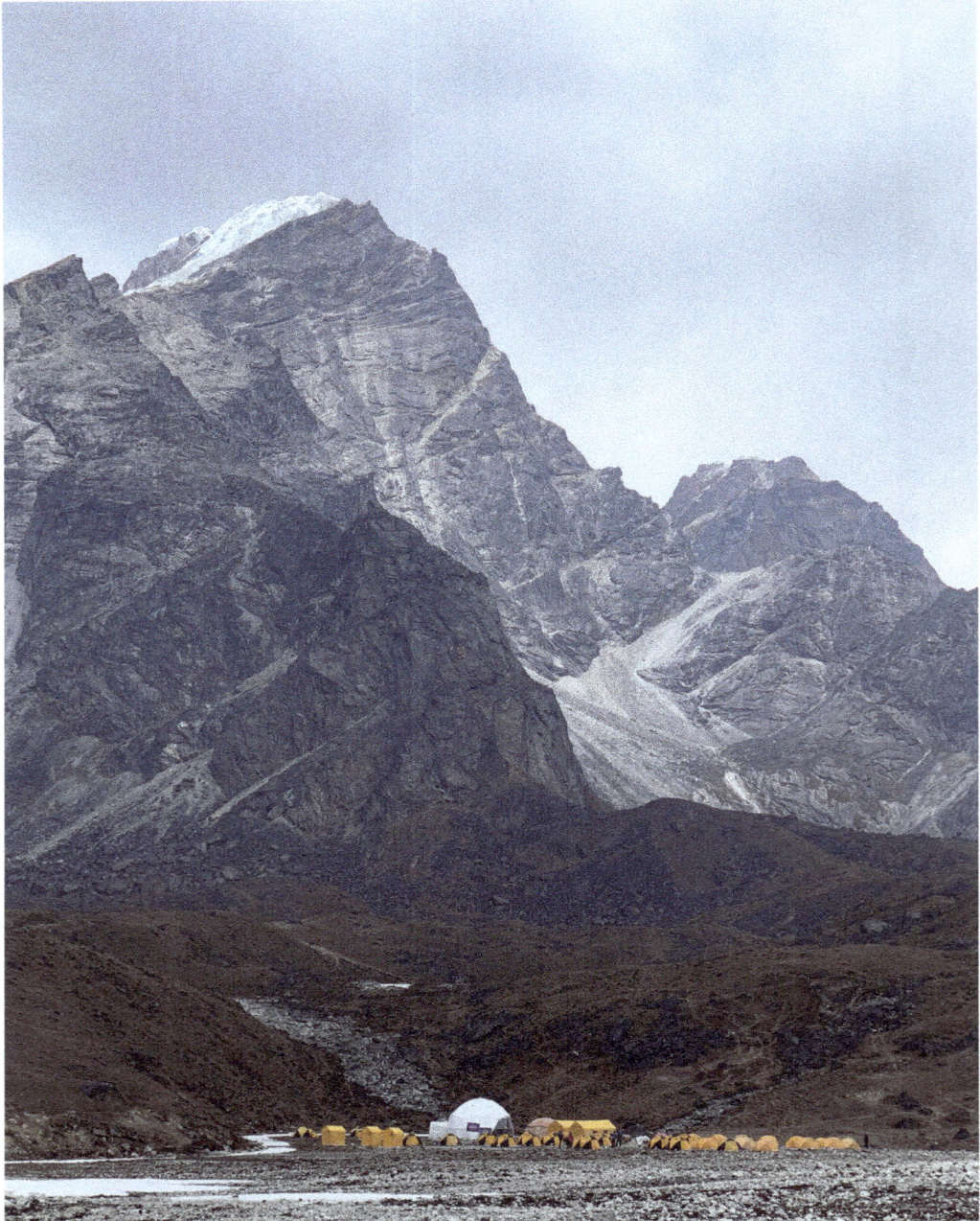

above Lobuche
Base Camp

It's snowing lightly when we move into our small shared tents. With the snow falling and the promise of a warm tent, Ryan and I rummage through our duffels and throw the essentials into the tent. Welcome home. Inside is nicer than out and my new sleeping bag is keeping up with the deteriorating weather. We have some visitors over. Six people in a two-man tent is a tight fit, but also generates some warmth.

A FILM of frost covers the camp, and condensation has crystallised in the tent. During the night I've fluctuated between warm and cold and my stomach feels squeamish. Sleeping on the ground hasn't done my hips any favours either. I've slept in a jumper, tracksuit pants and down booties, but need another layer to go outside. Unzipping the tent flap accentuates the crisp morning as I make my way outside. A slight headache is threatening, and my breath has shortened.

DISTANCE: 3.44km
TIME: 03:27 hrs
AVERAGE SPEED: 1kph
ASCENT: 454m
DESCENT: 432m
ALTITUDE: 5,265m
PULSE OX: 86%

Nobody is about, but I can hear some rumblings in the kitchen tent. The weather is calmer, the wind has stopped and, in the pre-dawn light, the camp is otherwise quiet. I'm not feeling great. Still, it's time to get some breakfast, which I don't want, and get my gear packed. I take off for a walk around camp. As my stomach churns, Big Tendi comes across to check my oxygen saturation levels.

'Drink at least one litre of water, now. Warm water. Go.'

Well, that's unexpected. I don't really want that much water sloshing in this belly, but best I oblige.

At breakfast I feel shitty, with a foggy head and no appetite. Still, I try the porridge. Nope. Maybe a piece of toast. Just a coffee and I'll have to be ready to go.

This morning we are to set off on an acclimatisation hike up to Lobuche Base Camp to drop some gear ahead of tomorrow's transition there. The climb to the peak of Lobuche, at 6,119 metres, is strenuous, I'm told. Although a short 3.44-kilometre climb, it's steep. It would be great if I could get into a rhythm, but I can't. My breathing is heavy and my heart rate higher than ideal. Labouring up the mountain, trying not to vomit, I realise my teahouse trekking is over and, although it's great to be scaling an actual mountain, the adjustment of altitude has no favourites.

There's a small section to scale on a vertical fixed line, then onto a ledge. Swinging through is no problem, it's catching my breath at the top that gets me. Then the going is mostly rock-hopping and traversing loose scree on a single-file track. Towards the top, there are larger rock formations that offer sure footing and the path to High Camp. It's windy on top, but not excessively cold. After a cup of hot lemon, a group picture and unloading our gear, it's time to descend. At least when I get back down I'm hungry. And while I'm tired, I no longer feel like I'll vomit at any moment.

At 3pm local Sherpa hold a climbing refresher session. Harnesses are checked, rigging inspected, and they run through preferred safety systems. It's a good opportunity to get rid of any gear that is not really required. Our small team will re-rig in an individual system, but this session serves its purpose.

Afterwards, we set off to a climbing wall just behind camp to re-run through the practical aspects of keeping safe while ascending and descending. This is a good opportunity to adjust my clipping system to mirror that of the Sherpa.

It's Ryan's fortieth birthday today, a big milestone for him, and after dinner it's time to celebrate. Mike presents a birthday cake, I pull out the Jack Daniel's, the music is turned up, and the partying begins.

Lobuche Base Camp to Lobuche High Camp

DISTANCE: 1.27km
TIME: 02:08 hrs
AVERAGE SPEED: 0.6kph
ASCENT: 372m
DESCENT: 11m
ALTITUDE: 5,200m
PULSE OX: 93%

I'll thank the Jack Daniel's for the clear head this morning. One of the trekkers was up vomiting with a headache all night. The opposite can be said for me; my stomach has settled and my appetite is back. With a few coffees and bacon and eggs, normality has returned. The sun has also returned to warm us. It's enough to hang out some damp clothes, hope they dry, and get my boots into the sunshine.

Lobuche is an acclimatisation rotation, and Big Tendi tells us we'll soon split into our small group to prepare for the main objective, Mt Everest. We have to split our gear into the essentials to move to High Camp on Lobuche. There's plenty of time, so I drag everything out of the tent and start sorting.

'Just go slow, enjoy this mountain. Time does not matter,' says Big Tendi.

Our tents have been vacated and the pack is ready to go. All that's left to do is farewell Mike as he too heads to Everest Base Camp. From there he'll continue to solely run logistics for all the many variables. Mike has plenty of experience on these mountains, having summited Everest six times himself. While not climbing this year, he has sixty Sherpa across his three waves of clients, and is confident any situation that arises can be accommodated.

From now on, Big Tendi runs the show.

Up the mountain we go again. We soon meet Clayton, who's on the descent from his Lobuche Summit. It's crazy that two people from opposite sides of the world first share a tent in Antarctica and then meet again in Nepal. But here we are.

'You're going to love the views from up there,' he says as we pass on the trail.

Slowly, slowly, we proceed upward. The clouds have moved in, threatening snow. With the breeze, you don't want to stop for too long or a chill will follow. The climb is rather uneventful, but we joke and laugh and keep a light-hearted spirit. I feel a lot better in any case, after yesterday's struggles. My pack has got a bit of weight bearing on my hips; I'm carrying a lot of gear to have at the ready should the weather turn.

Our tent position has been pre-allocated at Lobuche High Camp. The porters have beaten us up here, and our duffels are already at our tents. Despite the weather now closing in, the views from our tent site are sensational. We get out our gear, roll out our mats, and retreat from the icy wind. There's no dining tent here, and the guides want us to eat in our own tents.

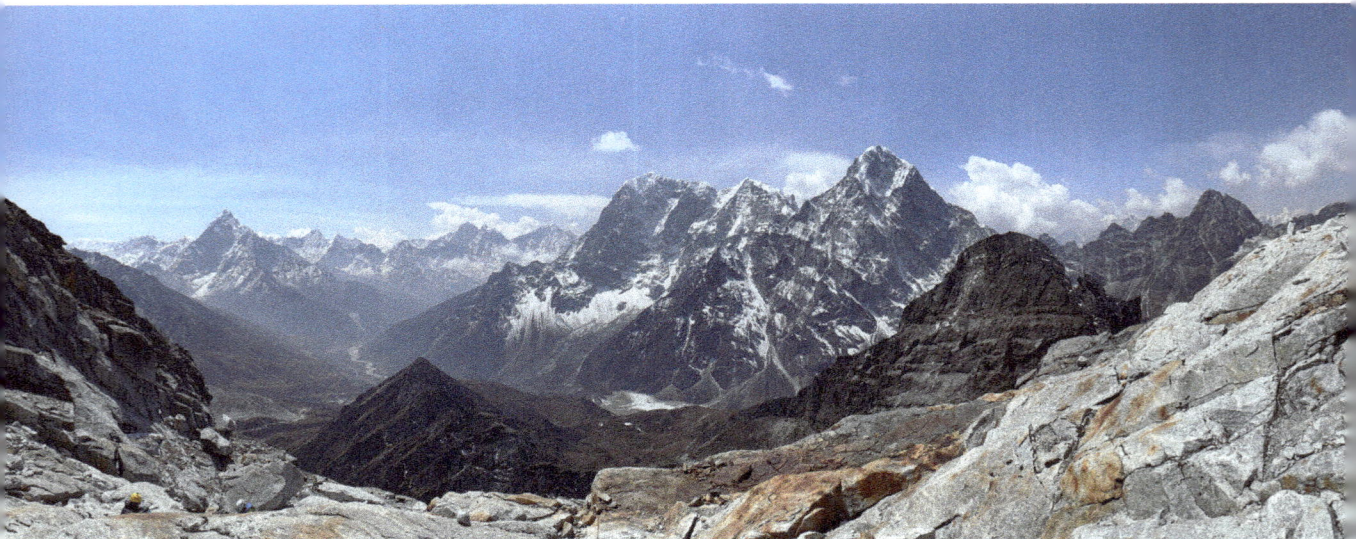

At this rate, I calculate we'll arrive at Everest Base Camp early on 17 April—just in time for my daughter's birthday. I've heard you can purchase wi-fi there. Thoughts of my daughter's coming birthday weigh heavily on me and travelling starts to feel trivial. That I'm not there for her big day feels like some version of homesickness. Missing home doesn't hit me often, but it's part of the experience to occasionally suffer when I'm literally on the other side of the world.

The clouds have descended, visibility is gone, and the mountains are out of view as if they too have gone to rest.

Lobuche High Camp to High High Camp to Lobuche High Camp

The mountains are alive and the sunrise is hitting their slopes against a backdrop of clear blue skies. Everything must be done a little slower, for exertion of any kind threatens shortness of breath. It's a slow start to the day before breakfast.

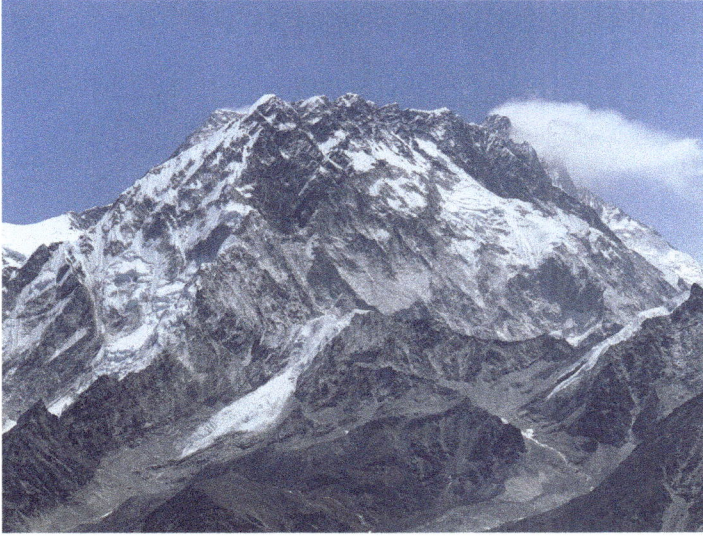

left A sneak peak

opposite The mountains are calling

Ryan and I are teamed up with Tenji for today's trip to High High Camp. As soon as we're advised that we need harnesses and 8,000-metre boots, I figure it's not going to be just another acclimatisation hike.

Once we're underway I discover my suspicions were right. It's actually steep going, and I'd forgotten how miserable these boots can be. It doesn't help that we're using them to rock climb. At first there are some guidelines to grip on the steep sections, then, not long after, Tenji ropes us up.

I wriggle my toes, kick them against unsuspecting rocks, and generally try to keep some circulation happening. Any distraction is welcome.

'Can you see Everest summit there?' Tenji points across the jagged mountains.

Immediately, my attention is focused on the mountain range.

'Is that it there, the far point?'

'Where the plume of snow is . . .'

A plume of sunlit snow streams from the summit of Mt Everest. There it is, the highest point on Earth, right in front of me. Well, in the far distance . . .

The mountain is now solid exposed rock, littered with boulders and with loose scree on the path. A lot of it is weathered and smooth, yet small lips provide perfect foot holds. Wriggling my toes no longer works, and only pain masks the pins and needles sensation. High High Camp is the saviour. Reaching the ice line, enough is enough—my toes are numb from pain. I wriggle them with the boots off, hoping circulation will return. As I slip the boots back on, it's much better. We've been climbing now for two hours.

There's not a lot here at High High Camp, just a couple of scattered tents. It's here we put on our crampons and pull out the ice axe. My crampons have a film of surface rust, ready to be stripped off against the ice ahead. It's been a long time since they were last used in Antarctica. But I lay them out, follow the ritual of setting them up, and tie them on. They fit perfectly.

Tenji leads us through the ice. There's no soft snow to speak of, so we kick our way to traction. It's a bit of fun really. Sit back, bend your knees, relax, and stomp your way around. Tenji finds the most challenging sections for us to practise on. We're actually not climbing any higher, but spend an hour essentially playing follow the leader. Up, down, across and climb up.

The steepest sections require kicking my toes in the vertical ice face and swinging my ice axe into solid ice for a hold to pull up against. We stomp around, take some selfies, all the while sucking big breaths in for our efforts. The ice can be sharp and concentration is always required for the next foot hold. Tenji uses an ice screw to see us safely down the last pitch. I've got every confidence in his mountaineering skills.

Tomorrow we'll pass through here en route to the summit in the near, but far, distance.

Reversing the process, we trek back to the edge of the ice. Off come the crampons and away goes the axe, although the three of us stay roped together for the descent. I'm in the middle, Ryan is leading and Tenji is our anchor man to the rear. The

opposite Finding the ice

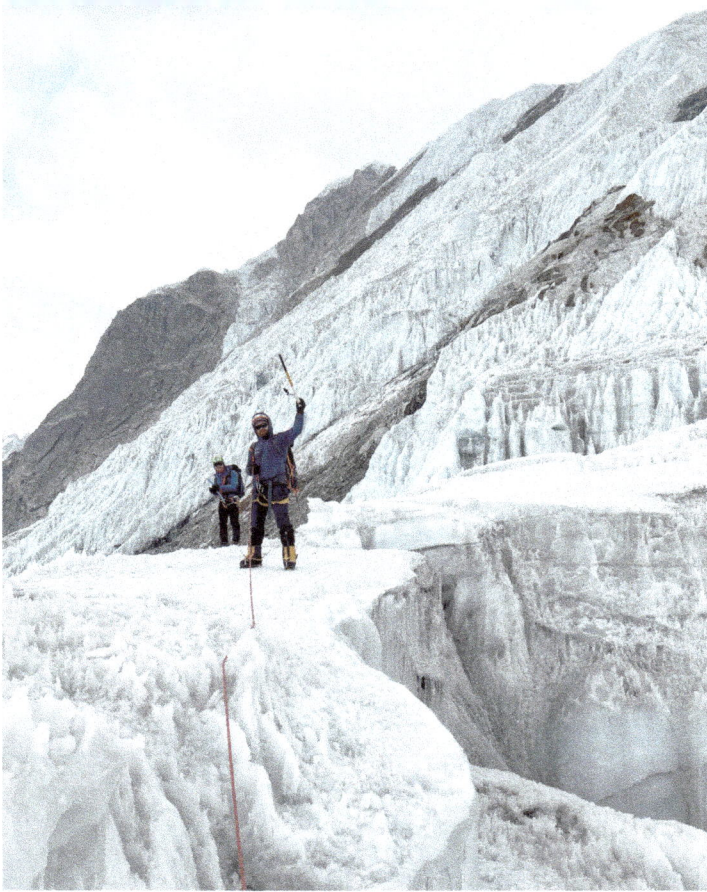

8,000-metre boots aren't ideal for this rocky descent, but my feet are faring a lot better than they were going up this morning.

At High Camp a hot cup of tea is delivered to our tent by the kitchen crew. I sit and cherish this small indulgence. The mountain views are all but gone, and the clouds are slowly settling in. Time to retreat to the comfort of the tent.

Later in the afternoon I emerge from the cosy confines of the tent to sit and write upon a rock overlooking the Khumbu Icefall. Snowflakes float past as I write. I can feel them melt against my warm skin. It's getting colder, and soon the snow starts to stream in. I retreat to the tent as my fingers start to go numb. There's no sunset to speak of, just creeping dark in the gloom.

DISTANCE: 1.65km

TIME: 01:26

AVERAGE SPEED: 1.2kph

ASCENT: 1m

DESCENT: 430m

ALTITUDE: 4,801m

PULSE OX: 92%

Lobuche High Camp to Lobuche Base Camp

It's 4:30am and snowing. We're set to walk in an hour, so the slow process of getting the warm layers of gear on begins. Snow slides down the tent wall, and we need to hit the door a couple of times to move snow so we can get outside. We can see that a lot of snow has fallen overnight, and Ryan and I debate the chances of heading off.

Big Tendi soon arrives with an update: 'Go back to sleep, far too dangerous to climb in this. Breakfast at seven.'

The clouds threaten to clear for sunrise so I venture out, set up the GoPro, then stumble back into the tent and my sleeping bag. Even this small amount of movement has given me a headache, and I have to pass on breakfast. In one way, despite the conditions, I'd rather be going for the summit. I know the smooth rock faces would be extremely slippery. But lying around camp, I'm being overcome by nausea.

The clouds close in and snow continues to fall. The instruction comes to get packed up and descend to Lobuche Base Camp. Packing up, I get a nosebleed for my efforts and an intense headache. It doesn't go unnoticed by the Sherpa that I haven't eaten. Nothing gets past them. One of the crew is vomiting, several more have had headaches. Altitude sickness in its infancy, no doubt.

Getting back to Lobuche Base Camp is a slow slog, and I have a persistent headache and unsettled stomach. It's slippery underfoot and two hiking poles are required. I feel rushed but determined to descend with the rest of the group. One of the guys isn't. Maybe I should be more transparent about how bad I'm feeling, but then again I know this will pass. I'm so fatigued when we get back to camp that I just sit on my bag. Back to that nausea, the silent suffering one does alone. After fetching my bags, I crawl into the tent. No longer bothered by the cold, I get my head down and rest as the snow continues to fall.

We hear news . . . another team went for the summit, only to turn around without success. Further, they got lost on the way down with the inclement weather. At least this puts to rest any doubt about whether we should have attempted a summit push.

Lobuche Base Camp to Everest Base Camp

Despite being able to use satellite phones and wi-fi to call home, one of the most difficult aspects of any expedition is being away from family—the people who accept me for who I am. I recall the enjoyment in their faces, the excitement of small moments, the warmth of an embrace. I can only visualise the laughter and the happiness that I hope continues in my absence. Only with perspective can I see that my children will always have each other—a brother, a sister, a family—long past my time. I rest easier knowing they're nurtured by a loving mum.

Our tent has been blanketed with snow overnight, and the entire camp is a white wonderland. The skies are clear again, and the sun casts long shadows on the surrounding mountains as the new dawn rises. The sun slowly emerges over the hill, promising warmth and bringing life to the mountains. I take a deep breath of crisp mountain air in its purest form and exhale it in a fresh fog.

I feel better, not instantly, but better.

It's time to do it all again . . . pack up our gear and get ready to walk. It'll be nice to unpack one last time at Everest Base Camp and skip this process.

It's only a half-hour hike to Lobuche Village at 4,940 metres, which is approximately 8.5 kilometres southwest of Base Camp. I've put in a request to stop here for a wi-fi call home. It's such a highlight to not only wish my daughter a happy birthday, but also speak with the family. It leaves me on cloud nine, though far behind the main group. No matter; they've left me a guide, Asis, to help me catch up.

Asis sets a solid pace, and I check my heart rate to ensure I'm not pressing too hard. We follow the Khumbu Icefall, only

DISTANCE: 10.74km

TIME: 05:00 hrs

AVERAGE SPEED: 2.2kph

ASCENT: 604m

DESCENT: 160m

ALTITUDE: 5,270m

PULSE OX: 92%

moving to the side for yaks to pass and the incredibly strong porters lugging our bags up the mountain.

Looking up I see the summit of Nubtse (or Nuptse), which lies two kilometres west-south-west of Mt Everest. Nubtse is Tibetan for 'west peak', as it is the western segment of the Lhotse-Nubtse massif. At 7,861 metres, it is big enough to hide Everest from our view. It seems unfathomable that we'll be trying to climb that high. Nubtse's summit is on view for the briefest time before the curtain of cloud hides her away again.

We catch up with the group before we arrive in the small village of Gorak Shep, the last resting spot for most trekkers before the final climb to Base Camp. Everyone looks fatigued. Gorak Shep was the site of the original Base Camp in the 1950s. Later Base Camp was moved closer to the base of the mountain, just below the infamous Khumbu Icefall. We've stopped here for a quick tea at one of the cafes.

'Tenji... Mt Everest whisky, is it safe to drink?' I ask. He doesn't even answer from the counter, just shakes his head and motions his hand sideways. That's a definite no.

Climbing time from Gorak Shep to Everest Base Camp ranges from one-and-a-half to two-and-a-half hours, depending on the weather and the acclimatisation and physical conditioning of each individual, says Tenji. At this altitude, few people feel comfortable and many start to suffer symptoms of altitude sickness or acute mountain sickness.

The scenery walking into Base Camp is like nothing I've seen before. There are crevasses surrounded by unstable rock and ice in unique sculptures, all with a backdrop of blue icefalls. Colourful prayer flags are suspended randomly, and as we get closer we hear water rushing from rocks in the afternoon heat.

Different camps with different languages are signposted and set up on any bit of flat ground available. The CTSS camp is the furthest from the entry, but arguably in the best spot. The Sherpa 'Icefall Doctors'—who each year carve out routes

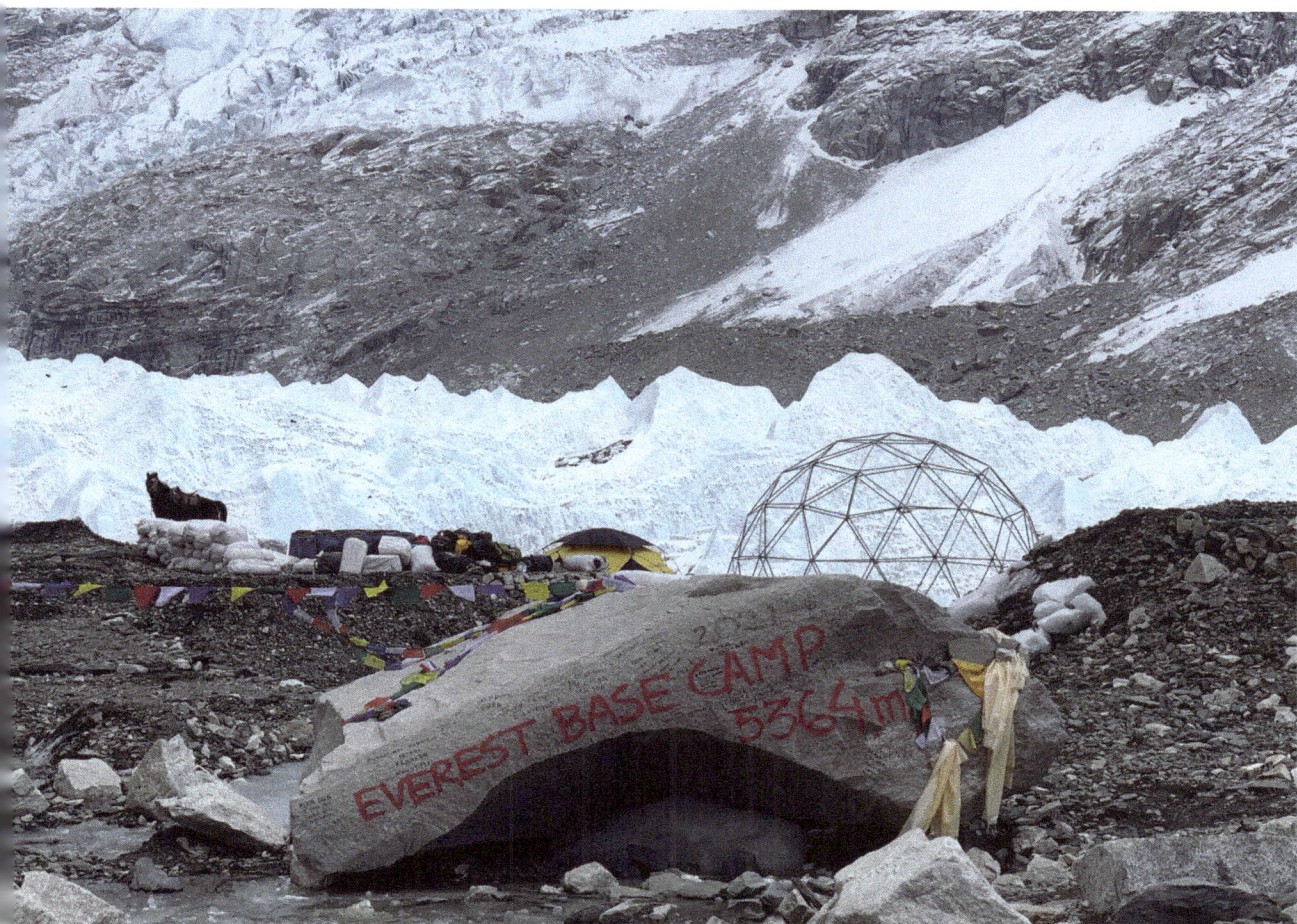

up the Khumbu Icefall, the gateway to the summit—are located just below our camp, and the Everest Base Camp Medical Clinic tent is just above our camp.

We're greeted by staff, then by Mike, outside our allocated dining tent. 'Welcome guys, great to finally have you here.'

Just as we take a seat in the allocated dining tent, an avalanche starts rumbling in the distance. Nubtse, I'm told.

Mike takes us on a tour of camp. It's a huge logistical undertaking they've built here. We start with the executive suites—top of the line, igloo-shaped retreats complete with double bed, single couch, table and chairs. Of course they come with a weighty price tag. They are seriously impressive, and the best on the mountain, I'd suggest.

From there, it's more about the functionality of camp. The heart of any camp, the kitchen, is hectic and employs twenty kitchen staff, who are turning out hot croissants when we pass. Then there's an additional mini city of Sherpa tents, with some sixty Sherpa part of the overall expedition. Solar power is the big investment at Base Camp this year, and panels that track the sun have been installed. No doubt a worthwhile long-term investment.

Next we're shown the crown jewel of camp—the heated 'Everest Big Tent'. This common area is just for hanging out, and comes with couches and two baristas who work the coffee machine. I'll be checking this out properly tomorrow. I feel dirty just standing at the door peering in, and after all the climbing I've done I'm sure the smell would not be welcome in a confined space.

Down behind the Big Tent, on a much lower area, are the people's tents. I get my own tent, which is small, but it's six feet to the centre and outshines my expectations. There's an insulating mat on the ground and a single six-inch mattress, too. More than enough room for me. All my gear fits, but in a disorganised fashion. Priority number one: have a shower!

After my shower I join a briefing in the dining tent led by a guy called Ossy. Some housekeeping matters are raised, we're given weather briefings, and groupings are discussed. Ossy then brings up the current Covid-19 situation.

'There are three confirmed cases in Base Camp,' he says.

It's already here.

Our camp is currently in lockdown, adds Ossy, and they're trying to implement the best policies possible. Cases are spiking in Kathmandu, so they actually prefer to have us here. Two of the confirmed cases from Base Camp are already in Kathmandu, and the last case is due to fly there by helicopter tomorrow. Everyone associated with those three cases is set to be tested. The risks may have been underplayed, but this is the situation we find ourselves in.

We're a closed camp. Nobody is to come in and we're asked not to venture to other camps.

Since speaking with the local doctors during the trek to Base Camp, I've sensed Covid is going to be a problem. To what extent, nobody knows. What Ossy also tells us is that we all accept some risk. He believes the social and economic impact of this climbing season not progressing would be devastating for this community—more devastating than Covid. Nepal is one of the poorest countries in the world. In 2020 the gross national income per capita was 1,155 dollars (Australia's was 53,730 dollars for the same year). Certainly, the economic disparity between this world and the one I come from is almost unfathomable.

I think we're all running close to the wire in our decision to be participants in this Everest attempt. Before a climber can even set foot on the mountain, they must pay for a climbing permit from the government of Nepal. That's 11,000 US dollars. Last count for permits to climb the mountain this season was 330. The government is set to close permits shortly, but the fact that it hasn't already speaks to the accepted risk. Knowing the pandemic has stopped trekking, and effectively siphoned off the country's other streams of tourist income, climbers may represent all that's left.

As I crawl into my sleeping bag, I hear the echo of another avalanche. Risks are everywhere, and always have been.

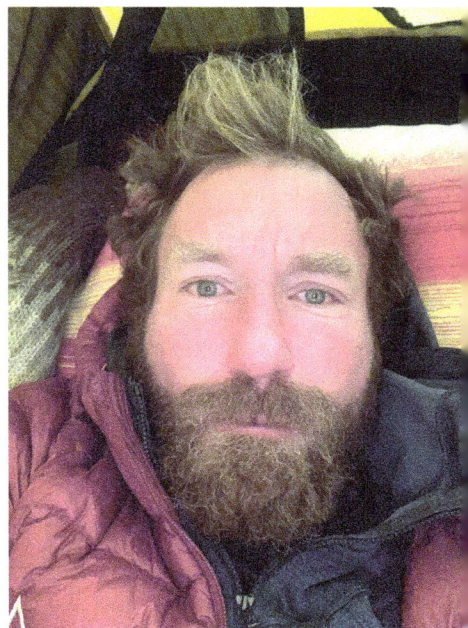

above Just me

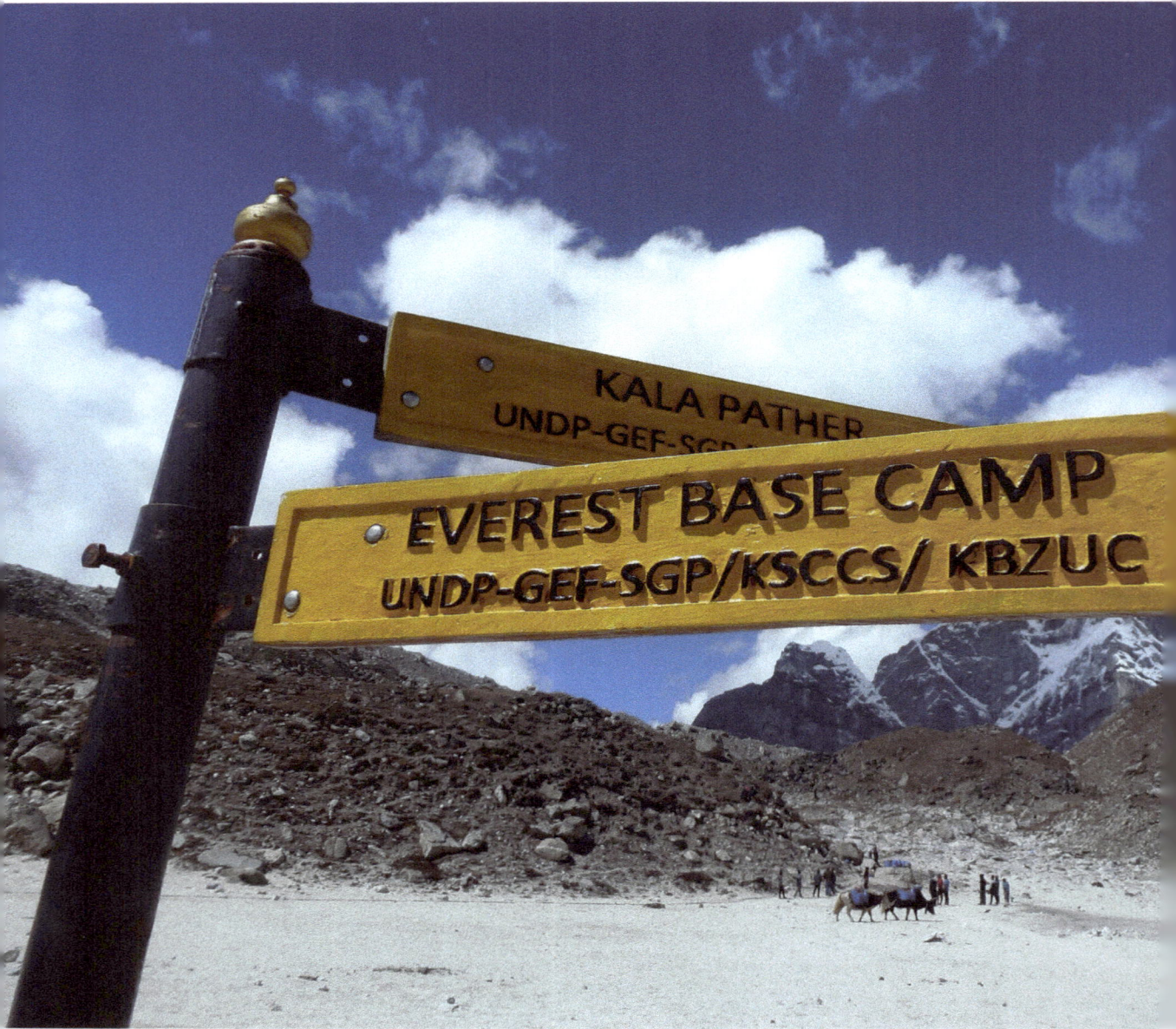

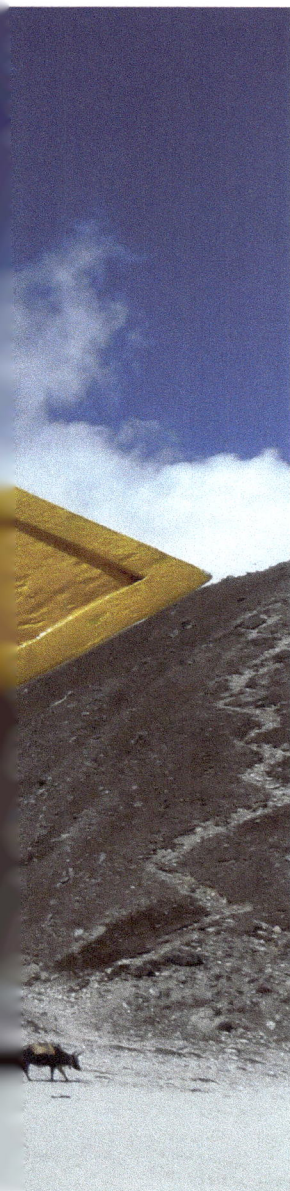

T'S JUST AFTER 5 AM, and I can hear a thunderous avalanche. Two more follow over the next hour. I never thought the presence of avalanches would be so acute. This is an intimidating place.

Today there's the blessing by the high lama—the puja ceremony. Several high lamas travel great distances to Base Camp to bless expeditions before they tackle the upper mountain. After breakfast we see the set-up beginning for what promises to be something special. Unlike the puja inside a monastery, this one is permitted to be filmed and photographed. Everyone can bring their climbing gear to be blessed by the high lama for a safe expedition. I like Ossy's suggestion to bring my boots—to keep walking—and helmet—to keep thinking. I've added my gloves—to keep my fingers!

Buddhists here don't distinguish between religious and non-religious beliefs; this ceremony is simply part of Sherpa culture—it just is, the way it is. It's a progression of prayer, chants and ceremonial processes that goes for hours. As the conclusion nears, prayer flags are rolled out above us with the colourful monument at its centre. Offerings are given, foods are received. At the signal of the high lama, rice is thrown for offerings of safe passage.

PULSE OX: 83%

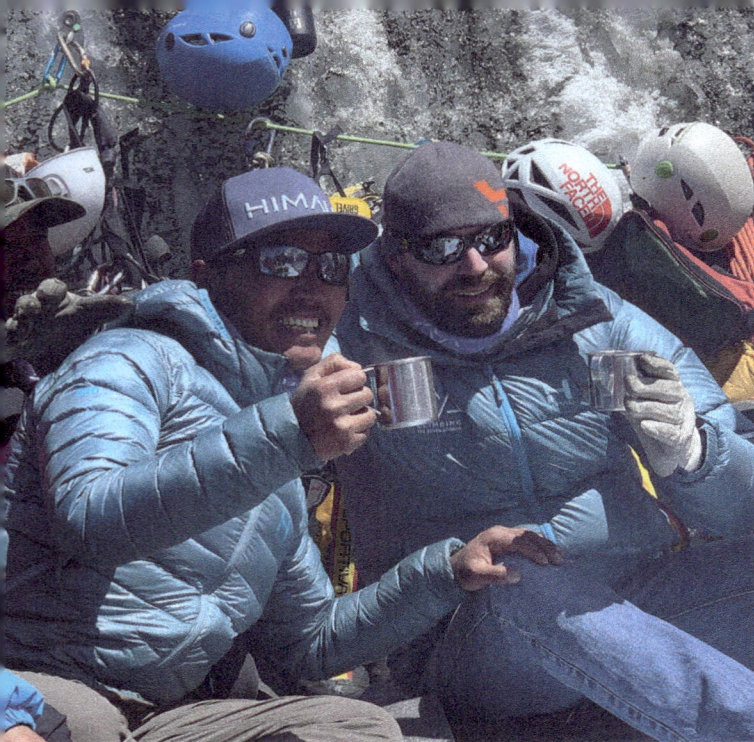

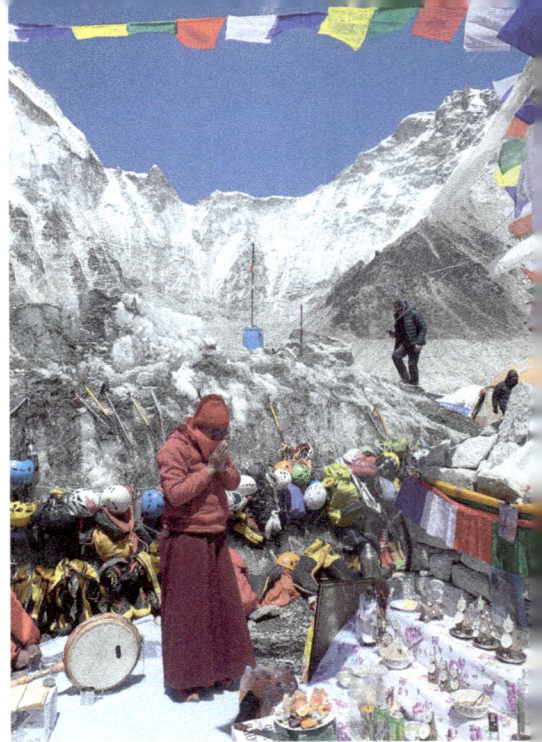

Acclimatisation day

Sneezing, I bring myself to life. The blood boogers I've been blowing out the last two days are just disgusting. One of the nearby tents hosts somebody with a relentless Khumbu cough, which does nothing for my splitting headache as I listen to it through the night. Condensation thawing in my tent promises that the morning sun is near. It's time to be motivated, for we're off on an acclimatisation hike shortly.

Leaving the tent, I see a helicopter headed towards the icefalls with a person dangling below it. Gee, that must be cold. I bump into Clayton, who explains that the ice supporting a bridging ladder crossing has collapsed on both sides. One of their Sherpa has fallen in the crevasse, breaking a leg and losing consciousness. Three people in total are injured. Sherpa later rescued the injured porter and stabilised him ready for helicopter transport. We're advised not to make a big deal about it.

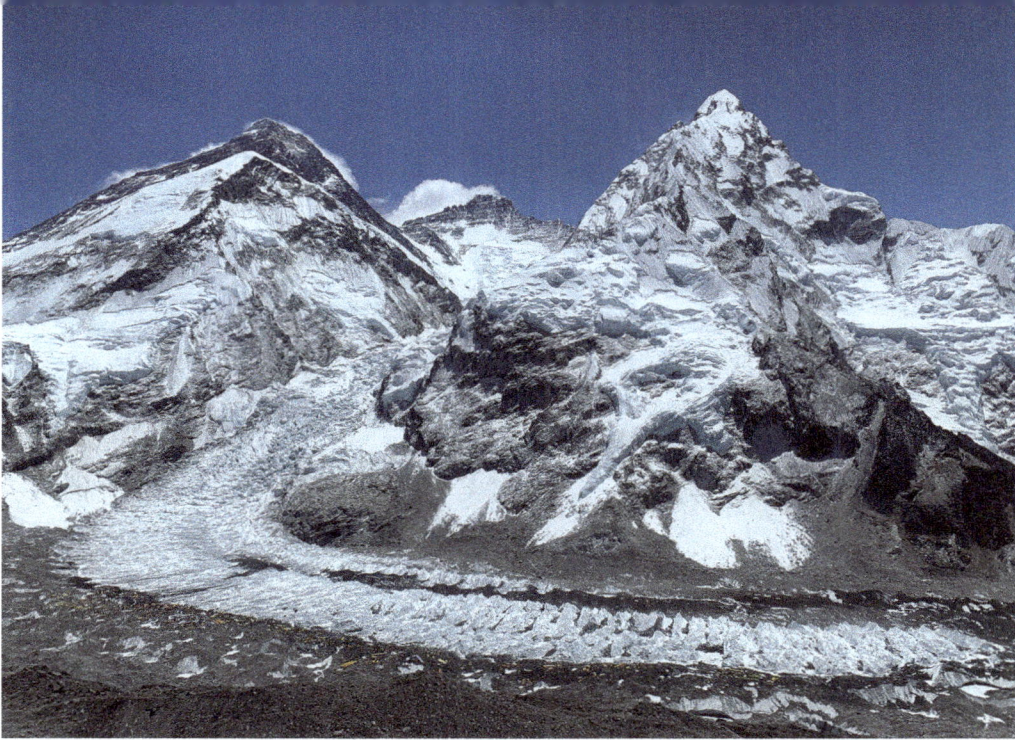

above High above Base Camp

'This is Everest, accidents happen.'

Our focus is to be on the acclimatisation climb. We stop at Pumori High Camp (5,700 metres). From here the whole Khumbu Icefall is in perspective. It's beautiful. Everest has a blue sky as its backdrop. Winds blow white plumes from the summit. Here I sit, looking at the highest point on Earth. In the foreground, yellow and orange dots indicate Base Camp and remind us how small we really are.

Big Tendi shares his thoughts on a summit assault and training plan that minimises our time in the Khumbu Icefall. 'Every second you put yourself in Khumbu Icefall, you're putting your life at risk.'

If we follow the ice doctors up, we can beat the crowds. While others are doing skills training, we'll be scaling nearby ridges, building our lungs and speed. If there's a pace gap, our group will split in two. The idea is to speed through the Icefall faster than others.

Ryan asks Big Tendi's thoughts on summiting without oxygen on the main route. His answer is unequivocal. 'No oxygen is just stupid, it just puts others in danger.'

Everyone needs oxygen to live, and you're just killing brain cells by limiting that need.

'No problem with people doing it, just don't be on the main route.'

The Sherpa and porters are trying to make their livelihoods, and while they welcome all climbers who bring money here, the selfish climber who endangers those around them isn't appreciated.

Training day

It's 20 April 2021. And it's my birthday.

I've risen early to ring home. Leaving my tent I find a calm morning; even the winds are still. It's cold, of course, and the shadows are creeping down the mountain's edge. But the sun will soon be here.

It's quiet in the communal tent. Nobody is around and the cold follows me in. I've made the call home, received my birthday well wishes and spoken with my family, thanking them for the card tucked away among my limited possessions.

Ryan and Mario track me down. They planned to bring me a coffee in the tent to celebrate my special day but settle for giving me a morning hug, which is more of a gang tackle with birthday wishes. We shiver through conversation until the sun finally breaches the mountains' height and filters into the tent, instantly warming us prior to breakfast.

Today we're on an ice obstacle course. Geared up in harness, helmet and big boots, it's time to throw the crampons on and get started. I've never done this much 'ice climbing', but settle into a rhythm as I kick my way higher. It's a long session, and around and around the circuit we go. We also try ladder crossings, which is something I've never done. In the Khumbu

Icefall the ladder is the only way to traverse the various crevasses. I've worked out how my crampons land between rungs, how to take my time, not to rush. We're not far off the ground on this training circuit, and I can only imagine looking into the depths of the crevasses to come. Exertion is easy to come by. The sun is out, we're climbing away, yet I'll be out of breath again if I can't slow down on the vertical climbs. It has been a good session.

The practice is fun, but in the background a huge avalanche brings the reality back.

As a birthday privilege, I've got the first hot shower after a late lunch. It's the small things that I've learnt to appreciate: the warmth of hot water, the steam, a feeling of cleanliness. Dry now, I can try to catch the kids before bedtime. There's no greater gift than their happiness. I miss these simple interactions.

With the kids now turning in for the night, I wander Base Camp in the direction of the exclusive 'executive' tents for a couple of pre-dinner nips. Some of the crew swing by and we settle in for a few stories, laughs and reflections. Dinner is a quiet affair, but Mike, Big Tendi and Tenji all stop by afterwards to turn out the lights and sing 'Happy Birthday'. Big Tendi presents me with a scarf for 'good luck' and his gesture is much appreciated.

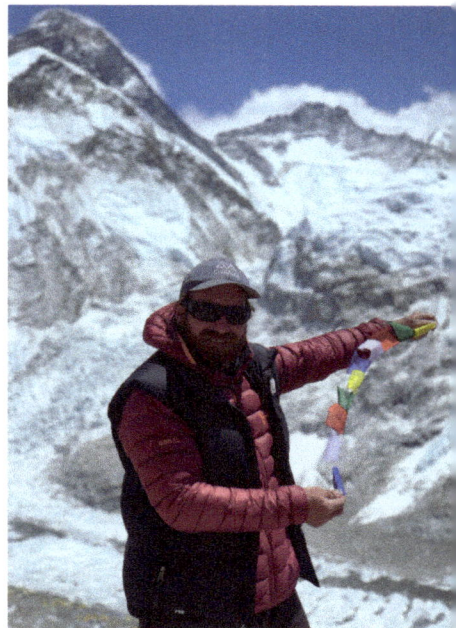

above Taking a moment

Rest day

The weather has turned to a snowstorm. About fifteen centimetres of snow has fallen so far and shows no signs of stopping. Not an ideal day to be in the Khumbu Icefall!

The sounds of avalanches roar in the distance. Some sound close, like thunder cracking above. I wonder how close they really are. There must be some lightning present too, such is the roar. Snow is continuing to fall and I don't think anyone will be moving far today. Crack! That one was definitely lightning.

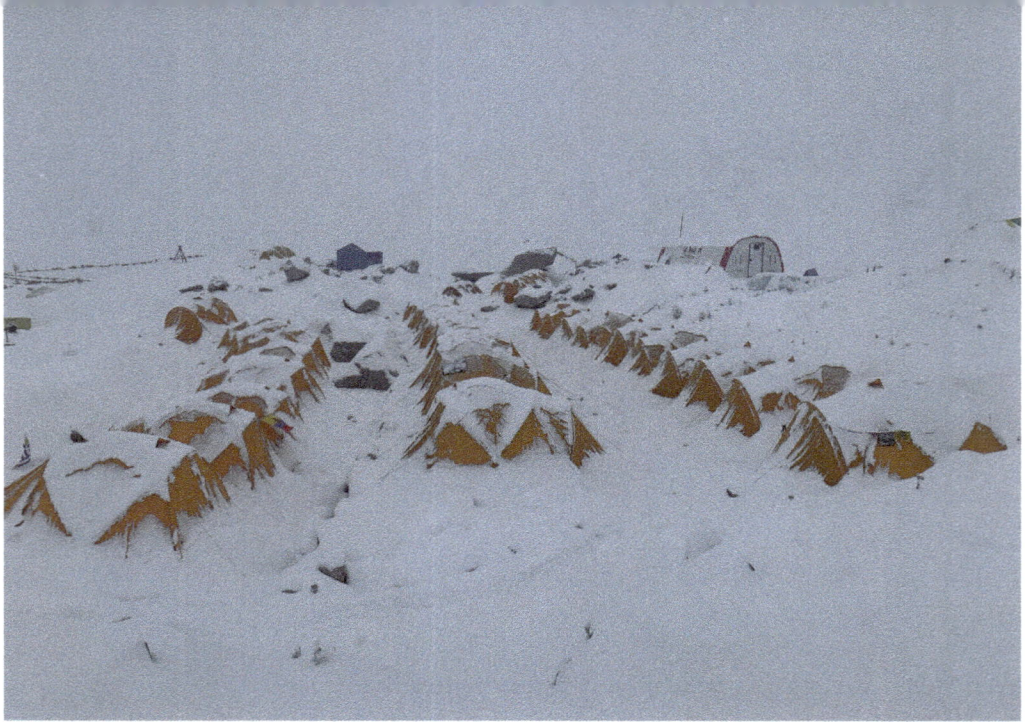

above Climbers camp

It remains cold, really cold.

With a constant dry throat, the famed Khumbu cough threatens to annoy me. Avoiding gastrointestinal distress in this often unhygienic environment is another constant challenge.

A presentation on oxygen systems for the summit push is underway in the common tent. Big Tendi and Tenji run through the gear checks and provide valuable insight on avoiding damage to the regulators and hoses that provide the all-important oxygen. Many tips and tricks cover everything from how to go to the toilet to where snacks go, how to stay warm and, most importantly, how not to freeze the masks. With their depth of accumulated wisdom, endless energy and practical know-how, these two Sherpa hold everyone's attention effortlessly.

Essentially I have been allocated eight bottles of oxygen. Ryan has opted for an additional three bottles as insurance. Individually all the items function well. But when you put oxygen mask, goggles, hat, helmet and down suit all together it's a little suffocating. Communication becomes difficult, visibility is restricted and breathing is laboured. But we turn it into a light-hearted session. There's even a little music and horse-play for the conclusion. Which helps us stay warm.

Ossy, who typically has been providing the briefings lately, has gone down with a fever. So Big Tendi delivers our briefing. Tomorrow we're to go halfway into the Icefall and become familiar with the conditions and route.

And a potential weather window for a summit attempt is opening.

Khumbu Icefall

DISTANCE: 3.14km

TIME: 03:55 hrs

AVERAGE SPEED: 0.8kph

ASCENT: 278m

DESCENT: 291m

PULSE OX: 83%

To acclimatise I'm typically drinking five to six litres of water per day. The consequences are obvious. Overnight, it's common practice to use a 'pee bottle', which reduces the need to venture outside to the amenities. On this occasion, discomfort and a mild dose of panic arrive when I discover my pee bottle is frozen shut. Banging it a couple of times in vain, I find myself out of time. The nearest boots are thrown on. It would have been a comic spectacle to witness me emerge and proceed to run past the tents in my long johns. Yes, it was freezing, but worth the eventual relief.

I notice we have clear skies just prior to sunrise, casting long continuous shadows across the ranges. I should go back to the warmth of my sleeping bag, but decide on getting properly dressed in anticipation of a magnificent sunrise. And I pick the perfect spot to capture this new day. I feel the first rays of warmth shining through as the sun rises over the summit of Everest. Despite freezing fingers, it's worth taking out my phone camera. The view is just spectacular. In fact I can't pull myself away even to enjoy the comforts of my tent, and instead watch the sun fully emerge well above the horizon.

I'm watching the sun rise over Mt Everest!

Then, disaster strikes—I've lost my iPhone. Before raising the alarm, I run back to my tent and throw my few worldly possessions everywhere. No phone. I scour the snow along the paths I've walked, but if it's fallen out of a pocket into the snow, chances aren't great it'll easily be seen.

Big Tendi is waiting to depart. 'C'mon, it's time to go!'

'I can't, I've lost my phone.'

I re-check my backpack, pockets and scratch around in the snow. Nothing—panic sets in.

When was the moment that this bond with an electronic device became more important than the adventure and discovery of a majestic place like the one immediately in front of me? But it's not until I'm presented with this reality that I realise how much is missing. My contacts, photos, notes and all the documents for travel abroad are stored on that device. Not to mention the connection it provides to family, business and all one's collected affairs.

It has got to be back in the tent.

The group leaves. I tear my small living quarters apart—again.

'David, David, come here!' Big Tendi bellows from afar.

I emerge from the tent. He has my phone.

Composing myself, I close the tent up and head in his direction as he walks off. Big Tendi hands me some rice as I catch up to him where the puja was held.

'This is for safe travel through the Icefall.'

I follow his lead, and throw the rice onto the monument. He hands me my phone. The phone had fallen out when I went to the toilet, but hadn't fallen *in* the toilet—thankfully. One of the ER workers had simply picked it up.

All seems well in the world again.

Walking slowly away, following in Big Tendi's steps, I contemplate how this incident is viewed by the Sherpa—how I came to have such an attachment.

'Now we can get back on track, no rush.'

It doesn't take long to catch up to the others led by Tenji. Into line we fall, wading our way through fresh, fluffy snow. We're all harnessed up and soon linked onto the fixed lines. Surveying the terrain, it's anything but flat, with either hard ice or soft snow underfoot. Vertical climbs have well-indented footholds from previous traffic, making ascending just a little easier.

With crampons fixed to my big 8,000-metre boots, they're starting to feel like an extension of my feet. Something's changed and I no longer dread their assistance. With the sharp metal points on the crampons, I really can venture anywhere.

The mantra of always being clipped on is now easily grasped as we bypass skinny ridges and wide crevasses. Staring down these huge cracks shows both the magnificent colours of blue as they darken with the depth, and also how fragile this environment is. Whole masses of ice, just existing in unique form, are created by the environment around them as the glacier moves.

In stark contrast to the previous days, the sun is out. With it the glare from the pure white surface penetrates everything. Huge sections of ice splinter into masses of tottering blocks called seracs, which can move and even fall over. They can look stable—some are as big as buildings—but they're not.

I've had good energy so far today, despite an aerobic work-out to our turning point. 'Good to see you're out of breath for a change,' offers Ryan, who is immediately behind me.

Descending is easier, faster and comes with a good dose of laughter. Mostly we hand-rappel down, always clipped in, but there are a few abseiling sections to navigate. Our Sherpa have us executing with a figure eight and self-belay—devices that create friction on the rope and allow us to control our speed.

April slips, lands like a starfish, and slowly circles down an embankment until kicking her boots in to stop. It looks hilarious, but the laughter won't come out. It takes my breath away. All I can do is gasp, which produces pains in my chest. It would have been great to film it. Luckily April is fine and sees the funny side.

Not too much further along, Ryan has difficulty managing his equipment and controlling his speed on one particular ledge. As he fumbles along, I chime in, 'Would you like some commentary?'

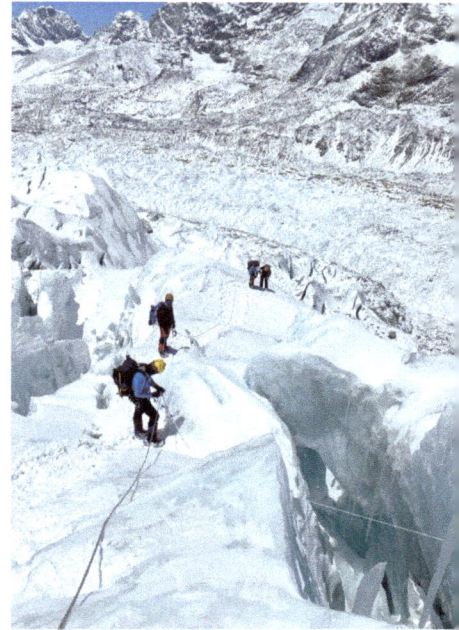

above Bottom of the Khumbu Icefall

'David, it is not appreciated at this exact moment.'

'I think that's his serious tone,' suggests April.

I'm having fun, but hopefully not at anyone's expense. It's always good to laugh at ourselves, and some of these situations can seem funny.

Down we come. And as soon as we finish the final abseil, something changes. I wouldn't say it was fatigue. It feels more like nausea accompanied by the re-emergence of the morning's headache. Focus on breathing. Find some rhythm. Why do I feel I could be sick? My muscles are fine, the body feels healthy, yet my head feels like it's under pressure. All I can do is descend back to camp and try to ignore the discomfort. Looking into the distance, I calculate I'll only have to tolerate this for half an hour. So, to not throw up for a halfa is my goal. Bending down to remove my crampons produces dizziness. Not too far now. I walk at the front behind Tenji, silent.

My tent's calling. I try not to think of bigger days ahead, of how I feel so miserable at the end of a relatively short day. What's wrong with me? Hiding my exhaustion, I head straight to the tents on arrival. My tent is hot, but I'm here. Slowly, I get my boots off. My harness comes off, then my climbing pants. I try some fluids. I feel like shit. Down I lie, for I know this will pass.

I doze off for half an hour. Waking, I feel groggy but know I should rise and get some fluids, and ideally get some food down. I sit up and feel even worse, but I'm determined to visit the dining tent. Shake it off. Could it be a little sunstroke? My eyes are stinging and watery.

The dining tent is half full, and I'm greeted at the entrance by Ryan.

'Bad news, mate. Three confirmed Covid cases. One of them is Clayton.'

It's news that no-one wants to hear.

I take a seat inside in time for Casey, one of the Western guides, to brief us. We're advised to wear masks and practise social distancing. Sitting in a packed dining tent, side by side with kitchen staff not wearing masks, creates mixed messages. Most people have a cough, a sneeze or some combination of cold symptoms, caused by just being on the mountain. Some, like Ossy, are still absent with a fever. Maybe it's a good idea if we all go to our tents for the afternoon and wait for more information.

The mood is low, speculation high. Given the day I've had, I'm worried about my own health.

We're told there are not enough tests available, but they're exactly what's required—everyone should be tested. The kitchen hands are supplied with masks, which they diligently wear under their chins.

Later we return for an update by Mike—our dining tent has returned three positive cases, including Ossy. There are now seven cases in total, and, yes, we've been exposed. CTSS is trying to get as many tests as possible up to Base Camp by helicopter. We're still dining together as the news is delivered, and it seems the horse has bolted.

We're told the new policy is that everyone who returns a positive result is to fly to Kathmandu. It'll be either to an out-of-town hotel, or to the hospital, with details still to be provided.

'It's early in the season, don't feel down, we'll get through this and do some climbing,' Mike offers.

It's been a big day and I'd like to rest as much as possible. Hopefully, I can start tomorrow energetically, in good health, and with a positive attitude.

Pumori High Camp

Our dining tent is half empty. The jokes about every cough, every sneeze are running thin. Our Covid tests should arrive today, which will no doubt divide the camp.

I'm happy to be hiking, and hopefully avoiding part of the circus. All rotations are on hold temporarily, which is responsible. We'll again be heading to Pumori High Camp at 5,666

DISTANCE: 4.65km

TIME: 05:17 hrs

AVERAGE SPEED: 0.9kph

ASCENT: 456m

DESCENT: 500m

ALTITUDE: 5,666m

PULSE OX: 82%

metres, which is fine. Keeps us fit and acclimatised. Nobody has been up there since the storms passed, so we'll also be breaking new trail. Looking up, I see that it's all white. The trek through snow-covered rock is going to be different from our last dry hike, which was mostly exposed rock.

The single-file track for our exit is frozen ice. Not slushy ice, but rock solid, hard blue ice. It takes two hiking sticks to stay upright, but that doesn't prevent a series of near slips, each one threatening to end in a hard fall. Where possible we walk in snow at the edge of the ice. The other worthwhile tactic is placing our feet on any bit of rock penetrating the ice, however small, for some grip. There's no way to admire the view; full concentration is required on every step just to stay upright. Mis-steps remind us how slick this ice really is.

When we reach High Camp, everything looks different. The view is enhanced by the white landscapes. Instead of setting up on large rocks away from the few tents, we stay close to them and use their makeshift rock walls as wind breaks. I notice prayer flags, relentlessly flapping, strung across a dramatic drop on the other side of camp.

There's no escaping the current situation, and the potential consequences play over in my thoughts. It's almost certain that a super spreader event is underway. I wonder how Nepal's Ministry of Tourism can continue to issue new climbing permits—the tally for Everest is currently 394. Considering that a lot of professional outfitters aren't on the mountain at all this year, there's speculation that less-experienced operations are taking advantage. This could mean less-experienced climbers too.

I arrive back at Base Camp in good time with Ryan and our guide to find that the elusive Covid-19 tests haven't arrived. But there's a little water in the barrel that feeds the communal shower. I haven't showered for days, so while everyone is still out I take advantage.

Positive

It's 25 April—Anzac Day. The sacrifices of those who have gone before us are not forgotten, even up here at Everest Base Camp.

'Lest we forget.'

Testing began this morning after the RAT kits landed with the first helicopter. Test positive, and down you go to Kathmandu Hospital. Test negative, and you pack your bags and leave for Camp 1 tonight. After breakfast we wait around to hear our fate, spit-balling the probabilities.

I heard the last wave of climbers leave in the middle of the night, untested. I'm torn trying to decide if they're lucky or if bad news awaits their return. Morally, everyone should be tested. There's a social responsibility not to spread the virus. The Sherpa are yet to be tested and seem unfazed by the process. As a climber, I just want to go up. Climbers climb. I'd prefer to skip this process.

The potential consequences of the test bend my mind. It seems absurd that a simple test like this will determine whether I can undertake the challenge I'm trying to complete up on this hill. Losing the ability to meet an expectation I have placed on myself could be imminent. Dread rushes in, as denial becomes hard to hold on to and thoughts of an undesired outcome consume me. Rapid antigen tests (RATs) take fifteen minutes to produce a result—and determine our fate. Pacing around camp after being tested, it feels like the longest fifteen minutes of my life.

A volunteer, in the nicest possible way, swiftly brings the crushing news.

'David Morgan—positive. Sorry.'

I've got Covid-19 ... I'll be on the helicopter out today. Ryan and April are negative and will proceed without us. Big Tendi and Tenji are also negative.

This is the way it is.

Some story, huh?

'He can't leave our team, he's our strongest climber. We need him,' offers April. But it's no use.

I'm shattered in every sense. I've felt okay the last two days, but that worrying question mark has remained—and now I know.

My chest feels tight, not for the virus, but for the disappointment. How dare this disease single me out! Why did this have to happen to me, now, when I'm so far into the challenge? What will I tell my family? Finlay?

Trudging back to my tent feels like a walk of shame. I'd always wanted the Seven Summits challenge to be about diabetes awareness and adventure. Slowly the narrative has become about Covid, the one thing I didn't want. I wanted to take the chance to finish the challenge while it was still there. It had become about more than mountains. It was changing my life and how I see the world.

As I look around this mountain range, I'm moved by the thought of how far I've come, yet frustrated that I can't complete the challenge.

In the coming days I will have plenty of time to imagine how Fin must view her unwanted diabetes diagnosis. But now it's time to pack up my belongings, expectations, hopes, ambitions and dreams. I don't even have a lot to take. My life here is all about climbing, all about Mt Everest. I relocate to a newly created isolation tent. The mood is depressing, to say the least. Now, despite my best efforts to stay positive, I feel something new for the first time—defeat. Slouched in my chair, trying to process the reality, emotions threaten to boil over.

Everything is on hold.

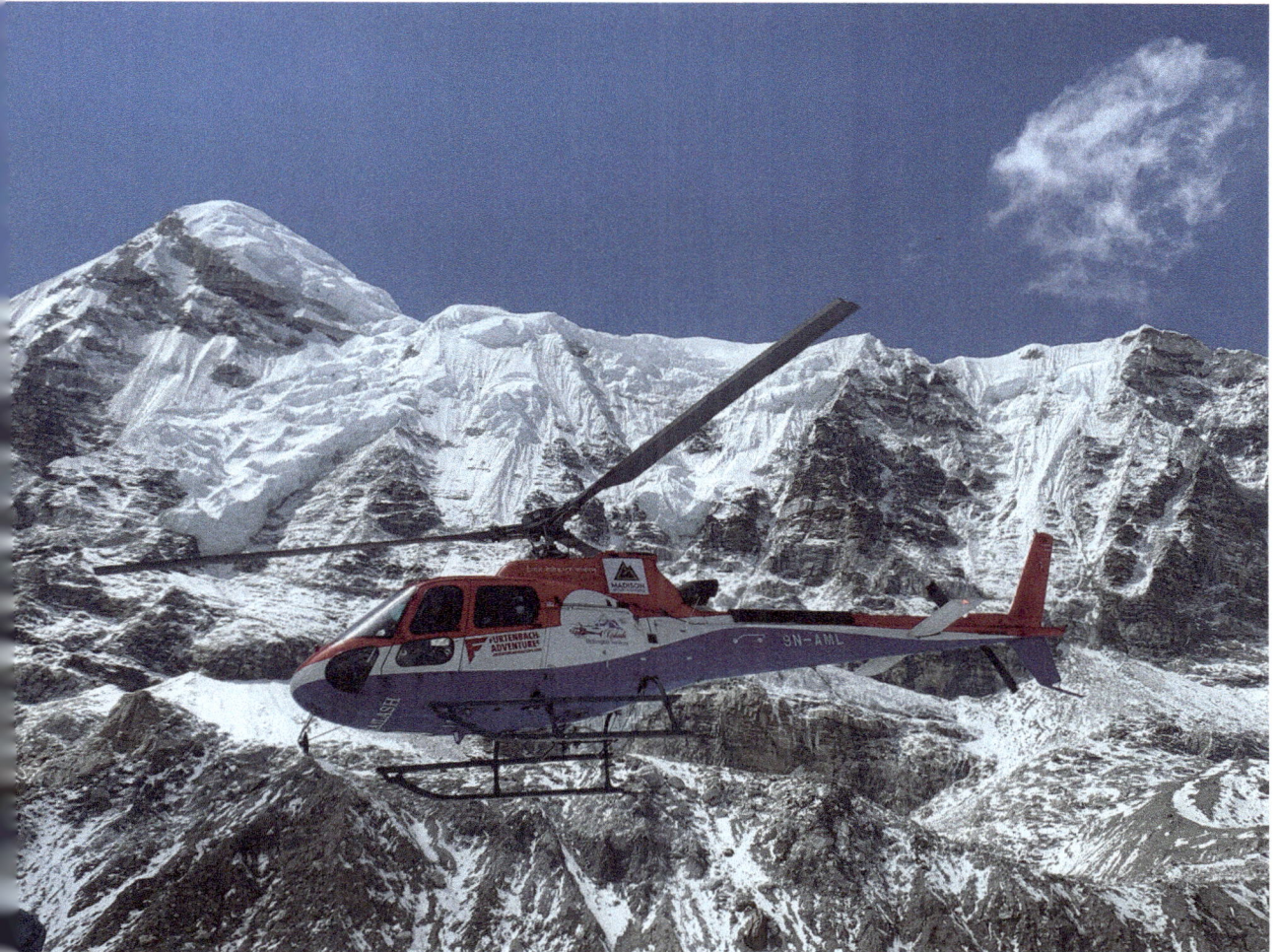

above Departing

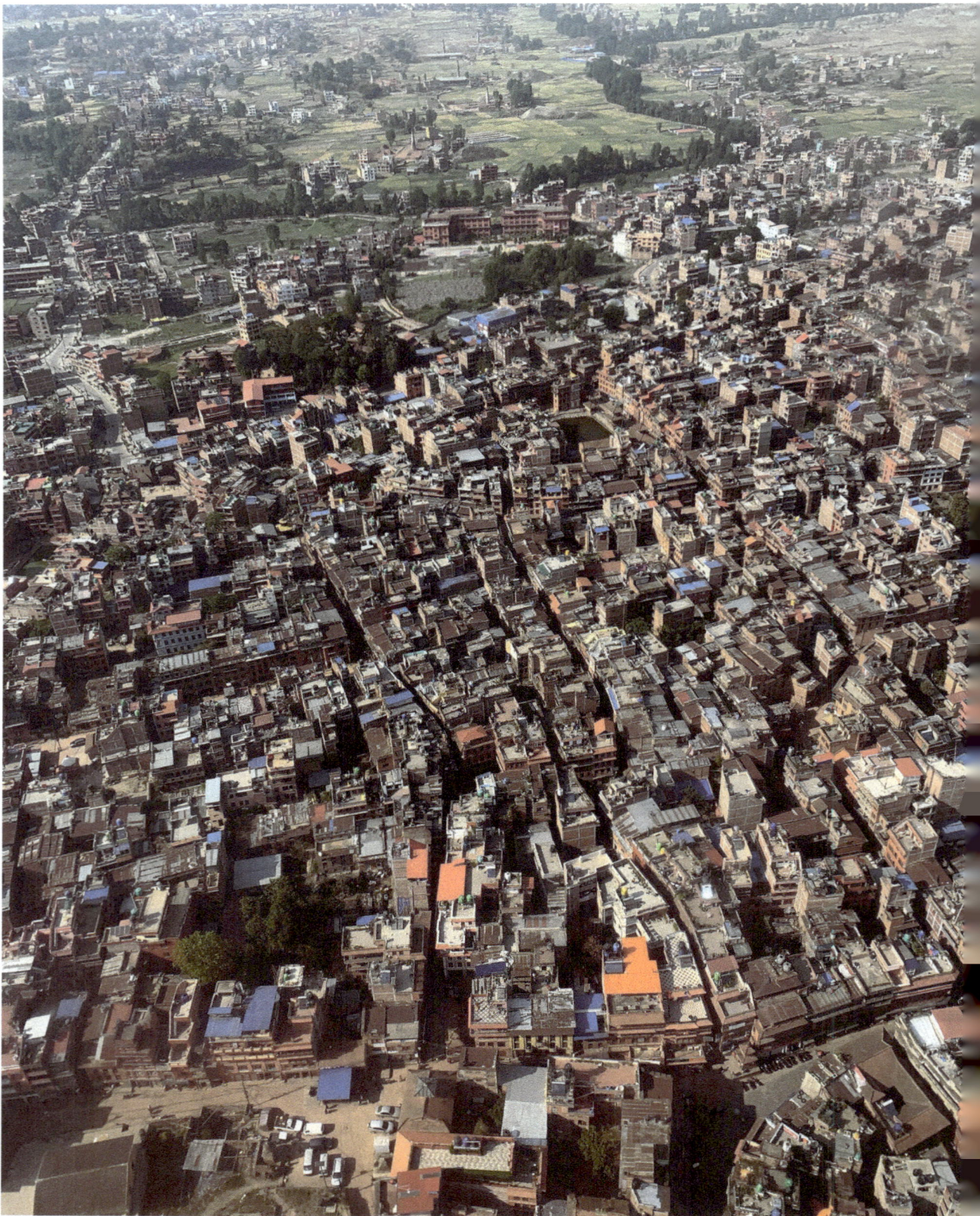

opposite Back to Kathmandu

WAKING IN a bed, warm, feels strange. Stranger still to walk into the ensuite and sit on the toilet, comfortable, for as long as required. I'm back in Kathmandu. Hotel Moonlight is our de facto quarantine hotel, where my mountaineering pursuits have landed me. I listen to the sounds of a city coming to life. Quiet, tranquil sunrises in the mountains couldn't be further from this metropolitan buzz.

What to do?

I can start by cleaning myself up a little. Sunkissed, red, hairy and tired, I look like I've just been dragged from the hills. Oh wait, I have. I apply hot water, scissors and soap. I'm not sure how the result looks, but I feel better. Next, two cappuccinos to start the day, and I'm awake.

Time to phone home. Heidi answers my call and offers assurances that it'll all be okay. Often the voice of reason in my life, she tells me to take it one day at a time and is more concerned about my health than some mountain summit. Hearing the small details of what's happening in my family's lives distracts me momentarily from the disappointment of my current situation.

I read up on the 'latest' reports from the Mt Everest climbing season. None of the articles reflect the reality of the current Covid outbreaks. I also hear that Ryan and April, the last two members of our climbing team, have headed to Camp 1 as a 'first rotation' in preparation for summiting Everest when weather permits.

Lou, one of the Three Peaks climbers, has turned up here at the hotel. He's also positive and is trying to get a negative PCR so he can fly out. That takes the numbers of positive cases from CTSS to thirteen, or about a third of that contingent.

Soon the highlight of the day arrives—it's time to get my brains poked at with another Covid test. Swacon International Hospital has set up testing on the third-floor lobby.

'Have you any symptoms?' our CTSS representative asks.

'No, nothing, never have . . .'

I'm not sure who I'm trying to convince. I'm healthy enough not to be in hospital, but 'nothing' is a stretch. Without the altitude, outside distractions, and exhaustion and fatigue-creating activities to blame, the fact is I can tell I'm not well. Common coronavirus symptoms bear a close resemblance to those of altitude sickness, but I'm no longer at altitude. I don't wish to share this, but I know I'm not going back to the mountains just yet.

The test costs twenty dollars. Results will be in this afternoon.

I'm full of energy, but there's real pressure on my chest and I puff out of breath taking the stairs. To be sure, I take the stairs again, and again, conducting some sort of self-examination. I feel pathetic. I should be climbing the world's highest mountain, not a hotel stairwell.

Hours pass. I can't take the waiting any longer and message the new 'handler'—Gobinda. 'Hi, if you get a moment can you please advise result?'

'It is positive results. So now the option is to wait for few days more.'

More waiting . . .

What is there to say? What can one do? Just wait.

Uncertain personal health dictating extreme outcomes is new territory. It's hard to navigate, let alone accept. I think we were all living in hope of different news. News that would allow us to plan for our return. Maybe the first tests were wrong?

Take me back to the mountains!

But all I can do is take myself back to my room, frustrated, and be alone with my thoughts. Settle in, this could be a long, boring yarn.

Testing positive for Covid prevents my departure to anywhere. There's literally nowhere to go. Except the hotel rooftop where, over a cappuccino, new conspiracy theories are already starting to whirl. Mario, also here and also positive, expresses the disappointment I feel while airing his frustrations.

Given this miserable state of affairs, it's hard to see something positive developing in the background—friendship. Mountain climbing connects us, even in the most unpredictable of circumstances. We're under no obligation to be the person we were yesterday. Here we are, present in this experience, which will surely define us somehow.

Grievances are freely shared about all the promises that were broken. What did they expect to happen when people mixed in confined tents, including sick and newly arrived climbers? And what about the hotel? Have all the staff here been briefed on their infected guests?

'My dream, two years, for this...' Then a silent climber stares at the ground.

I cling to the hope of climbing again, and for a negative Covid test.

We call Mario, the Croatian celebrity. He and I are from completely different cultures and came here for very different reasons, yet we share many similarities. This isolation has allowed us to learn of our mutual desire to continue, that our willingness to suffer isn't as rare as we might think. We're just a couple of adventure enthusiasts trying to make our way in the world, talking it through over one coffee at a time.

Overnight, Mike has emailed some further requirements that must be met before we can return:

1 You must be ten days from initial onset of symptoms.

2 You must have a negative Covid PCR test.

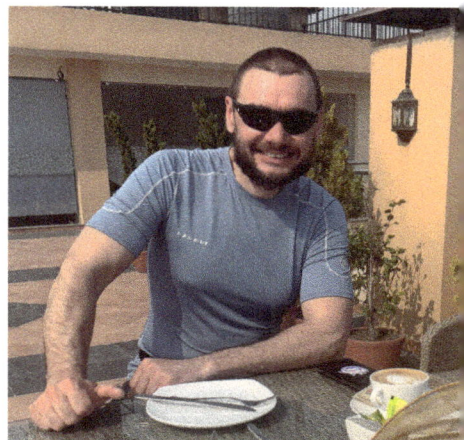
above Mario

3   You must be asymptomatic and without fever for at least forty-eight hours without use of meds like Tylenol or Motrin.

Furthermore, we require you to get checked out by a local physician and will help you arrange this. They must sign off on paperwork that you have:

opposite Day's done...

1   Normal vital signs

2   A clear EKG and proper heart function

3   A clear chest X-ray

4   They feel you are fit to climb at high altitude.

It seems a lot, but reasonable in the situation. My hope lives on.

If only they'd been testing at Base Camp earlier, this virus may not have infected so many. But reality is here and now, and there's no point becoming negative and playing the blame game. It is what it is.

'This too shall pass,' somebody once said.

I've emailed Mike with my own concerns on how long viral shedding can last. I understand they have 'consultants' to help navigate this difficult situation and seek some clarification if a negative PCR test isn't forthcoming. Will considerations be made to isolate at Base Camp, instead of Kathmandu, after a period with no symptoms? I think it's a reasonable enquiry, given that we don't know exactly when we were infected.

The sun is setting on my first day back in Kathmandu, with me as its witness. It fades behind the same mountains as yesterday and the night before.

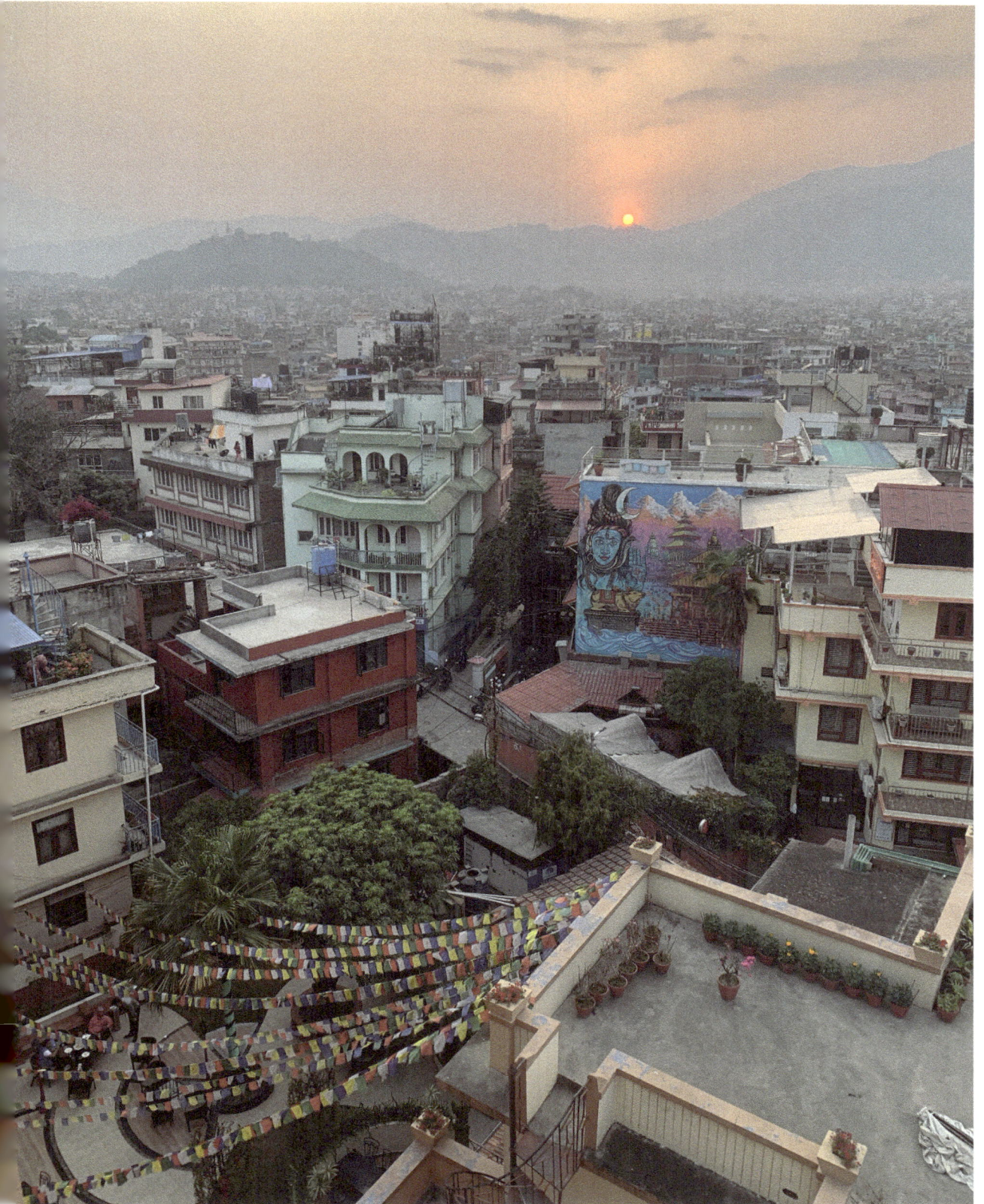

Day 2

The good news begins to filter in. Taylor has received her negative PCR test and can fly out tonight. Then Lou messaged from the airport to say he has also received a negative PCR test today and is on his way home. I run into Nicholas in the hall, who tells me his PCR test is negative. He's moving to the Marriott Hotel. He adds that he threatened to get a private test, and believes this is why his is negative. The CTSS guide who came down has also received a negative test and headed back to Base Camp today, we're told.

All tests are negative, on the same day, after recent positive tests. Coincidence?

I'm uncertain now. How are my circumstances different from these guys? It's not like I was running around licking door handles or sharing different germs with random strangers. Nicholas and Lou are from my dining tent! There's concern about missing a summit window that's opening on the mountain, should we even be able to get back. The weather seems it's going to take a turn and we might already be on the wrong side of it. I can only request, through Gobinda, to be tested again and hopefully receive my results the same day.

Day 3

One of the climbers has been transferred to Norvic International Hospital overnight. Unable to breathe properly, he has been admitted and has sought help from the Thai embassy. Those well enough to be out of bed gravitate to the roof to share and process the limited information.

Seven Summit Treks has the contract for line-fixing above the Icefall this year. Someone from the company texts Ossy: 'Everyone is sick. The Sherpa, the cook hands, the clients.' Yet they have nowhere near enough RAT kits for everyone.

We discuss the predicament of being in Kathmandu. The general consensus is that if we are past the infectious period (ten days) and we feel capable, it should be our decision to return. This is what the current global health information supports.

Many other infected climbers and workers may indeed still be at Base Camp. Without sufficient testing, it's impossible to know how many people have been infected. Because everybody lives in close proximity at Base Camp—sharing tents and other facilities—it's assumed that the virus is spreading rapidly and that operators have serious health issues among their people. Ironically, the types of sickness that have always been common on mountains can be similar to Covid symptoms.

Another problem is that nobody is being open about the situation. Alan Arnette, while not on the mountain, is a respected mountaineer who runs a blog on all things Everest, and is reportedly trying to break any news on the current situation. He is exhausting every contact trying to find somebody to speak out. Nobody does, and relationships are tested.

If not enough people are tested up there, it stands to reason there will be either a low success rate or high death toll—a result nobody wants. Some outfitters are reported as advising that a positive Covid test means your attempt at climbing Everest is done. This in itself would change a lot of clients' self-diagnosis. Or their willingness to take a test—if one is available.

There's still hope for a summit bid for us—I think.

Gobinda has scheduled a trip to the hospital for those in need of medicine, examinations and testing. It's great to get out of the hotel. Kathmandu is going into lockdown tomorrow due to the increasing Covid cases, which is reflected in the organised chaos in the streets. Roads will be shut for a week to all private and public cars. People are to stay home, or they 'will be punished'. Travel for medical reasons and to purchase limited groceries is exempt. This is being called Nepal's second wave and is now clearly visible in a graph of active cases, from a low of 550 on 21 February to nearly 20,000 by 26 April. How things change in two months.

'Both the government and the public ignored all the warning signs, the government did not respond in time, and the people got complacent and gathered in crowds without masks,' explains Sher Bahadur Pun, a virologist. 'We are already experiencing what we did during the peak last year. It is anyone's guess what will happen in the next few weeks, but one thing is for sure: it will get much worse.'

Our van pulls up at Swacon International Hospital after hours, and we are not that impressed. Every procedure is old school. First they photocopy your passport and create a hand-written 'patient card' on paper. Although staff are certainly prepared, and wear head-to-toe protection suits, glasses, shields and masks. To save coming back, I may as well request my examination while we're here. Permission is granted.

First stop: the famed PCR test, plus a rapid antigen test for good measure. It looks like the administrator is the same guy who previously visited the hotel. Full pink gown and gloves, plus booties on the feet. From behind his shield, he gestures for me to lift my mask.

Up the nose it goes . . .

'Too far mate, too far!'

It's not considerate, but I have to pull away. I've had a few of these now and that was rough. Worse, he still needs to do the other nostril for the rapid antigen test, then again for the PCR test. Tears stream down my checks, and he gives the slightest smirk.

Yeah, funny, grown man wipes cheeks.

Next, the x-ray room for a chest x-ray. It's a small, tiled room, filled with the oldest of medical contraptions. A small computer, housed in an even smaller cubicle to the side, shows the results. You could film a horror movie in here just by dimming the lights.

'Stand here, when I leave the room, take a deep breath and hold.'

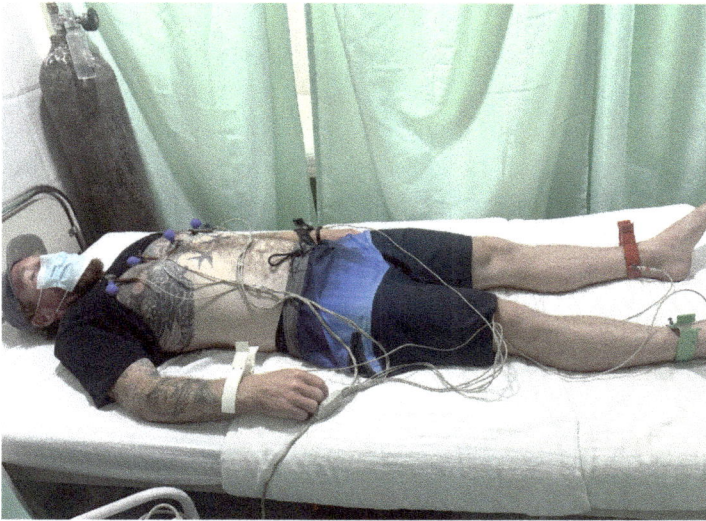

For how long?

Back to the waiting room. The owner, or maybe manager, addresses us and provides information we mostly know.

'You can have positive results for weeks after symptoms have passed. No need to get PCR test if you're already positive results lately. It can just risk my staff and other patients because you've all got the Covid here.'

Tonight, however, I've paid for both a PCR test and a RAT.

Gobinda emerges from the testers' room shortly after the testing.

'All positive—except David.'

I can't believe it. I'm shocked. Astounded. The rapid antigen test has come up negative.

'Can I get that in writing?!'

'Sure, it will be in your file with results tomorrow.'

I share high fives with Clayton and he can tell I'm stoked.

'Told ya it could happen...'

I have to go back to talk to the doctor, who diligently takes notes before I head in for an EKG test. Some of these rooms make me feel like I'm re-entering the horror set. This place, and the equipment, is not just dated—it's a little creepy. Pulling back some curtains, a simple bed sits next to a massive oxygen tank. Sleeping here would freak me out. It's sterile, cold and quiet. This is one 'out of the box' experience.

Test done, I'm glad to escape to the refuge of the reception area, clicking my heels as I go. This moment is what happiness feels like. It's sinking in that I've jumped through all the hoops to return. Back to Base Camp for me. Perversely, I feel like my family would be proud of me.

I consult with Gobinda, asking, 'Am I a chance of being on the next chopper out then?'

'Yes, with Clayton, there's one spot left.'

It all sounds too good to be true, so I try to dial down my enthusiasm. I'd be shattered if there was somehow a mistake.

Outside we wait for our return transportation. A guy carrying a fridge on his back passes by. He's using a head strap for balance—how bad must that be for your neck? How about a tree on a scooter, or a ladder? There's always something to see.

Day 4

The situation in Nepal is dynamic, as are all Covid-19 issues here. Lockdown restrictions went into effect at 6am. With 4,774 new infections recorded in the past twenty-four hours, the active case count stands at 30,209, according to the Ministry of Health and Population.

While Kathmandu hospitals turn away even serious Covid patients, we're told to stay indoors and I'm uncertain how we'll travel back to Base Camp. Even with my new negative test results, which are hopefully being included in my file as promised, travel is a challenge. Restrictions have the potential to force travellers into isolation.

On the rooftop, it's quiet, almost too quiet. Missing is the buzz of the morning commute, the constant beeping of vehicles, the sound of people in conversation. The haze is even worse than it has been lately, adding a gloomy start to an otherwise warm morning.

Gobinda messages me: 'Just quick update, your PCR got positive. So what you decide from your side. You can plan. This is different results than yesterday.'

It feels in an instant that I've slammed into an emotional brick wall. I now have a negative RAT result, but a positive PCR result—which is the more accurate of the two. Most people infected with the Covid-19 virus can expect to experience mild to moderate respiratory illness. I should recover without requiring special treatment, and generally have felt better lately. But does this mean I'm healthy enough to climb the world's highest mountain?

My thoughts vary every day about the risks and opportunities. I feel better, then I feel sick—confusion in between. Last night I was elated at the possibility of returning to Everest Base Camp. This morning I feel like I'm on a roller coaster that's destined to de-rail. I'll receive a hard copy of my results this afternoon, but I'm not sure my path forward is any clearer.

The weather, like my day, has turned. Rain, thunderstorms and quiet contemplation are all that remain.

Later, 'Gobinda hour' has arrived. It's time for a briefing. The group gathers rather formally. Hard results are in. My cover letter states, 'Covid Ag test was negative.' All supporting documents that I require are there and everything else is fine. My PCR test, however, is positive. Probably only just, but still positive. The Ct values are at a low to non-contagious level.

Quickly, the conversation changes to insurance, the cost of helicopters and hotel charges, and the debate begins. The risks are many and varied. Ultimately, it's us who have to deal with insurers and the individual who has to understand their own risks, and to that end our own insurance or exposure if something goes wrong. Opinions are varied and enquiries passionate. Everyone has so much invested in this; not just in terms of money, but emotionally. Tensions that have been simmering away now pour out. Moral standings are challenged, the value of life is discussed, and there's that question that's not going anywhere—who can prove when the infection period ends? Gobinda is reduced to tears.

As for the chance of us infecting anyone in Base Camp, Clayton has his own summary, stating, 'Okay, it's already all baked into the cake.'

Anyone from our camp who was going to get sick already is. There have been enough of us here, so the thinking goes.

Our destiny is in our own hands, but still Gobinda is upset. It must be taking its toll. He hasn't returned home himself because he has a seventy-year-old grandmother, so he has been living in a hotel nearby.

'Have you tested yourself yet?'

'No, but I will soon.'

I'm still included in the group to fly, and Gobinda has had to arrange a special permit for us to travel to the airport tomorrow, given this lockdown. Apologising on behalf of the company for any of its shortcomings, or where he may have let us down, he is again overwhelmed by emotion.

What an impossible situation. This predicament, this climbing season, is surely like no other. The frustration here at times borders on unbearable.

Ossy will go to the doctor tomorrow and wants to climb, positive or not, given that his ten days will have passed. For me, given that I have permission, the time to go back is now. I'm past contagious (the accepted research suggests), we'll be isolated on return, and acclimatisation should hold if I return now.

I know Clayton is a strong climber and I would be happy to climb with him again. What are the chances the guy I got stuck in a tent with in Antarctica is the one I'll be sharing an isolation tent with in Nepal?

All there is to do is send Mike a copy of my results and negative antigen test. My fate is in his hands. It's a nervous wait, but the reply finally comes.

'You are the man! That is exactly what I want to see. Yes, you will be returning with that crew... Fly safe!'

It has got to be a tough gig for Mike. Sick himself and stuck in Lukla, he's responsible for one of the only teams testing on the mountain, and the only team I've heard that is allowing climbers to return after being infected with Covid.

But it's time to get my head out of the politics and into the mountains—I'm flying tomorrow.

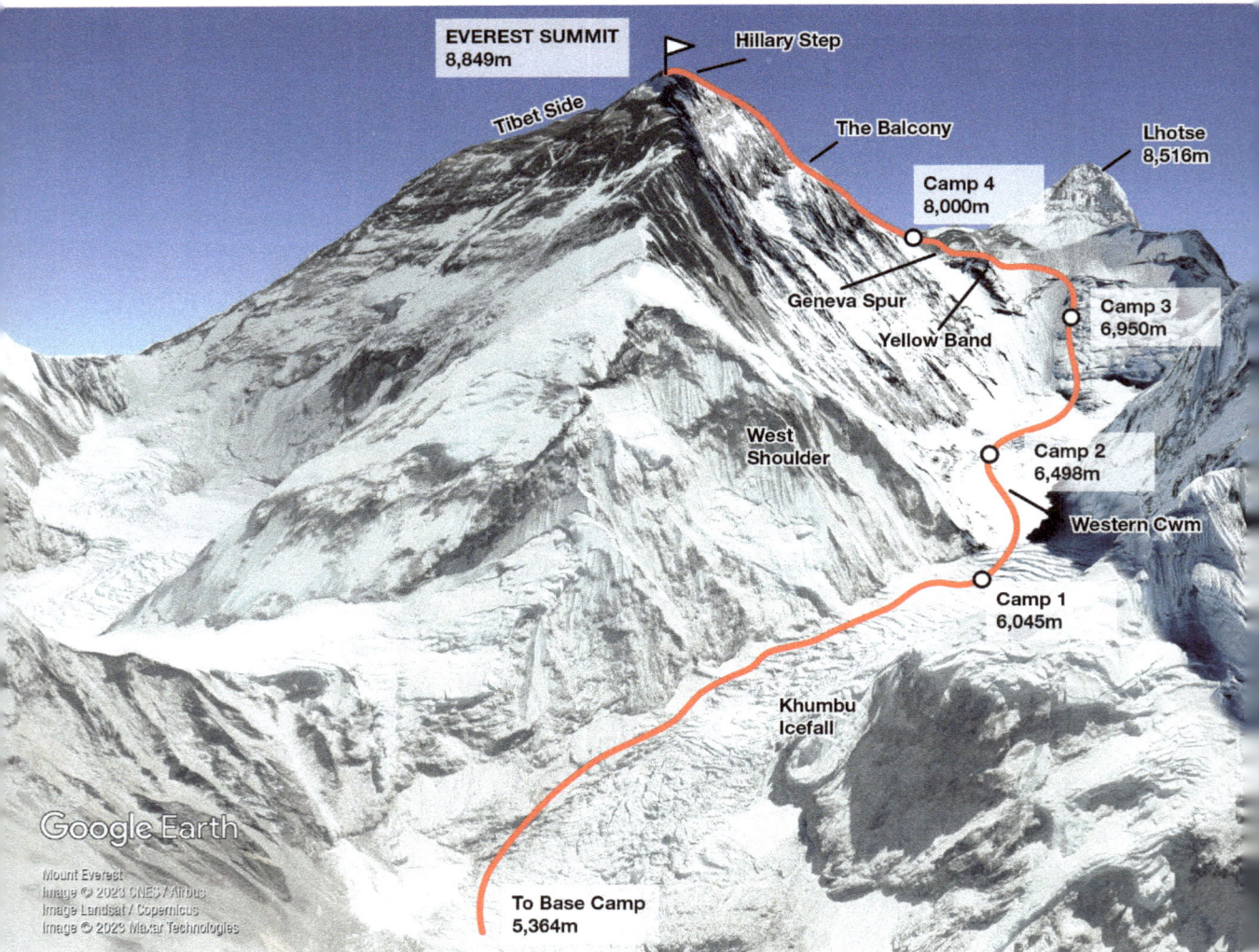

EVEREST SUMMIT
8,849m

Hillary Step

Tibet Side

The Balcony

Lhotse
8,516m

Camp 4
8,000m

Geneva Spur

Yellow Band

Camp 3
6,950m

West
Shoulder

Camp 2
6,498m

Western Cwm

Camp 1
6,045m

Khumbu
Icefall

To Base Camp
5,364m

Google Earth

Mount Everest
Image © 2023 CNES / Airbus
Image Landsat / Copernicus
Image © 2023 Maxar Technologies

MT EVEREST

9,467km from Home

ELEVATION: 8,849m

COORDINATES:

N 27 98.830

E 86 92.446

Nuptse
7,861m

EVEREST BASE
CAMP—TAKE #2

10

I<small>T'S JUST BEFORE</small> 6<small>AM</small>. Lights are off and I've taken the stairs, as the lift seems to be hibernating. The hotel foyer is dark as I approach the lobby. Simply asking to check out has flustered the male receptionist. But it's time to leave.

The Kathmandu streets are dead. Armed army personnel, posted at multiple checkpoints, enforce the lockdown orders. Travelling through three checkpoints with a printed permit on the windscreen and accompanying lanyard, Gobinda explains, 'They are very strict—that's why we need these.'

He's right. An otherwise quick trip to the airport is delayed each time we go through an armed checkpoint. Officials are thoroughly checking the paperwork.

The airport also lacks the usual chaos. We walk straight through the front doors, only slowing down to offer our hand for a temperature check. The lady waves continuously to motion she has done her job. Nobody is stopped. Bags go through an x-ray machine and we continue through the metal detector. Again, nobody is stopped, despite the machine beeping at every individual.

Ten metres in, our group steps over and onto the bag weighing platforms, taking a shortcut through the check-in counters. Arriving at our helicopter 'check-in', we pay our four per cent merchant's charge (1,250 dollars each way) and receive our boarding passes.

It's straight through the lounges, then time to say goodbye to Gobinda.

We shuffle into a van, then navigate the airstrips, circle around the aircraft and arrive where the helicopters depart. It's a forty-minute flight from Lukla to Kathmandu.

'We're doing rescue from Camp 2 every day—mainly Sherpa but clients too,' the pilot tells us. 'Be careful of the Covid up there; people are coming down in the choppers every day.'

Winding up the valley, hills are dusted in recent snow. Fields show as patches of white rectangles where crops would grow. This raw environment is more beautiful than I remember.

opposite Lukla Airport—take 2

Our chopper pilot is Canadian through and through. He says, 'It's a shit show up here.' The tower tells them to hold altitude heights they can't due to the mountains, so there's a culture of lying. Problem is, they don't always understand where other aircraft are. They fly through clouds, unassisted by radar. They shouldn't, but it's unavoidable. Every day aircraft are off the tarmac is considered 'fair weather flying'. The pilot takes pictures of the instruments, and is sick of telling the Nepalese, 'The helicopter needs maintenance!' Often, the pilot will call back to Canada for diagnosis assistance. Today, he has assessed that the blades need to be rebalanced, there's not enough power, there's too much vibration and we're slightly overweight. My uneducated opinion, in looking at the dials, is that we're flying at or near the chopper's capacity. The pilot constantly runs power diagnostics as we climb, reducing power over every new mountain ridge.

Lukla Airport appears in the distance—hidden between the mountains, but there. It really is a tiny airstrip in the middle of nowhere. Whoever chose this place as the ideal location for an airport was certainly creative. We approach quickly and the chopper spins into the landing direction. We've arrived, for the second time, at this remote, essential destination.

Out we hop. This time they're taking fuel out as we're too heavy; overloaded, according to the pilot. We also swap pilots. It's the same guy I had on the way down.

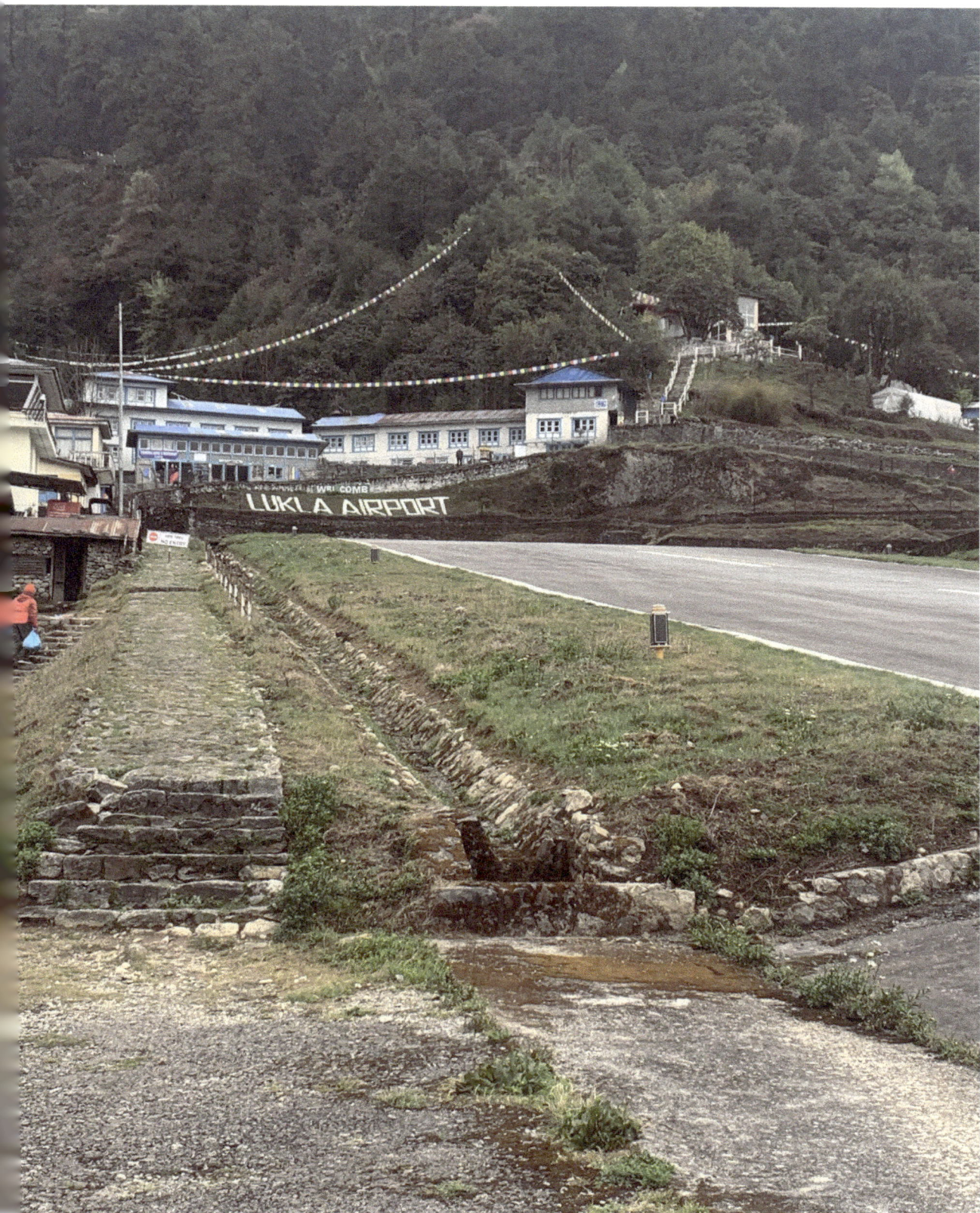

'I remember you,' he says. Another climber vomited in his chopper on the last trip down. 'It won't be as bumpy today, so don't worry,' he reassures me.

Whenever someone says that, I can't help but both wonder why and worry just a little. I know that to fly in these mountains these guys have to be great pilots, but machinery failure can happen to anyone.

Our new helicopter pilot manoeuvres quickly after take-off and we roar back into the mountains. We fly close to the mountains' edge, close enough to admire where the greenery changes to snow caps. Quickly, my attention is drawn to the centrepiece. The mighty Mt Everest. It's still there, it hasn't changed. My impression of it has, however. I stare, a little more focused, a little more serious.

I wasn't the first to leave with Covid, but I'm the first to return. This somehow, intuitively, means something to me. None of this would be possible without the systems Mike is trying to create. Whatever policies were missing that allowed us to be infected and forced us to leave are being compensated by this very precedent. For this I'm grateful.

Touchdown.

The flight from Lukla back to Base Camp takes just fifteen minutes. The doors open and after the luggage piled around us is removed, I take my first steps back on the ice. Moving to a safe area just outside the rotor blades' span, I plant my feet back where I left as the helicopter powers back up and lifts off.

Picking up my pack, the Sherpa enquires, 'You know your way back?'

'Yeah, I'll be fine.'

Wandering back, it's quiet, really quiet. No need to rush. I stroll through the fresh snow, which crunches under my weight. I gaze upon the ER station as I pass through. There's no movement there. Not a soul in the Sherpa section, either. I continue on towards the central area. Nobody's here. Frozen clothes hang behind a tent. A wash bowl lies abandoned, still with frozen water and cups inside. Even footprints that define the path are absent. It's a little eerie.

Fittingly, Big Tendi, standing at the puja memorial, is the first to greet me.

'Welcome back, man, you feeling better? Did we see Mike in Kathmandu?'

'I thought he was in Lukla.' Signs are he might have the virus, but nobody will say.

Big Tendi is not too well himself, I observe, as he coughs and points to his chest.

He gives me a few updates, which are appreciated. Ryan and April are touching Camp 3 today. Everything must be working out for them and some positive news, while welcome, somehow goes against the grain. The entire kitchen staff has been tested and are free from Covid. But—there's a big 'but'. Everyone who went up the mountain for a rotation before testing commenced is due to return to Base Camp soon. And testing is set to recommence. Returning climbers dine separately for now, and our 'quarantine tent' might be a sanctuary.

Early morning snow is starting to fall lightly, and it seems the fog is descending with it. We're probably lucky with our timing, as soon flights will cease.

My tent is exactly as I remember, and almost welcoming me back.

A wave of climbers is on the way down. Clayton gossips that at least two of them are not vaccinated, maybe three. This wave of climbers has an advantage: 'Doctor Mike', a sixty-five-year-old American ER doctor. This guy sounds incredible. He volunteered in Africa at the epicentre of Ebola when it plagued the continent. Without enough supplies, he had to reuse his mask every day while operating and no doubt placed his own life at risk. Here, Clayton says he has already assisted twenty people, with everything from giving advice to emerging, bloodied, from helping a Sherpa with a compound fracture. You'd be forgiven for forgetting that Dr Mike is a client intending to summit both Everest and Lhotse without oxygen. If successful, he will be the oldest person to do so.

The wave of descending climbers will be here soon, and will be required to take a Covid test at some stage. Fingers crossed that another of the exiting helicopters isn't required for them.

I learn that Mike is in Kathmandu—and positive. Worse still, he is staying at the hospital, so the symptoms can't be good.

News here is like that—good news is received in one hand while negative news passes through the other.

Protocol still hasn't taught our friendly kitchen hand that the mask needs to be over his mouth and nose, but I try to compensate by putting on mine when he enters our isolation tent. Sitting alone and drinking fluids, while letting my body adapt to the radical change in altitude, is all I can manage today. Headaches come and go; it might be a rough night. But this is what the human body is designed for—adaption. It's cold early in the evening and I shiver, even with the additional layers. Being in Kathmandu has done nothing for the temperature shock.

Come dinnertime, Big Tendi sticks his head in, asking, 'David, tomorrow we walk to Pumori High Camp, yes? I haven't been for a walk in ages.'

It's good to be back.

PULSE OX KATHMANDU: 92%
PULSE OX BASE CAMP: 82%

Base Camp to Pumori High Camp to Base Camp

Hygiene hasn't changed in the toilets. I'm disappointed to find they're still filthy this morning. No soap, water or sanitiser in either of them. Simple things like this could be addressed for the benefit of many, surely. Not how I wanted to start the day. I keep my mask on.

Breakfast is rubbish. We're served last, which is fine, but one piece of cold toast and some sides that look uneatable—not cool. Regardless, I'm happy to be up early, sorting my gear and packing my pack. Be back hiking soon.

Time to get moving, and Clayton is joining us for our trip to Pumori High Camp.

At first the hike is hard to settle into. Lots of snow has melted and underfoot it's mostly dry, making it a different journey from last time. My heart rate skyrockets, as if it has forgotten physical activity altogether. But I've trained for this and insist my muscles move. By the first water break I'm dropping an energy gel. The calories I had for breakfast can't sustain this.

Big Tendi is also moving a clip faster, presumably to see if we'll bend over and gasp for air. 'This is a test,' he would say. One thing's for sure, however: we're all happy to be out getting fresh air. The mountain still produces an occasional avalanche to draw our attention. The choppers are buzzing in one after the other.

Big Tendi has been in charge of Base Camp since I left, only handing the reins over to Little Tendi today. 'I didn't want to be in charge, I wanted to go up. So did Tendi, so we flipped a coin for it—I lost.' Sometimes the big decisions are as simple as that.

I ask Big Tendi what the hardest part of his job has been since he was put in charge.

'I sent down eight of our alpine workers. They are my friends and don't want to go. They know they might not make it back.' It's an insight into his incredible and selfless struggles.

He tells us that since we left, 200 people with Covid have been flown out, including thirty-eight from Camp 2. That's almost a quarter of the estimated total number of people here. Yet the government continues to issue permits. At last count, 408 Everest permits have been issued, smashing the 2019 record. That year was the last time climbing was open, and eleven people died on the mountain, with ten of those deaths occurring on the Nepal side. But this year climbing has changed. There are no gatherings or celebrations. People are wary of each other. Separate camps retain roped boundaries. Signs are erected: 'KEEP OUT', 'CLOSED CAMP', 'WHERE'S YOUR MASK?' All these are new additions to a changing landscape.

As we trudge along this now familiar route, Clayton and I have time to reminisce about Antarctica. It starts to snow as we arrive at Pumori High Camp, adding to the attraction. This time we don't acclimatise for long, just have a drink and a quick bite to eat. Soon it's time to descend.

'Did we pass the test?' Clayton asks.

'Of course. You are both very strong.'

Tomorrow all the 'Moonlight Hotel survivors' will take a rest day. Except me. Big Tendi wants me to climb at 3am with the two speed ascenders. I've not met them, let alone climbed with them. But he says I'll be fine; they're really strong climbers. The advantage is that the earlier I get through the Khumbu Icefall and onto the slopes of Everest to complete a high-altitude rotation, the greater the chances of re-joining Ryan and Tenji. But I have mixed feelings about this. I just assumed I'd be climbing high with Big Tendi—and now I know I'm not. To be fair, his health isn't great and he says he needs time to be strong again.

The great divide continues.

I just have to trust Big Tendi's advice and go, or I'll have to wait three or four days for my next shot.

DISTANCE: 4.10km
TIME: 06:11 hrs
AVERAGE SPEED: 0.6kph
ASCENT: 676m
DESCENT: 44m
ALTITUDE: 6,045m
PULSE OX: 77%

Base Camp to Camp 1

It's the nominated waking time of 1am, but I've already been getting changed for half an hour. I slept rough, if you can call it that. More accurate to say I napped infrequently. My body is drained. I execute one task at a time, then reward myself with a small sip of hot water from my thermos.

At last I stand dressed in climbing gear, harness and pack in place, but I'm far from ready. A coffee is all I can manage and have to pass on the full cooked breakfast. I take an energy gel, as I feel depleted before I've even started.

At 2:21am we're off, led by Sumon Sherpa and his two clients.

It's a cool morning, not too cold. The stars are out and I'm feeling buoyed. But my chest doesn't feel great, and I pant in the cold air just leaving Base Camp. The snow glistens in the dark, like glitter flickering everywhere I look, creating an almost magical scene. Dotted headlights form a trail on the slopes up high, beacons that remind us we're not alone. The stars and moon provide enough light to see the form of the ice, but not enough to see a path without a personal headlight.

Half an hour in, on go the crampons, and this is where the work begins. There are not many on the trek, but the first vertical climb brings all teams to a standstill. We have to pause and wait our turn for this vertical rise, which gives me a chance to just focus on breathing. Hopefully my heart rate will come down. As it snows the chill can be felt on one's cheeks, and the patience of some climbers wanes.

I can recollect sections we've scaled before. But soon I look down, and there's something else. We're skirting the edges of huge crevasses. Bottomless to the eye, I know from seeing them in daylight the horrors some of these offer. Gone is the safety of ladders and double ropes offered as security. Nobody tells you the magnitude of some of the jumps you'll undertake.

'Make sure your carabineer safety is screwed up before you jump!'

Thanks, Sumon. Great advice.

Of course, I look down before I jump and see walls of darkness plummeting without end. Here goes; momentum ensures I'm fully alert.

This is something else, the ice valley parting in irregular and sensational fashion. This unique place demands your attention unlike any on Earth that I've seen. Unique, yet

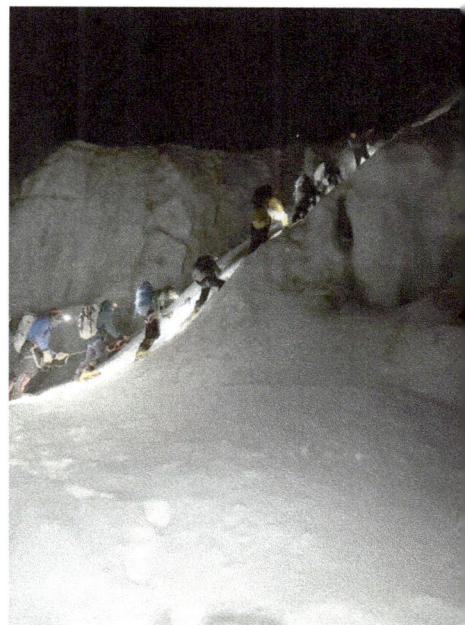

above Back climbing

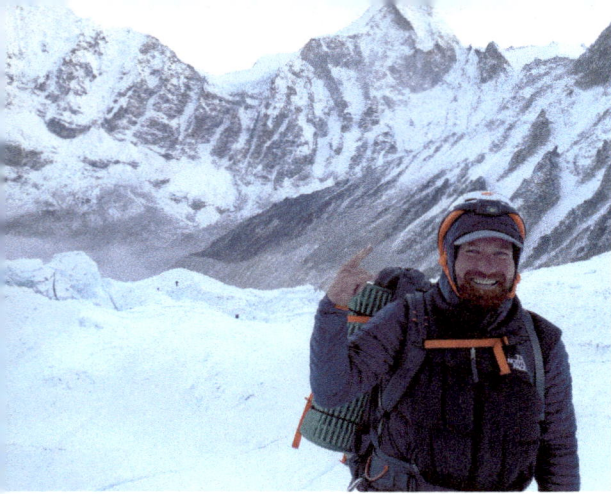
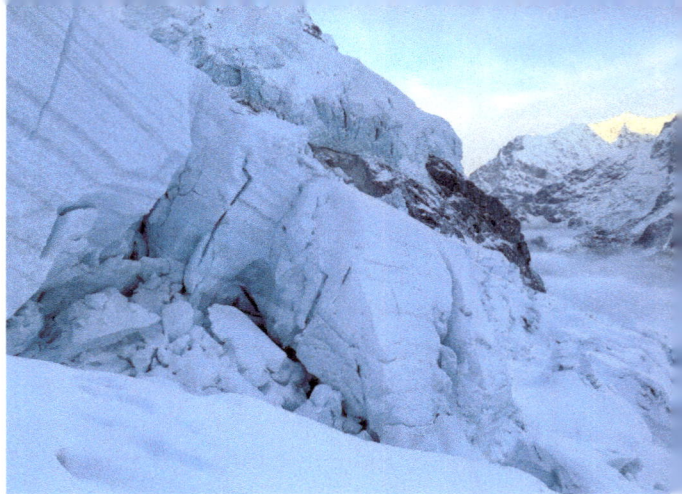
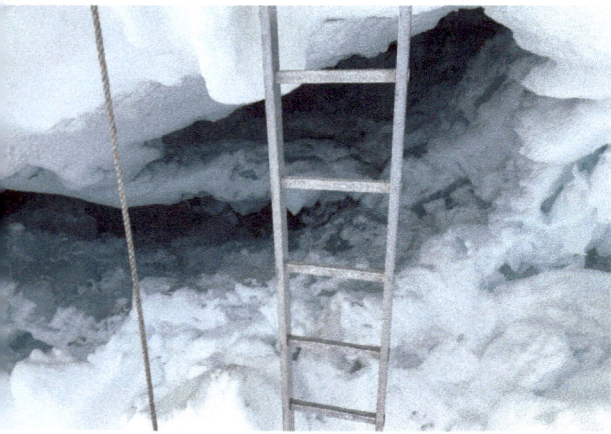
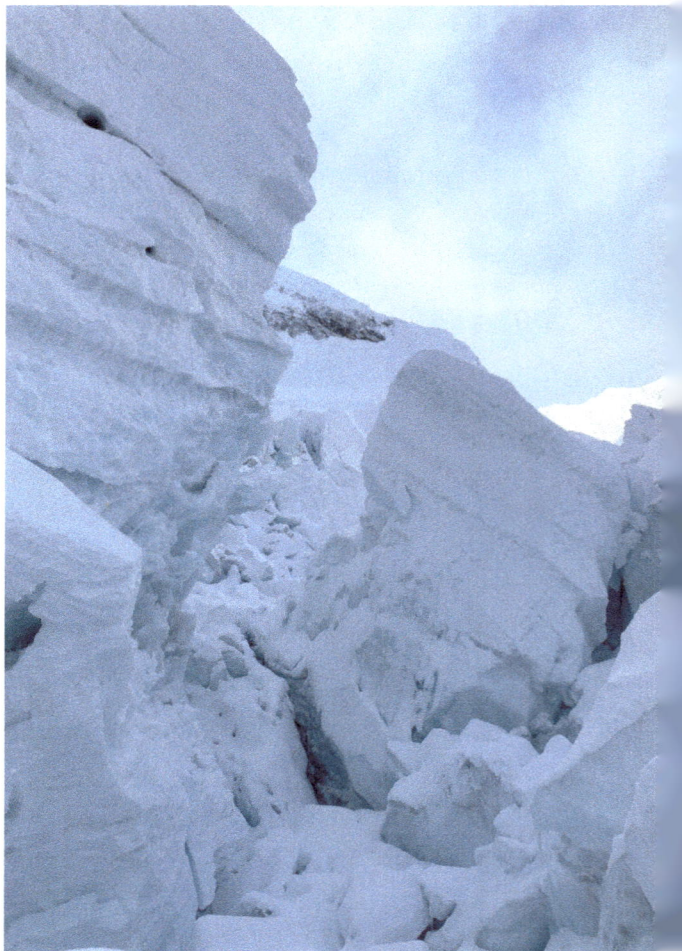
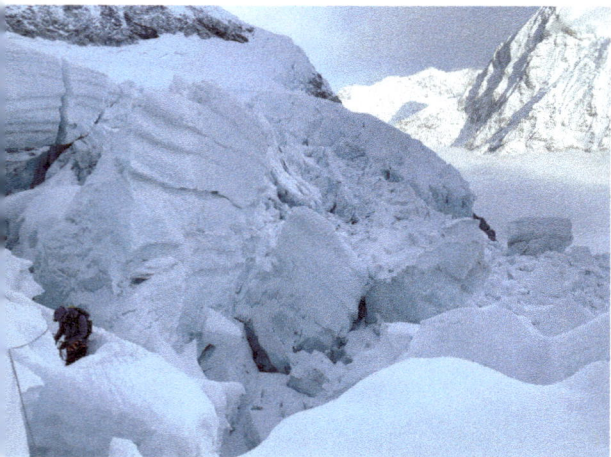

dangerous. Fascinating and captivating, yet dangerous. I get it—this is no place for complacency.

The new dawn highlights the tips of the mountains with blue skies stretching forever. Famous mountains: Nuptse, Pheriche, Lhotse.

We pass the 'football field' and enter the 'popcorn fields'. Here you're not only ascending the Khumbu Icefall, you're also at times descending into dark crevasses with overhanging ice formations. We traverse a crevasse, then scale the next section of ice. Then we cross a ladder, and make it onto another section of ice.

Lines are never really an issue. In one section we hand-rappel down and wait at the base, surrounded by sheer drops and looking sideways through a gaping hole in the ice. Maybe we should have abseiled down. It's a lot of pressure on the hands and slips are not acceptable here.

To get out of this 'hole' there's a ladder to cross, two ladders immediately afterwards to scale, then an almost vertical side of ice to kick your way up. It's taxing, and a few people have to wait their turn here, but this is understandable. Everyone wants to be safe and it's important to take your time. Still, I don't like waiting at the bottom, peering into another bottomless crevasse.

I suspect the dark has disguised some of the most harrowing drops and dangers. Panting and tired, I'm happy to kick my way out of this section. At the top I'm elated to see the top of the Icefall—or should I say the end of it! The sun is out and beats on us. From freezing cold to this. How I would welcome something in between.

The final slog to Camp 1 has begun. Only this single track we follow breaks an otherwise pristine environment of smooth rolling snow. Winding around the mountains, up, down and across, there are still awe-inspiring cathedrals and sculptures of ice everywhere I look. I'm enchanted by three sections that lean towards each other like multi-storey buildings. The

opposite, top left The rollercoaster of emotions

opposite, top right The maze of ice

opposite, center left Ladder crossing over the abyss

opposite, bottom right Constantly moving and changing icefall

opposite, bottom left Making our way through

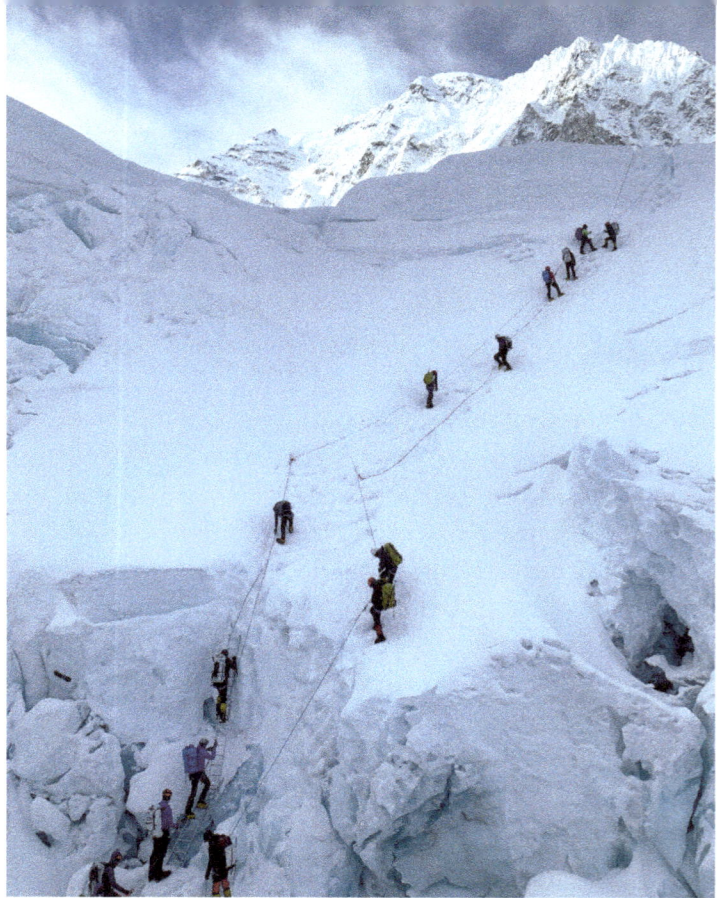

right The one and only, Khumbu Icefall

over-reaching ice defies gravity in its strength and weight.

A quick self-assessment only confirms what I suspect—I'm deteriorating rapidly. I try a little water, and feel worse. I try taking off some layers, and the sun reaches through me. My gaze is stuck with every step, my head hangs a little too low. All I have to do is walk, yet my body tells me I'm done.

Then there it is. Vomiting!

The last altitude check before keeling over to spew was 5,496 metres. Just to be clear, this wasn't a spew where food comes up and you feel better. No, this was gut-wrenching pain where a little acid comes up and your stomach is in knots as you dry retch again. This is altitude at work, demoralising the visitor. My head spins, my body collapses, and I dry retch some more.

Now sitting, Sumon passes me some tissues. I don't even care to wipe my face. Deep breaths, this will pass. With the sun ripping any ability to bounce back, all I can do is warily stand. This will pass. I wipe up my chin, disgusting bile soaking the tissue. Backpack on, I can move. In discomfort, but I can move. Certainly can't stay here.

The climb to Camp 1 becomes a blur.

Next thing I know, I'm staring at the CTSS tent, then staring at the ground, almost motionless. Nobody is in front of me. I take a few more steps, look up, and there's someone running at me. I'm greeted by a bear hug from Ryan.

'Good to see you mate, you made it.'

I'm spent, but take the final steps and am met with a hug from April too. Tenji is here, and they're just about to depart. We only have moments to get reacquainted and I tell them that Mike is in hospital. They didn't know, and I inform them how bad the Covid situation really is. With a last embrace, they have to go. Tenji wants them climbing down through the Icefall to Base Camp.

'See you guys real soon. Stay safe.'

The boost that seeing my friends gave me quickly passes and I need to sit. Have to sit, now. A warm cup of tea is received, my stomach growls. I drag my seat into the shade and drop my harness off, also removing my crampons. This takes every effort as I watch people moving to their tents. Time to do the same.

I'm overwhelmed with my inability to move. Raising my head, it just wants to fall back down. It took all my strength to roll out my sleeping pad and I've collapsed on top of it. Sumon Sherpa tries to get me to come out. 'Tea, soup, anything?' I can't. I'm in struggle town. I've been here before and I need to get my head down.

The sun beating down makes it hot inside the tent and I eventually strip down. A sip of water here, a gulp there, and I'm back horizontal. An hour passes. I try to pee. The Sherpa offer me more water. 'Drink and pee-pee, drink and pee-pee.' I try.

Another hour passes.

That tipping point has arrived when the sun and its warmth vanishes and the snow and cold move in. I put layers of clothes back on. At the same time I try half an apple, pee, and curl back up in my sufferance. It's getting cold. I've somehow lost several hours in my hibernation, but now I need to think of the evening. It's coming and I'm lying here cold, immobile and feeling miserable.

opposite Camp 1

There's discussion over the radio about an accident in the Icefall. Two people are injured and need a helicopter. I stay engaged long enough to hear it's Sherpa, not Ryan and April, before curling back up.

I need more clothes. I need my air pad blown up. This takes half a dozen of my best efforts. Then I need to rest. I get my sleeping bag out. Then I need to rest. Warm at least, I curl up in misery.

Am I napping, hallucinating, or is this whole day sliding by? I haven't left the tent all day, and now that day is gone.

'We really want you to come get something from the kitchen. There is dinner ready now.'

I brace myself. I should try.

Rugged up, I must look like death dragging myself a whole ten metres for some soup. I try a little rice, but can handle no more.

'The accident—is there any news?'

'This is alpinism, it could be a friend, so I don't want all the talking, don't worry about it, not serious accident, just some ice fall.'

I need to crawl back to where I came from.

Has this day been a success or not?

I made it to Camp 1—who really cares?

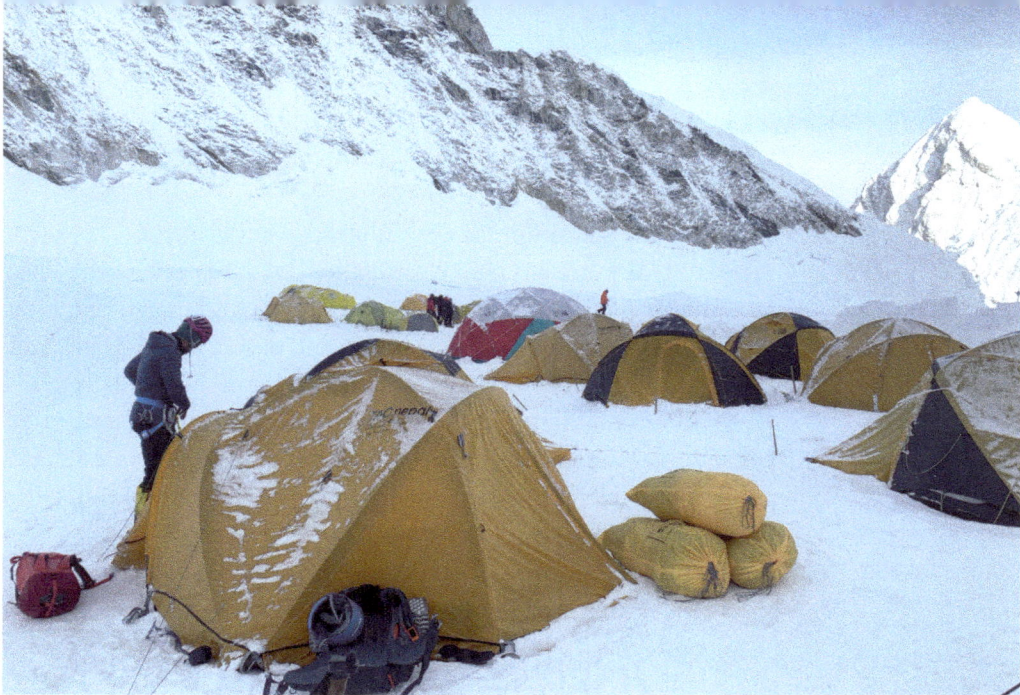

Camp 1 to Camp 2

Spew, spewing. Gasping and dry retching any balance of fluids and acid into that plastic bag I prepared earlier. This is how I start my waking hour.

It's 4:30 am. I've got to pack this tent up, get in my climbing gear and accept that this is what I've got to climb with. I get some light to inspect what's running from my nose, and confirm that it is indeed snot, not blood. On top of the snot and the headaches overnight, I've found a new problem. Packing my sleeping bag up, which involves more or less jamming it into a bag, my hand feels like it's broken. Inspecting it, I can see that it's swollen and probably just bruised, but it's hurting nonetheless. At least my nose is fine.

Time to get my big boy pants on and keep moving, I'll just dry retch one more time.

Okay, the inners of my climbing boots are frozen. Best I bang that ice off first.

6,045m—6,498m
DISTANCE: 2.85km
TIME: 04:05 hrs
AVERAGE SPEED: 0.7kph
ASCENT: 386m
DESCENT: 22m
ALTITUDE: 6,498m
PULSE OX: 83%

Sumon Sherpa brings a cup of tea around.

'What is this?!'

'Just the contents of my stomach, don't worry.'

One job at a time. The strenuous jobs are packing the sleeping bag and rolling up the air mattress and mat. Then I just have to drag all my gear together and pack it into the backpack. After this, I can drag my sorry arse to breakfast and pretend I want something to eat while I try not to vomit in the cook's tent.

My body accepts coffee, so I start there. Aware that I've not kept much food down and it's going to be a long climb, I also try a small porridge.

'Sorry yesterday was a little fast, but Icefall very dangerous at moment, so I tell you we have to go fast, sorry,' Sumon explains. 'Today you can go a little slower, not so dangerous and maybe better for you.'

I excuse myself and wander around camp, hoping in vain this will help.

My head spins as I put my harness on, my feet are already frozen in the big boots, and I grimace as I squeeze on my glove. Perfect, I'm ready to go.

Dorje Sherpa is short-roping two of us up from here while Sumon Sherpa is with two other clients. I'm to the rear of the three of us, so when we transit downhill I lead. Initially, I presumed being roped up might be a bit precautionary. Then we had to jump over the first crevasse. Then another, and another.

Once we get past the most severe of crevasses, the long stretches of zig-zagging through the gently undulating glacial valley basin that is Western Cwm begins. The sun comes over the mountains, promising warmth, while the glare from the white fields' smooth surface is instant.

Being roped up forces the pace, and I actually welcome it to help me keep moving. Because I want to stop.

One step in front of the other.

Our three-man rope team has no rhythm, and two things happen on the long climb to Camp 2. The sun becomes

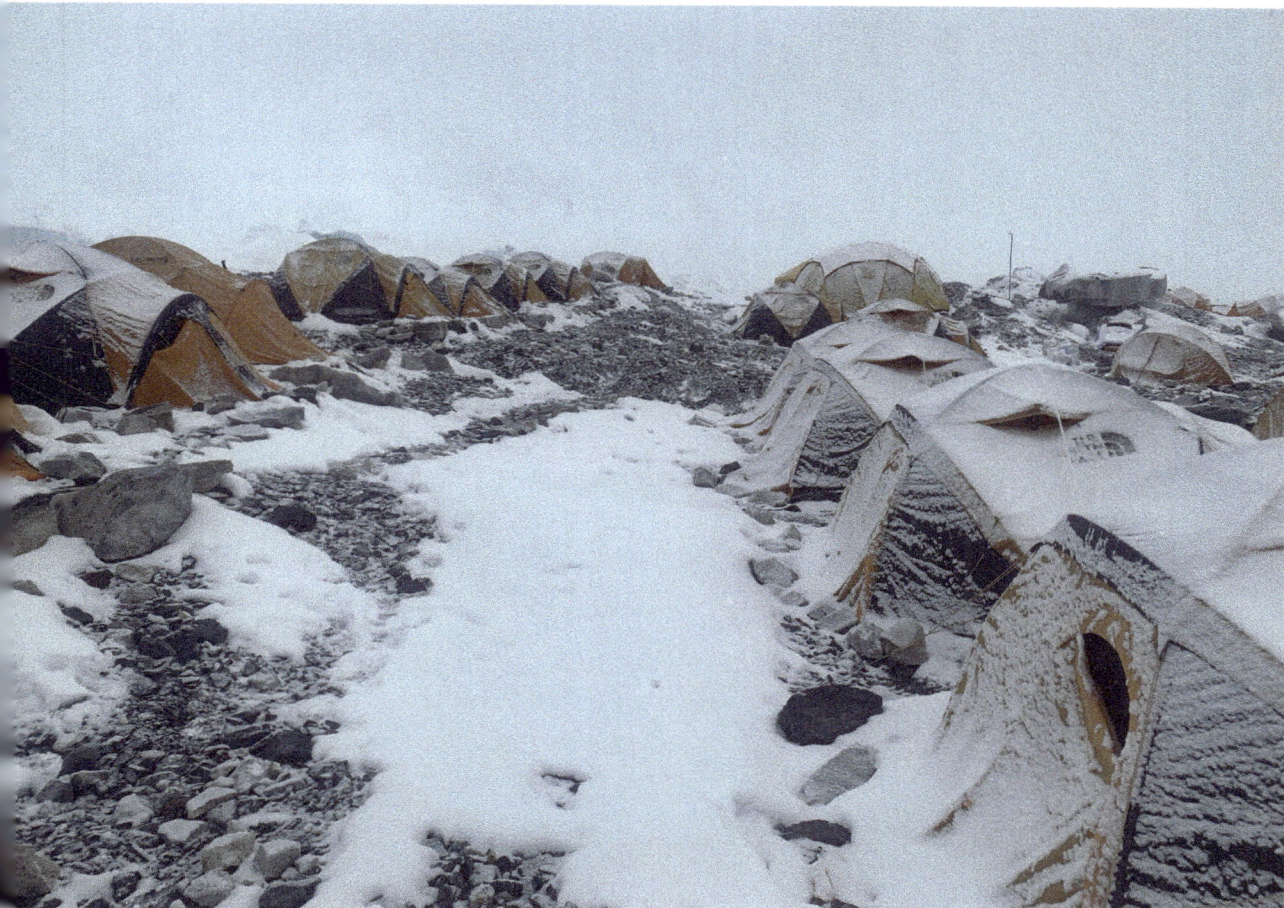

above Camp 2

piercingly hot, offering glare that gets into your head. And Dorje Sherpa slows. Taking regular stops, I too need to suck in big breaths. I'm not alone in my struggle. Sherpa bend over regularly, gasping under their loads, occasionally vomiting. Everyone rests intermittently. This is a long, slow grind ever upwards.

I can see the camp up in the distance, but that's where it stays, in the distance, as the sun beats on us. A small avalanche holds our attention temporarily to our left, seemingly closer than our destination.

Okay, time to push on.

The single narrow route to camp never eases, and climbs steeper on the approach. It's so hot, and there's one more push before, here at a group of rocks, we can remove our crampons and lose the rope. I'm exhausted, and camp is yet another push. I drift behind the others as my heart rate climbs and my enthusiasm for camp wanes. We stop outside our dining tent. I want to drop, but unload my gear instead. Small congratulations are exchanged, but I'm not in much of a mood for high fives and socialising. I just need to sit, catch my breath, let my foggy head relax.

I'm still tenting alone due to a mix of precaution and suspicion. Getting settled once more, I sit in my tent in contemplation. Snow falls. Yesterday's inability to function weighs on my thoughts, even worries me a little. I feel I've just survived the days, and not conquered anything. It has been a long road back and I'm still paying the price of having had this virus on top of trying to make the huge altitude adjustments. Some sleep is what I need.

Active rest day

6,498m—6,745m
DISTANCE: 2.85km
TIME: 03:07 hrs
AVERAGE SPEED: 0.9kph
ASCENT: 252m
DESCENT: 258m
ALTITUDE: GAIN: 247m
PULSE OX: 86%

The head is still foggy, but at least I haven't tossed and turned dreaming of sleep. The sun here is early and I can feel it radiating from every surface. It's time for our 'active rest day'—a hike across the fields that glare all at once. I pack light, sensing dehydration is going to be a close companion today.

Sumon Sherpa has rushed us right to the minute for a 9:30am departure. I can't work it out. Every other day he has always been less than punctual. Now today—precision.

And we're off. Onto the mountains covered in pristine snow, sun beating down from above and heat radiating from all directions. I'm already thirsty, and exposed skin is starting to burn. Here we go, that sensation of feeling terrible while I move uphill one foot at a time. Crevasses are still present, but mostly unseen in this crazy environment; we remain roped. My chest thumps, head banging to the sound of irregular breath. Lots to work on here. I can't say I'm enjoying any aspect of this. A day without suffering would be good about now. I can't help but wonder if Covid has left permanent damage.

It's a two-hour trek to the starting point of the Lhotse face. Tomorrow we'll make the push up from here in search of Camp 3. If I can just reach Camp 3, say hello and descend all the way to Base Camp to recover a bit, that'd be great.

With light snowfall, the radiating sun has given way to increased fog. The descent is somewhat easier. My heart rate calms, I find some rhythm, and there's fresh snow to stomp through. We move fast and, without the sun beating on us, this remains my favourite part of the day.

Snow continues to fall through the afternoon. Back at camp, everyone has been called outside to help 'dig' the tents out. I can't believe how quickly the snow has built up. I've got to push snow out of the way just to get in and out of my tent. While I'm at it, I may as well do the perimeter and get the roof coating off so I don't suffocate in here.

Rest day

PULSE OX: 77%

Weather is just a prediction. With Mike still in hospital, the 'expert forecasting' is another absent tool that can't assist us up here. So we wait for first light to reveal the Lhotse face conditions and if we should touch Camp 3. The first twenty-four hours after a snow dumping is the most risky period for avalanches. All that fresh snow is yet to be exposed to radiation and heat to assist it settling. Nobody can be seen 'kicking in' new trail. So there's no departure to Camp 3. Today is a rest day.

'That's the most snow I've seen in all my trips here,' one of the Western guides claims.

It's a welcome delay for me. Yes, I want to keep moving, but not with the headache I faced this morning. Struggling to motivate myself, the inside of my tent is ice, including a coating over my sleeping bag. My drink bottles are frozen and I can feel dehydration in the mix of my sorry affairs.

Eventually the sun hits camp at around 8am. Every ounce of my body insists on staying put, and only the promise of hot coffee raises me. I've lain awake, dormant, for three-and-a-half hours, wondering if we'll still climb or if the ice will melt before I rise. Neither happened.

There has to be a tipping point when I get better.

With time comes plenty of reflection. I think often of Fin and her burden of diabetes. I try to draw parallels between not quitting my quest and her inability to put this disease behind her. One day will it be possible? Will this mountain be the one that'll get the better of me? Unlike Fin, with her diabetes, I signed up for this... voluntarily. Unbelievable. Yet disappointment and failure feel uncomfortably close. I ask myself if my time would be better spent with her in the comforts of the perfectly good home I've left miles and miles away. There's so much about myself I wish I could change. I'm sure Fin feels the same way at her tender age.

The first avalanche can be heard in the distance. I suspect it won't be the only one today. This is where I'm at: in the tent, at the mercy of the weather, alone. The thunderous chorus of snow crashing down the slopes continues.

I've made a rookie mistake and left my boots under the tent fly. Which is fine, except there's a section missing in the fly and my boots are now full of snow. I focus on digging the snow out of my boots with a hiking pole before defrosting them.

Camp 2 to Camp 3

It's 2am. The sound of the dedicated porters marching past the tent cannot be missed as they lead the charge for Camp 3 like a line of stormtroopers—driven. Our departure time is 4am, so getting back to sleep seems pointless. But I'm not nauseated, I'm not tired, and I've got a good sense I might be off to a better start to the day than I anticipated.

Outside my tent, the camp is already abuzz with climbers making their preparations. Kitchen tents are turning out hot water and breakfast, teams are getting ready to depart. It'll be a busy day on the hill. A long line of head torches can already be seen on the route further in the distance. It's the porters, no doubt, efficiently weaving their way up the mountain.

My two companions are fumbling around, still not ready. I ask Sumon, more than once, why I'm waiting and we're late, yet on the rest day we were rushing for departure. It's too cold to be standing around, but my point is made. Now I wait.

Quickly, quietly, we depart camp and the only sound is crunching fresh snow under our crampons. The night sky is clear above us and moonlight highlights the top of the mountain, but shows no visible details. I watch the snaking line of head torches winding up the track in the distance. The vertical nature of the mountain makes the lights look like they're stacked on top of each other.

I'm jumping the crevasses, tromping through fresh snow, breathing the crisp mountain air as first light reaches us. Is this enjoyment I'm experiencing as I gaze upon the mountains' summits, now highlighted by the dawn?

There's a fog chasing us up the valley. We have clear views of the trail ahead, but a dark grey cloud is intent on catching us from behind. In no time it has consumed us, and visibility is lost. We can't even see the mountains anymore, just a small section of the trail we're following.

UP

DISTANCE: 1.53km

TIME: 04:53 hrs

AVERAGE SPEED: 0.3kph

ASCENT: 452m

DESCENT: 4m

ALTITUDE: 6,498m—6,950m

GAIN: 452m

DOWN

DISTANCE: 1.85km

TIME: 02:11 hrs

AVERAGE SPEED: 0.8kph

ASCENT: 1m

DESCENT: 547m

ALTITUDE: 6,950m—6,498m

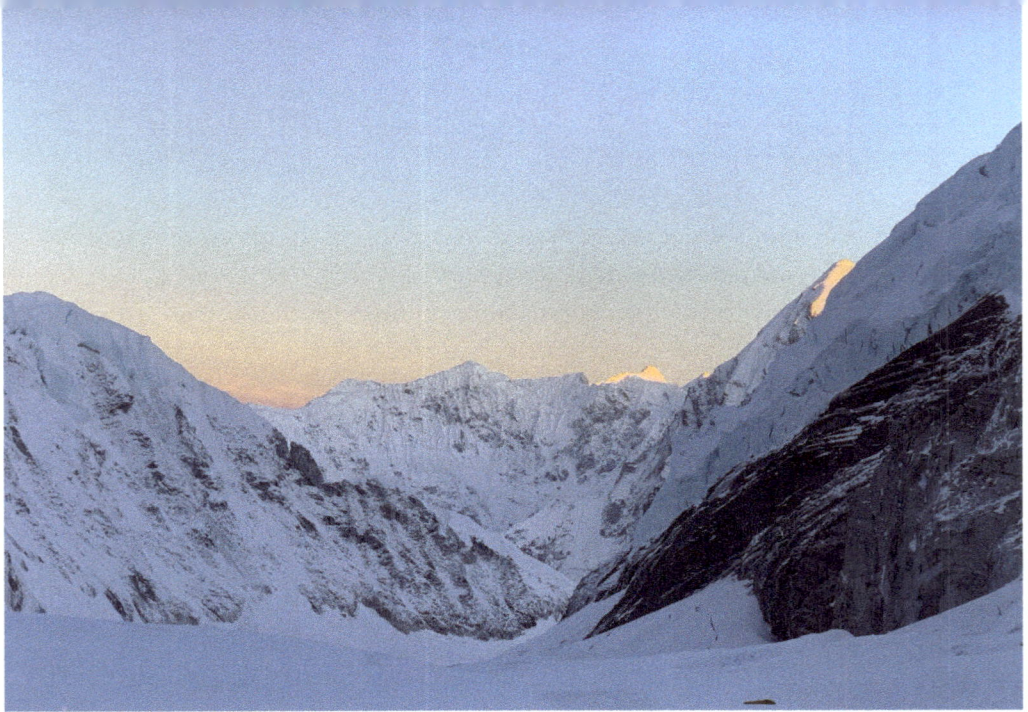

Once we've climbed the long, continuous incline to where we were two days ago, I find I've got more energy and some excitement to press on.

Lhotse is the fourth highest mountain in the world and plays an integral part in the ascent of Everest. At the start of the Lhotse face there's a huge crevasse to transit via a small shelf. Of course, we're clipped onto fixed lines the Sherpa have dedicated their time to installing here, but even so I feel a new dose of uncertainty.

'It's collapsing under me, get ready to hold!' The shelf gives way and I slide down until the ropes rake up.

My feet scramble at first with no footing, dangling over a deep void. Then the only thing to do when panic subsides is to kick new footholds into the mountain's edge and climb back up, boosted by a healthy rush of adrenaline. I didn't drop far, but I'm unnerved by how much further I might have fallen without the safety rope. Fine snow is blowing across the mountain's icy and hard-packed surface, building to a layer of ice on my beard. It floats like a cloud passing by, only to return again.

Ascender in hand, still on the fixed line, the morning's work now consists of one steep step after the other. It's about two hours of near vertical climbing. Since the storm some new 'steps' have been kicked into the ice, but there are sections where it's easy to fall knee deep in soft powder. It's a slog, but there's something soothing in its simplicity.

opposite New dawn...

The last section to Camp 3 is a nasty vertical ice wall to deplete you of any reserves. I take the lead; I want to get this done. Kicking ice for twenty metres is enough to leave anyone gasping for the end. And finally it comes.

With my chest thumping, I clip onto the safety rope that leads to camp and savour the exhaustion. I finally can see tents pitched on platforms, chipped into the mountain's steep slope. Yes, now my legs are tired and I welcome a break, knowing I gave that climb everything. Watching another climber vomiting repeatedly into the bank of snow, I sympathise. I know how he feels. Here the oxygen density is approximately forty per cent of what's available at sea level. Yet today I've pulled through. And he'll soldier on, because it's time to go down.

Camp 3 with a view.

The summit of Everest, however, continues to hide. But it's enough to just sit here, contemplating the journey. I'm grateful not only to have made it this far, but also for the break with my health that has enabled this success. Plagued by doubt, I've just tried to tackle one day at a time, sometimes one hour at a time. Sitting here feels like I've overcome those doubts.

It's time to go down.

Rappelling down is certainly way easier than climbing up, and I fly down alone with confidence. Aside from pausing to swap my rigging at anchor points, momentum has me at the bottom in no time.

But nobody's at the base of the crevasse. Do I really need help to get across? I figure the worst thing that can happen is that I'll fall, but somebody will come. I'll just sneak across safely. I can't let any old crevasse panic me like earlier. I need redemption. Cautiously, I use two safety carabineers and lower myself onto a newly formed ridge with the figure eight rappel. I'm on the ledge, but now the ropes are too tight and I can't release my figure eight.

A porter shouts from the top, 'Are you okay down there?'

'Sort of, just going slowly.'

'Can I overtake you?'

'If you want, I'm not rushing.'

He jumps down, seamlessly landing on the ledge without breaking it.

'You should short clip here, very dangerous.'

Instinctively, without asking, he short clips me and notices my issue with the figure eight. I don't complain as he pulls on the lines, releases it and clips it on my harness.

'Thank you. Sorry to have held you up.'

'It's no problem.'

I move along, and he leaps around and continues downward. I've still got some room for improvement, but I gave it a shot.

I know the guides won't be happy if I continue any further, unroped, across the crevasses, so I wait. Sumon eventually emerges with his client and is happy enough to rope me in so we can all continue. I like their descend speed and we motor down, around the crowds, at times knee deep in snow, and soon enough camp is before us.

It dawns on me that tomorrow I'll be walking into Base Camp. The purpose of this rotation is complete. A shower awaits. I can only hope that tomorrow I wake and the day works out as well as today.

Sumon tells me in the dining tent, 'You were strongest today, so strong, I didn't realise you were so strong from other day.'

Let's see what tomorrow brings.

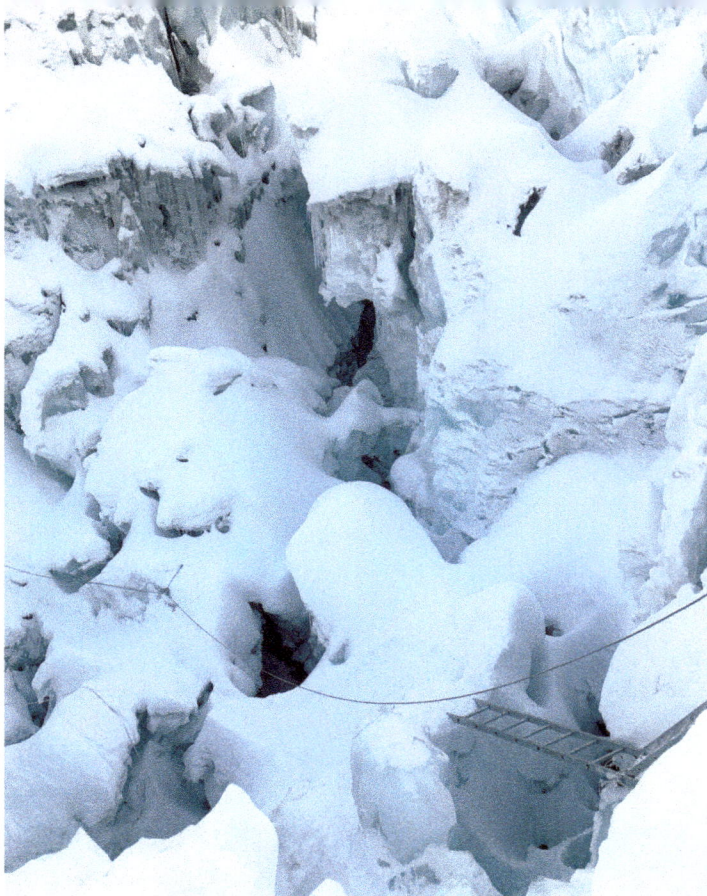

Camp 2 to Base Camp

My alarm tells me it's 3am. I have a splitting headache. How is it my head feels so heavy I can barely lift it? I drop a couple of headache tablets and convince myself I'll feel better as we track lower down the mountain.

First light hovers on the horizon and a mix of colours forms the backdrop to the mountains. Light's filtering through and it's time to rope up again.

Climbing feels different today—enjoyable, despite the headache—and not just because I'm leading. I can appreciate the scenery, the spans of white fields with nobody yet

DISTANCE: 8.20km
TIME: 04:59 hrs
AVERAGE SPEED: 1.7kph
ASCENT: 112m
DESCENT: 1,292m
ALTITUDE: 5,395m

transiting. The huge rock faces to my left could be art on a wall. The snow is still too fresh to settle into pace, while the going is all downhill and isn't too taxing on my strained muscles.

In an hour-and-a-half we've casually arrived at Camp 1. Big Tendi is here and asks why we're so early.

Time to push on through the Khumbu Icefall while it's cold—before the ice warms up too much. My pace is slightly faster than the others, and in any case we have to go independently due to the rappelling and the crowds coming upwards. Dorje Sherpa gives some instruction, yet always tells me to keep moving where I can. This gives me freedom to take some pictures of the environment, although no picture can truly capture the magnificent blues that form the bottom structure of these unique ice formations.

Going the opposite way, and in daylight, is a completely different experience. Some things I recognise, others are completely new. There's a particular new 'double ladder' crossing which is essentially two ladders tied with rope to span a large crevasse. This must have been the remedy for the recent collapse.

'Please move fast, this is very dangerous here,' Dorje expresses. He never has too much to say, so I heed his warning.

I soon see why it's so dangerous here. Large vertical ice walls, storeys high, are to my right. To my left sections of ice hang overhead as I first descend under them and then quickly rise up the other side. The ground doesn't seem stable, and on some sections I don't even consider pausing. Best to keep momentum up and pass the dangers that surround me. The jumps I remember clearly, yet the distance to jump seems further. Maybe the dark distorted the task, but missing the landing is not an option.

I'm getting further in front of the others and have to wait. As the sun rises, this place becomes more dangerous and the heat more dehydrating. There's no real safe place to stop, so I continue to press on. There's a nearly continuous safety

opposite Down, down, down

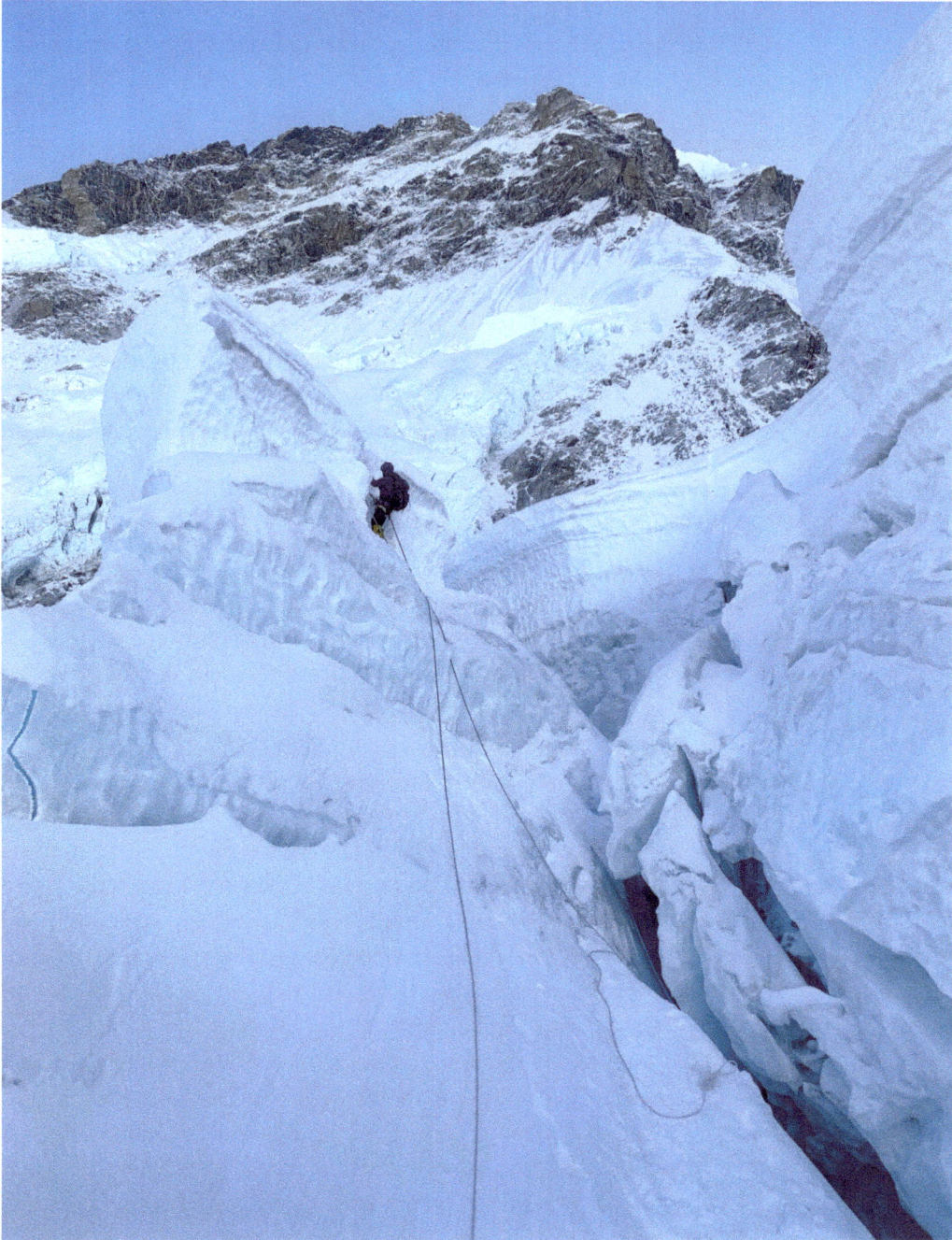

line, so it's almost impossible to go the wrong way. Generally, where there's no trail, crevasses or walls of ice make it impossible to veer off it.

I can clearly identify the 'football field' this time.

Moving solo now, I eventually catch Sumon and his client, who are taking a break. They don't object to my passing, so I continue along.

Meeting two porters, they claim to recognise me from Facebook.

'But I'm not on Facebook.'

'Ahh, the CTSS Facebook. You were leading and have the beard.'

Okay, I'll take their word for it, and compliment them on having good memories.

Time to push on, it's heating up.

My rappelling is now getting fine-tuned, with no oversight required. I watch the occasional porters come scurrying down from nowhere. How they navigate this environment is worth trying to emulate. Quickly, they tend to disappear.

I can see Base Camp slowly coming closer and, still solo, press my own pace to get to the lower sections and navigate my way out. But nothing looks familiar anymore. So much snow has melted and the trail is unrecognisable. What was once snow underfoot is now rock and flowing water. Landmark ice structures are gone. Glaciers have been reduced to streams. I have to pay attention to what footprints I can see to keep picking up the trail. Careful to not 'cut through' anybody else's camps, I take a longer trek before arriving back at Base Camp.

It's taken less than five hours to get from Camp 2 back to Base Camp. I'm content with my efforts.

Now, hot water, that's something else. When you can't remember your last shower, it's cold out and you have to wait in line for it . . . wow, it becomes special. After filling the drum with the help of a stranger, it's time. The hot sensation over skin that hasn't seen the light of day for ages. The steam that gets in your face. Soap that promises to remove the smells of many days' worth of sweat. It's so good. I feel like a new human.

I hear that the lines to the summit were laid today, and the record holder on his twenty-fifth ascent was the first to summit. This significant event allows everyone else to follow, as weather permits. And there's a weather window opening for 12—13 May that has everyone talking. It would be tough for me to turn around and climb again tomorrow, but missing it could result in another week at Base Camp.

Other news is that Mike has left hospital and is waiting in a hotel to get back here, which is great news. Then there's that old chestnut—Covid. Everyone who didn't have Covid has had a four- to five-night stay in Lukla to refresh and prepare for the big one—the summit push. Slowly, as helicopter logistics allow, all those climbers return, including Ryan.

Around and around the rumour mill runs on the smallest update, with weather being the favourite subject for speculation.

Tendi addresses our dining tent at length over dinner. Everything is discussed, from clarifying the weather opportunity to how they'll allocate the oxygen. It looks like a large portion of climbers from CTSS will try utilising this first weather window. It would be great to get back up there and try for summit. In my view, any small inconvenience now isn't worth postponing an attempt for another week. Besides, the second weather window will be busy. Not many camps or climbers are actually ready for this window. Although that could, in fact, include me.

I've discussed it with Ryan. We both think we should go. Tenji has to talk it over with Big Tendi, as he'd be guiding us. I believe Tenji is happy to take Ryan and me, but April has said that she's ready to go too. I'm unsure how this sits in practice and will have to see how it plays out.

I've had an appetite since getting down, and begin to bank some calories. Hopefully a good sleep will follow.

Decision day

A yellow glow lights the inside of my tent. It's first light gently bringing me back from a deep slumber. Headaches, in varying severity, have come to define my waking hours. But not today. Warm, in no rush, I get to lie here in contemplation. I can feel the sun hitting camp. It's a new day.

A call back home is a welcome break from the mountain's constant demands. The stories Heidi tells me, my kids' voices and the sounds of our normal, chaotic family life are all the motivation I need to get to the summit and, more importantly, get back home. Just explaining to Heidi what I'm up to brings my ambitions back into focus. The opportunity I have to climb this tough mountain, and to be here a second time, is a gift. To have technology that enables this conversation via satellite is another gift. That I have a family back home who support me regardless of any summit—priceless.

Yet my son simplifies it, asking, 'Can you make it to the top this time?'

The weather has been updated. 12 May—summit day, with very little tolerance. All those who were hoping 13 May would be an option have had to postpone their attempt. That has reduced the number departing significantly—to seven, I think.

Ryan and I have decided, with the Sherpa's permission, that it's our time to climb.

First on the to-do list is receive our oxygen mask, which we check for fit, and regulator. Packing has to be extremely well thought out. Miss something and there's no getting back up the mountain. Pack too much and your pack becomes a burden for you, or, worse, for some poor porter.

I'm as ready as I can be.

As we sit in the dining tent, a thunderous avalanche can be heard. It's loud, the type that gets you off your chair to inspect. Rushing outside, we see that it's to the right of the Icefall. High up, an accumulated section of ice and snow has let go and continues its long and destructive path towards the bottom of the valley. It's a big one and I momentarily wonder if it could reach the bottom of the valley, or indeed cross it.

I try to assess how I feel about departing so soon. Nothing there, really. I just want to get back onto the mountain and give my all for better or worse.

We have the destination firmly set in our minds. The weather is confirmed as ideal, if only momentarily. It's time to double down to make sure we get to the summit, experience it, and get back to our 'safe lives'. If successful, and when we return, we'll celebrate.

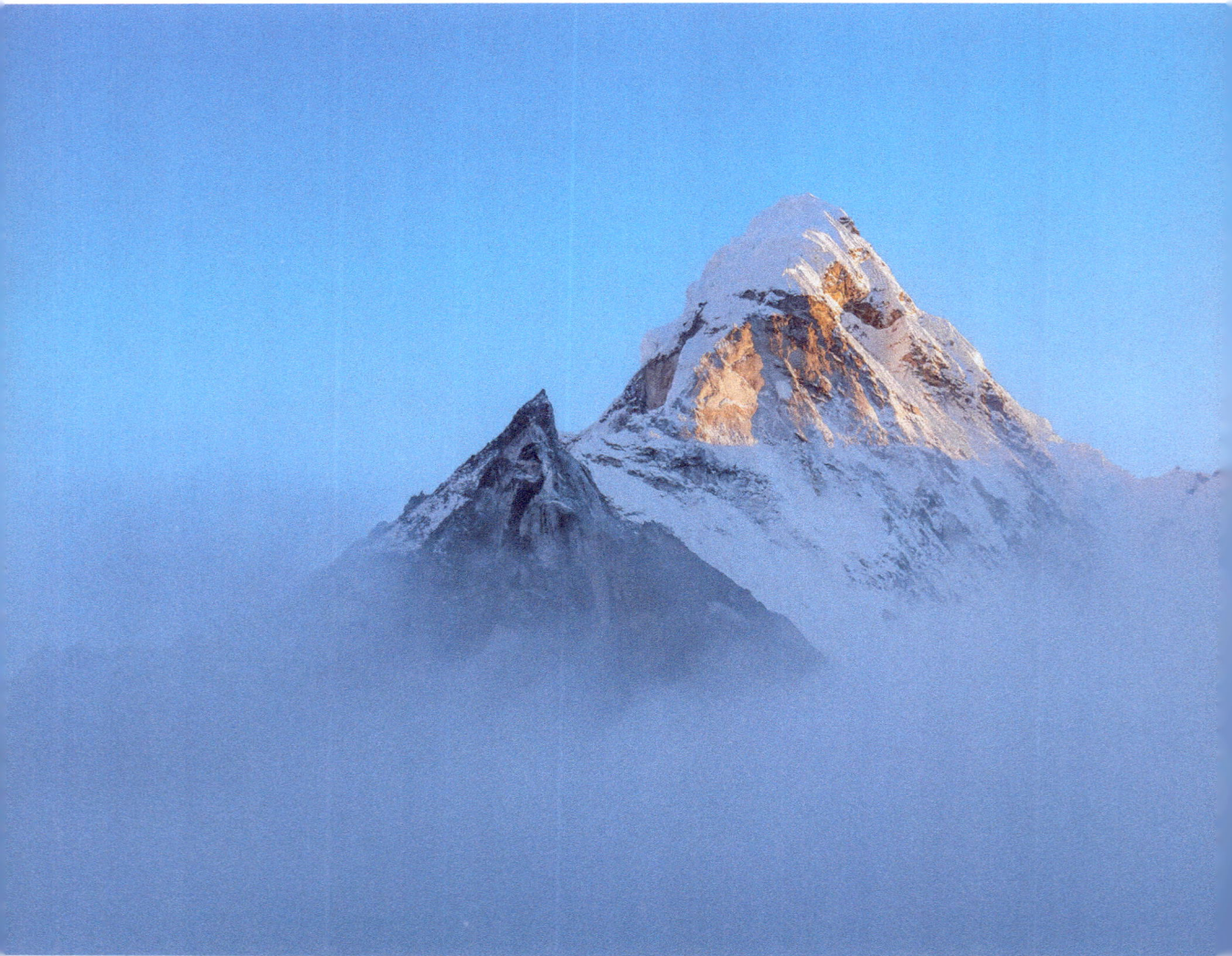

SUMMIT

11

I'S MOTHER'S DAY.

To manifest change in this world, Heidi supports and uplifts those around her, and is a mother in every instance first and foremost. This day belongs to her.

To have a strong woman supporting my undertakings demonstrates strength and character that our children can learn from. Heidi has supported this challenge from the start—excluding Everest. She is never afraid to share her thoughts, regardless of what people think, but those thoughts are always delivered with poise. She has picked her battles over the years and could be forgiven for knowing I would still attempt this hill.

It's 1am—time to rise, and make those final adjustments to my pack.

This is it, a continuous program to the top of the world. I'm excited just to get back out into the mountains, to see the beauty. Every time there's something new to see or experience, and that's what gets me up on time.

At 2am I'm standing ready, rugged up, harnessed and sipping hot coffee.

There was little sleep last night due to party music at a nearby camp, and there also seemed to be more avalanches than usual rumbling their way down the mountainside. But the morning weather has never been so still and clear. When you have a long day ahead, they're the conditions you dream about.

A small fire is burning at the puja and smoke drifts straight up, leaving a distinct smell in its trail. Our small contingent

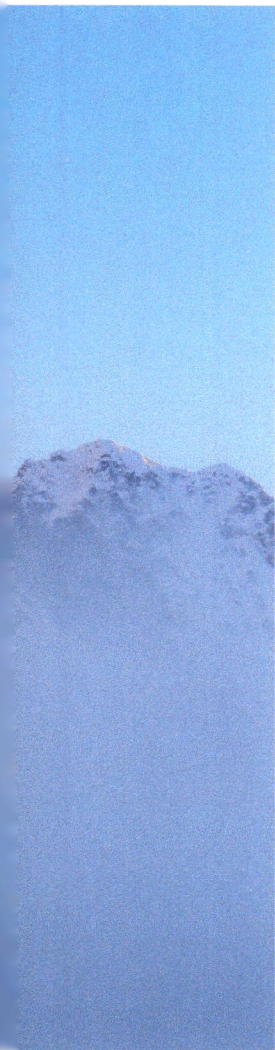

DISTANCE: 7.33km
TIME: 10:41 hrs
AVERAGE SPEED: 0.7kph
ASCENT: 1,123m
DESCENT: 97m

circles briefly. Some pray, and we give rice offerings before our departure. Silently, in reflection, we exit camp with hope in our hearts and our purpose in front of us.

It has just occurred to me that I'll be the first person in the world to have been evacuated from Base Camp with Covid and subsequently returned to summit—should we be success-ful. While I'm optimistic, I've come to expect a lot of twists, turns and surprises in this journey.

The ice is melting. Where icy surfaces once threatened to slip us up, rocks now lie bare. Our 8,000-metre boots are sturdy, but traversing the rock paths in all our climbing gear is still tricky. Running streams and fragile, semi-melting ice have replaced the glacier travel we first experienced.

After a half-hour hike, it's time for crampons. We've once again entered the frozen environment that is the famed Khumbu Icefall.

I'm tucked in behind Tenji, who's leading, but he doesn't allow me to push the pace. At every turn we'll wait for Ryan, who's behind me. April is behind Ryan, and Dorji makes up our small team to the rear.

The first vertical climb doesn't have the crowds we had to manoeuvre through last time. It's a great test for the lungs in the early morning air, and helps us to gauge our confidence. I scale it with relative ease, which sets the tone for my morning climb through the seracs.

Hours seem to slide by in the dark, one at a time. The morning light reveals spectacular scenery and fog that hov-ers below us, weaving its way through the mountain range. A ladder in our path always creates a sense of occasion. Sunlight highlights the tips of the mountains, which I could never grow tired of viewing.

At the top of the Icefall, ascending together, I suddenly no longer feel like it's me against the mountain. I feel part of something inclusive, a team. These guys believe in me and I have trust that they'll be there when it matters.

opposite What a morning

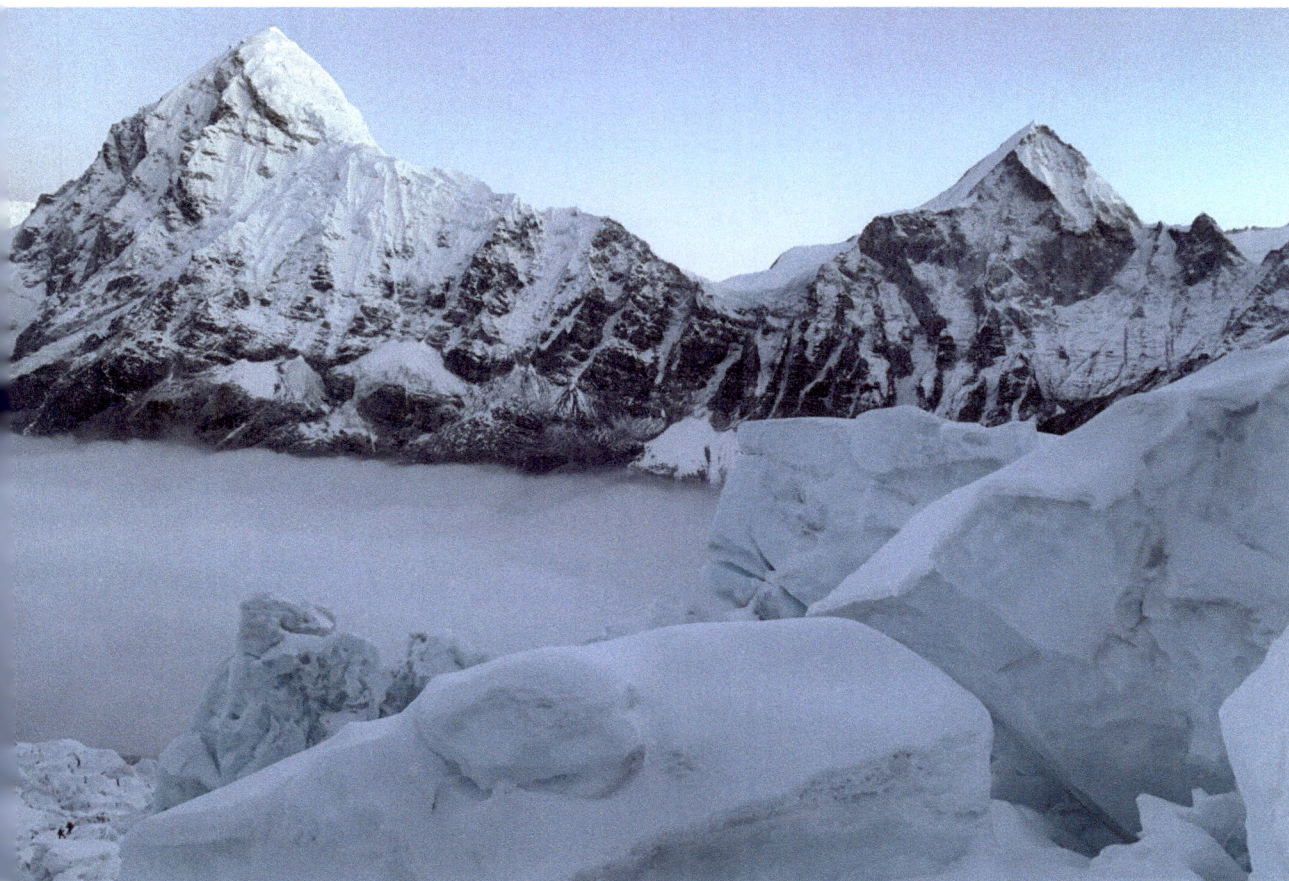

Before exiting there are steeper ladders and sharper grades to navigate together. Then it finally flattens out. We pass Camp 1 and continue steadily into the Western Cwm.

With these clear conditions it's hot—really hot. It's not time to be complacent, as 'snow bridges' can hide deep crevasses from unwary climbers. Other crevasses have already been identified and rigged with ladders.

The last hours coming uphill towards Camp 2 under the relentless heat and glare are soul-destroying. You can see it in everyone's faces, hear it in their voices, and witness it in the slow march that still hasn't finished. I close one eye at a time, trying to focus on where the next step goes. The glare penetrates my sunglasses, and any exposed skin is burning despite the frequent application of sunscreen. My lips cannot be protected enough, and shrivel.

The pace is slow, but set by Tenji.

It feels like longer, perhaps unnecessary exposure to me, but he's insistent the slower pace means we will retain more energy for tomorrow. So under the beating sun we absorb all the radiation a white field of snow can offer.

At Camp 2, I sit on the first available rock. Ryan lies down, his body slumping. The kitchen hand serves lemon water. It stings my lips at the touch, but the healing process has to begin. Big Tendi is here on a separate rotation and welcomes us, which is always a pleasure. The positivity of the guy can cut through the most depressing circumstances.

As soon as we can manage, it's time to get horizontal for the required rest. The process has become all too familiar. Roll your sleeping pad out, check for any sinister-looking rocks, throw your pack in, and strip down some layers. Ready to sleep. As the afternoon cools, I'll blow up the air mattress and rummage for my sleeping bag so that I don't catch a chill.

My nap is a good two-and-a-half hours. That's a long nap for me, and it felt great. No headache, got some fluids in and generally just enough energy to comfortably get myself up for dinner.

DISTANCE: 2.98km
TIME: 05:34 hrs
AVERAGE SPEED: 0.5kph
ASCENT: 549m
DESCENT: 0m
PULSE OX: 80%

Camp 2 to Camp 3

For the first time I don my technical, one-piece, down summit suit. I'm leaving all the climbing gear here that has served me so well: my climbing pants, big jacket and favoured puffy vest. Reducing weight now is a priority.

For the first time I'm introduced to my personal guide, Lhakpa Tsering Sherpa. What he lacks in English-speaking skills is more than compensated by his experience, including multiple summits of Everest from both the south and north.

Leaving Camp 2 at 11am, I fully expect a brutal grilling by the sun, but it's short-lived. Cloud covers the entire valley, offering some reprieve. Conditions remain warm but not debilitating. But by the time we're strapping crampons on, the only base layer I have underneath my summit suit is drenched in perspiration. There's nothing that can be done except drop the top half off to be tied around my waist and open the leg vents. This offers some reprieve. Then the wind picks up again and the chill follows, and just as quickly the top half of my suit goes on again.

Moving across the approach to Lhotse face, Tenji again insists on a slow pace to preserve energy.

Chaos is waiting on Lhotse face as we catch the crowd in front. Wind sweeps snow off the mountain's face and clouds all but cover the afternoon sun. Climbing now becomes slow, real slow. The terrain is steep, and this is a mammoth mountain face to scale. Leapfrogging a few people here and there doesn't actually get you any further faster. All one can do is follow the pace of the chain of people, and we find we are all one. It's too steep and risky to overtake, although some porters do. Most of us just accept the situation and exercise patience.

Standing still on the slope turns out to be the biggest challenge. There are some great footholds, but when you get caught without them for extended periods it's just brutal on the muscles. The spikes of crampons surely weren't designed to be balanced on for extended periods. It would be nice to move a little faster. Bloody crowds.

We come over the same vertical ice climb to arrive at Camp 3. Dropping our bags for a drink, I notice a lot more tents have been set. Looking further up the hill, on the outskirts of everybody's camps, I see four tents standing on a slight ridge. I somehow know they will be ours.

After a short break, we continue the slog upwards to the outskirts of Camp 3, at what seems like the highest point. Exhausted, Ryan and I are shown our tent by Tenji.

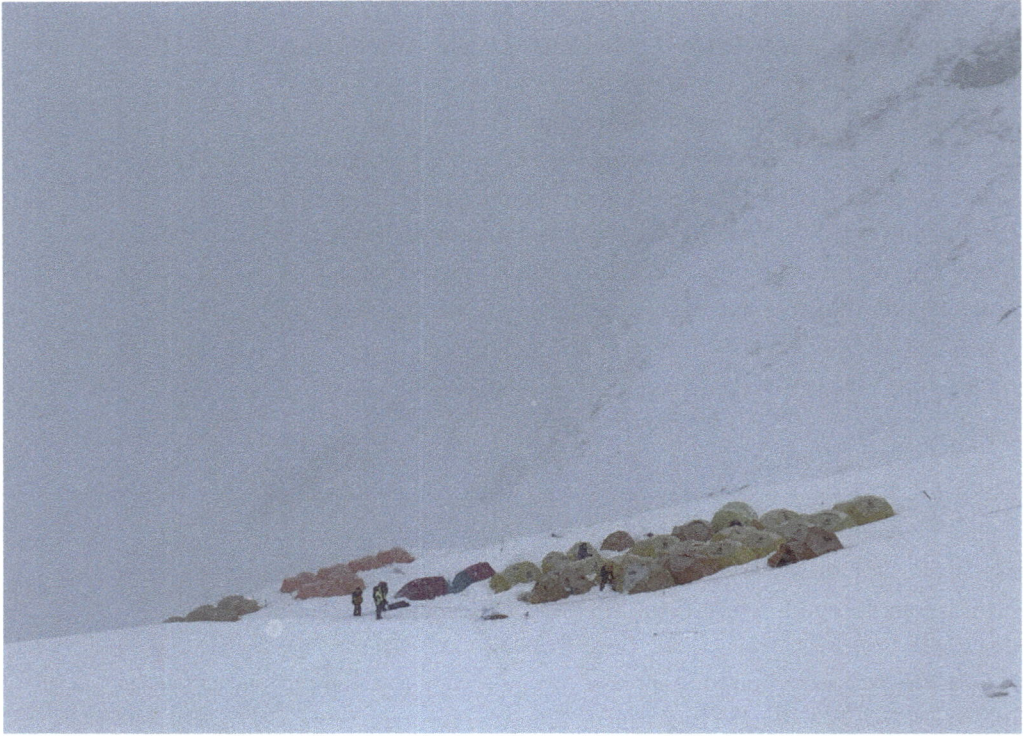

above Camp 3

right Two tent mates

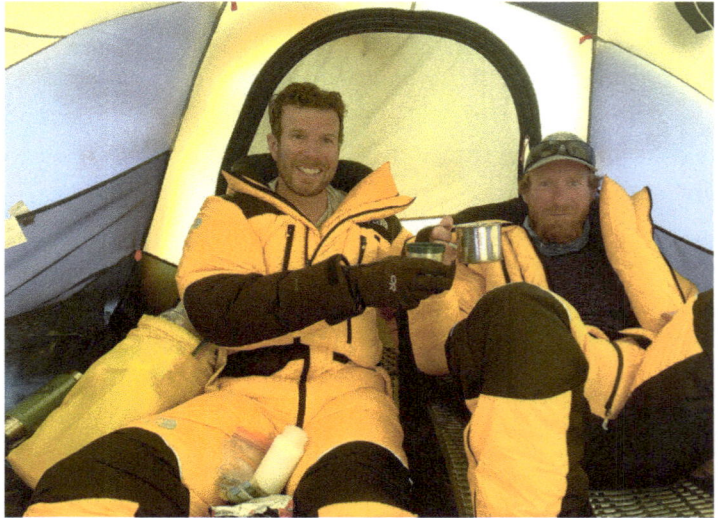

'Don't forget to take your crampons off before getting in the tent.'

Silly things happen when you're tired, but we worked efficiently to get sorted in that tent in record speed.

Arrived.

An hour after arriving my chest is still thumping. Our bodies will only continue to deteriorate. It was a taxing day yet again, but when all the work's done, you have to admire how high you've pushed. Looking over the camps below, I try to view the situation differently. We've got less climbing to do tomorrow than others. If only marginally.

Food is hard to get down. Fatigue has set in. The body is in knots, bracing itself for sleep on an uneven tent surface. But tonight, in another first, we'll sleep on compressed gas, which will hopefully help our bodies to adjust within these nylon walls.

Camp 3 to Camp 4

Spending the night on compressed gas was a little claustrophobic, and has left me staring at a significant dribble patch. But that's normal, right?

Our tent walls are covered with a thick frost, yet we are warm. The blizzard that circulates as we knock the tent's walls to dislodge the snow does nothing to distract our preparations. Ryan and I have made sharing a tent seamless. Both of us shuffle at about the same speed, go through nearly the same order of tasks, and are prepared for an on-schedule departure. There's no such thing as an 'on time' departure.

Out we shuffle together, crampons on, at the ready. Lhakpa Tsering is waiting patiently just outside our tent door for some personal gear to take to Camp 4.

But while Ryan and I are ready, April is not.

So I stand there in the cold morning air, stomping my feet to try to warm them, staring at the hill ahead and getting

DISTANCE: 0.97km

TIME: 8:25 hrs

AVERAGE SPEED: 0.1kph

ASCENT: 496m

DESCENT: 5m

colder and colder. Climbers are already on the track in numbers and ascending the ropes. The first section looks like an ice climb, then the route just appears to continue going up.

With a fresh bottle of oxygen rigged up, we're ready, finally. All the disappointment of waiting around vanishes as we climb.

The views from up here are amazing. There are deep crevasses to glare into. Ledges, once traversed, have magical views to look back from. With these clear blue skies I can see all the way back to Camp 2 with its rocky exposed ledges. Features of Everest are discussed as her legendary topography comes closer into view.

A lot of the climbing is mostly, well, up. We're on Lhotse face, which is steep. The track is narrow and passing frequently difficult.

My feet have been ice blocks for four hours now because of the waiting around. I inform Tenji, who replies, 'C'mon, man. Really stomp and kick them in. They should be warm by now.'

As we started to the rear, we encountered minimal crowds. It was a little slow as we climbed the yellow band—a strip of limestone that is more like clinging to smooth rocks with fixed ropes than stomping into hard-packed ice. The thirty-degree angle and slippery nature slows everyone down, but after this it's a long sweeping walk to our left in fresh snow. The climbers before us have left their mark, which defines the path.

Late in the day the wind uncomfortably picks up. Clouds have combined to remove any view. Then a 'what the?' moment. A guy's coming down with skis on his pack. This track is hard enough to walk on, and I wonder where they could be used.

It's a steep, unclimbed bank to one side, with a ridiculous drop off the other. Hence we're always clipped onto a safety rope, or each other. One tricky, vertical ascent to go. The Geneva Spur, an anvil-shaped rib of black rock, has been reached. This long day's climb is done.

Eight-and-a-half hours after departure, we take an easy walk around to the right and we're here—South Col, Camp 4.

It's a harsh place. We have to navigate decades' worth of discarded tents, gear and detritus. The wind blows harder here. As I walk through camp, looking for our tents, there are plenty of signs of destruction. Many tents have been ripped apart by the wind. Some are half standing, some flat to the ground, and some just reduced to parts. Yes, there's rubbish too, and discarded oxygen bottles.

This is the death zone—a place of survival—and unfortunately that means the area isn't maintained well. A place of transition, climbers and Sherpa alike urinate and defecate wherever is easiest in this inhospitable habitat. Normal standards of human behaviour are simply too onerous to apply in this harsh environment. But while using walking paths is one thing, relieving oneself around the tents or while still 'clipped on' raises eyebrows.

It may be a harsh environment, but it's surrounded by majestic mountain views. And there it is, as the backdrop—the pyramid-shaped summit of Mt Everest with a plume of snow streaming off her as fierce winds roar.

The weather is really turning. Wind here strips the rocks bare.

Our tents are of course isolated away from the main camp, and are the most distant. The largest of rocks anchor the tents to the ice, where we hope they will stay. Before I hunker down, I stabilise my GoPro behind the tent and point it towards the view we came to see—Mt Everest. Hopefully it captures the coming and going of clouds as dusk settles.

April, Ryan, Tenji and I are to share what's typically a two-person tent. Add all the climbing gear we don't want to freeze, plus all our oxygen bottles, and it's tight. We're really just lying all over our bags in a disorderly fashion. But we only have a few hours' rest here, so no point in worrying too much.

Dorji has wedged himself in the tent's door to cook and melt water, which boils at lower temperatures at higher altitudes. It's produced from snow and ice collected from a dirty plateau, and isn't pleasant. There are visible 'floaties' to contend with.

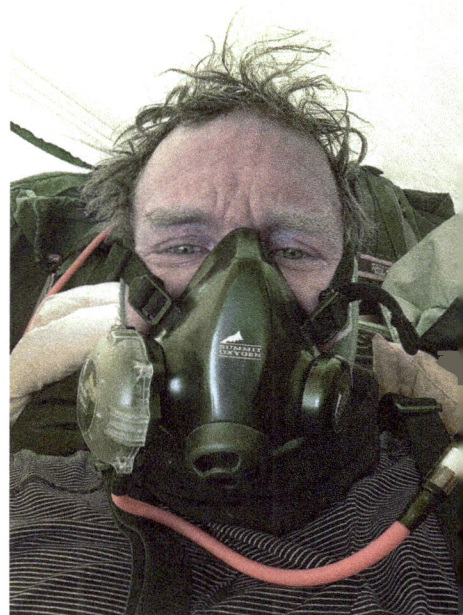

above Life at Camp 4— 'The Death Zone'

'Guys, sleeping bag on!' Tenji announces.

We laugh. Yeah right, five of us in here and we'll (try to) nap before a bite to eat? The tent continues to shake violently. Nobody sleeps—not even Ryan, who's normally great at fitting in a power nap.

The priority is to shuffle all your main summiting items around so that you know where everything is. Then the nerves and anxiety over what's to come settle in. This is it, the real deal. Soon we'll tackle the highest peak on Earth, the reason we came. Training's over, it's game on.

Out of the tiny tent's quarters we emerge, oxygen bottles always connected. Just five minutes disconnected here leaves you uncomfortable and short of breath. Shuffling around, in full climbing gear, it's headlamps on. The smell of burning incense fills the air as we attach our crampons firmly to give these boots the traction required. I look around. Nobody is still, everyone is in the zone. We're in expedition mode.

The atmosphere fills with suspense as the night darkens and everybody jostles to ready themselves. Gotta move to be warm. The wind has abated, the environment feels calmer, nobody rushes or stresses, and every step and precaution to depart has been taken.

I'm ready. Taking a few departing photos of nothing in particular, Lhakpa Tsering Sherpa (Cherry), my companion and personal Sherpa, has found my side. With a couple of head waggles, we take the first steps to depart. Ryan is directly in front, identifiable by the pink flamingo hanging out of his backpack.

Harmoniously, we form our single trekking line at about 10pm on the night of 11 May.

Camp 4 to Summit

I thought the man sitting with his backpack on might be taking a break, so I'm puzzled that he's not far from our tents. Then I realise he's breathless and lifeless, and the first corpse I've seen on the mountain.

From the start I just want to settle into my breathing and be at one with my altitude worker's pace, or have him be happy with mine. But the incline from South Col up the Triangular Face provides an opportunity for nimble teams to push past on the single track and chop in. Though we're independent with personal Sherpa, until now we mostly moved as a group. But from the very first hour, I can tell Cherry isn't happy with this position and we become ruthless in the 'overtaking'

SUMMIT BID

DEPARTURE: 11 May—10:03pm

DISTANCE: 2:23km

TIME: 14:28 hrs

AVERAGE SPEED: 0.1kph

ASCENT: 901m

DESCENT: 876m

ARRIVAL C4: 12 May—12:31pm

50 people, including Sherpa, summited

CTSS: 17 summits

below In awe of Everest

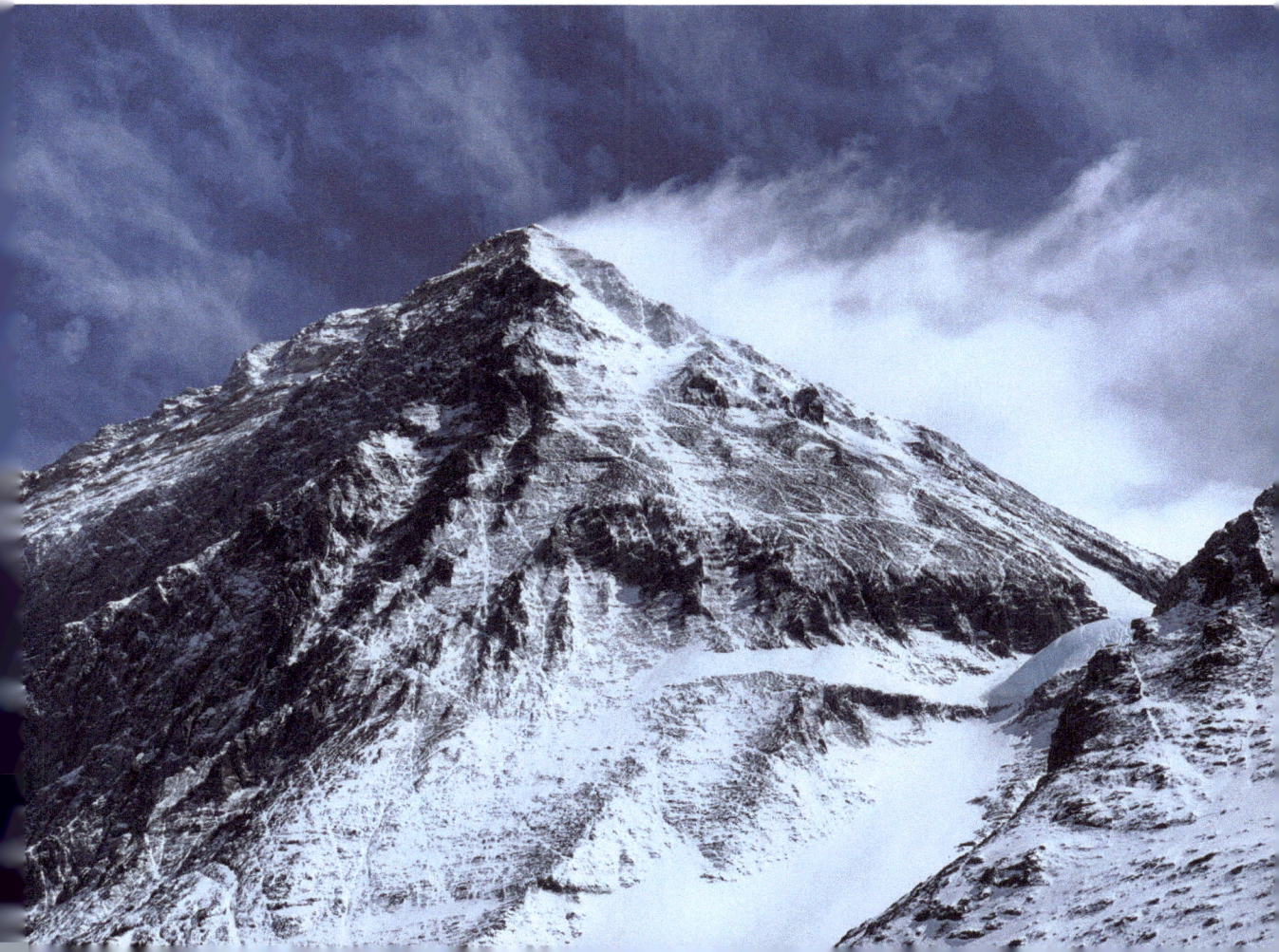

shenanigans. Stepping out from the single ascending line, we stomp up the hill at a pace that feels unsustainable. I'm gassed. And we have hours upon hours to go.

But I also want to get it done!

Cherry either doesn't understand too much English or doesn't want to, although I have picked up that a rattling of the harness means we are overtaking. I press hard to keep up a uniform pace. When not exhausting myself, the constant lightning storm that flashes through the sky can occupy my attention until the next gasp and we move again. But I soon learn that Cherry too is only human. Progression ever upwards is extremely taxing on both the body and the lungs. It's cold and it's hard work. Cherry frequently makes some ground, then we pause. We both gasp, he rests his weight over one knee, then we push on.

What is this? Up ahead there's a huge piece of rock, which the few climbers in front of us seem puzzled how to scale. Yep, you can't go around it, you must go over it. It's dark, really dark, but I recognise this landmark from previous days.

I think it can't be too far to the summit from here. How wrong I am.

One particular gentleman is struggling to scale this section. In turn, people have to wait. I wonder how he has trained, how he'll continue—he doesn't look in a good way. Eventually he pulls out to the side, exhausted, three-quarters of the way up. Now every other climber has an additional challenge—to clip a spare carabineer around this exhausted guy and back onto the fixed line above.

The fixed line nearly every climber relies on is simply a rope that is anchored to the route and left in place. Used correctly, it allows safe, quick travel up and down difficult or dangerous stretches, which is most of this mountain. Just one climber, however, can stop or slow many others here. Worse, any time you're not 'clipped on', which is essentially attached to that rope via a personal carabineer tied to your own harness, safety is compromised.

The Balcony is a small platform at 8,400 metres where we take our first real break. We've passed all but a handful of climbers and here swap in a new bottle of oxygen. My water is frozen, and barely a drop comes out. I'd taken all the precautions and used insulation sleeves, but it's too late, so I opt for some gummy bear sweets instead.

We've transitioned the South Summit at 8,750 metres, but are now forced to descend several times along the undulating ridge, losing hard-gained altitude. The true summit remains elusive, always further than I think, and I'm somewhat surprised how much further we still have to go. From here the iconic ridgeline view is truly spectacular all the way to the true summit.

We're following the knife-edge of the southeast ridge along the 'cornice traverse' that leads to Hillary Step. Snow is covering intermittent sections of rock. One minute you're rising, the next looking straight down. There are some really exposed sections here on the southeast ridge. It's some 8,000 feet down the southwest face to one side and 11,000 feet down the Kangshung face on the other.

Suddenly there's a crisis.

We have one spare bottle of oxygen, two guys that need it, and Cherry has a broken regulator. Is this what will turn us around? Cherry tries to troubleshoot the immediate issue and imminent danger.

Is this the end?

We're standing here alone on this dangerous ridge, clipped onto a line that narrowly separates disaster from survival in the event of a misstep, yet something else has my attention. For the last half hour, before this oxygen-regulator crisis struck, I've been watching the star scattered pitch-black sky give way at the horizon to a long, thin, light blue strip as far as the eye can see. I look to one side of Everest's ridge and instinctively know that sunrise is coming. The other, darker clouds are set lower than the mountains. We are truly above the local weather.

So as I stand, anchored, on the ridge, it's the sunrise that provides the 'wow' moment.

I don't even take a picture at first, I'm so awestruck. Then it dawns on me that I must. Without a doubt, it's one of the best, if not *the* best, sunrises I've witnessed. The sun pierces the horizon with a bright, shining presence, drifting into full display and lighting up the sky. Patches of orange leave highlights on the clouds beneath the sun, while a thin band of light is reflected above it. The snow is no longer cold and hard, but looks softer and shimmers in a new shade of white.

Now the new day has arrived, what are we going to do to move from here? Which direction will we go?

'Wait here, I'll be back...'

And with that Cherry is gone and I'm truly alone.

For me, oxygen at this extreme altitude is non-negotiable. In this temperature of some minus thirty-five degrees Celsius my mind is lost to the horizon, yet I intuitively know my body is slowly dying. I've suffered a lot to be here. Those hardy souls who insist on climbing without supplemental oxygen attempt a feat that remains rare and was once considered scientifically impossible. I have concerns. Not just for my breathing, but for Cherry, who hasn't had oxygen for some fifteen minutes now. I can see the concern and panic written across his face as he returns.

Frantic, he asks people as they pass, 'Regulator?'

He's constantly on the radio, but eventually scurries up the nearby pitch and, unbelievably, returns with a regulator.

Our summit bid can continue.

Depleted by lack of sleep and food, and with water bottles frozen, my perceived limits are officially shattered. Left with a single objective, nothing has any significance at this point except to reach the destination. And when what is in front of you is the biggest thing in any direction, it's an easy but painful mistake to assume you're close to the top.

The dawn is motivating, mainly because the bitter cold is thawing.

opposite, left

Admiring the view

opposite, right Sunrise!

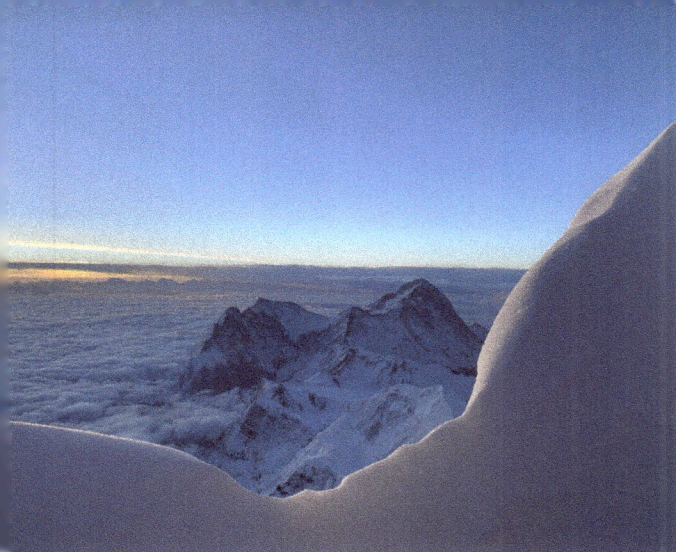
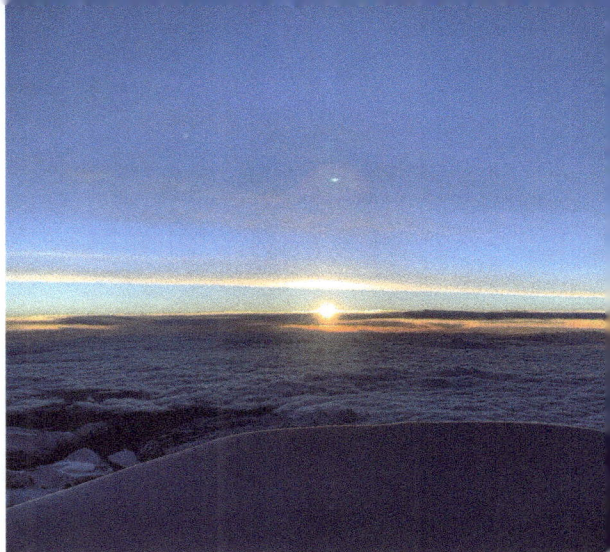

I can't find words for the landscape before me. All my senses leave me with just emotions of gratitude. There's a joy to simply be still moving forwards and upwards.

We arrive at the famed Hillary Step, a twelve-metre wall of rock. It's a dominant section that presents us with a fixed rope to trust, a perilous drop to our left, and a singular pass to shuffle along.

Hanging off the edge, still connected to the safety ropes by slings, is a dead man. I'm told he has been here since 2019. After the initial shock, I wonder if he's real. From a distance you can't tell with full climbing gear, goggles, masks, and so on. A group is gathered near him, and people try not to stare. There's a delay going up the steep, rugged section, past where he appears to have come to grief.

One by one, people shuffle past. Waiting my turn, I can't imagine his final thoughts, looking down at the continuous drop. Out of respect for the Nepalese government's wishes for this season, I don't take pictures. Regrettably, plenty of other people do.

This season there's an independent film crew doing a documentary on the attempted recovery of two people who died on the mountain in 2019. Three alpine workers are tasked with the impossible challenge of muscling one of the bodies

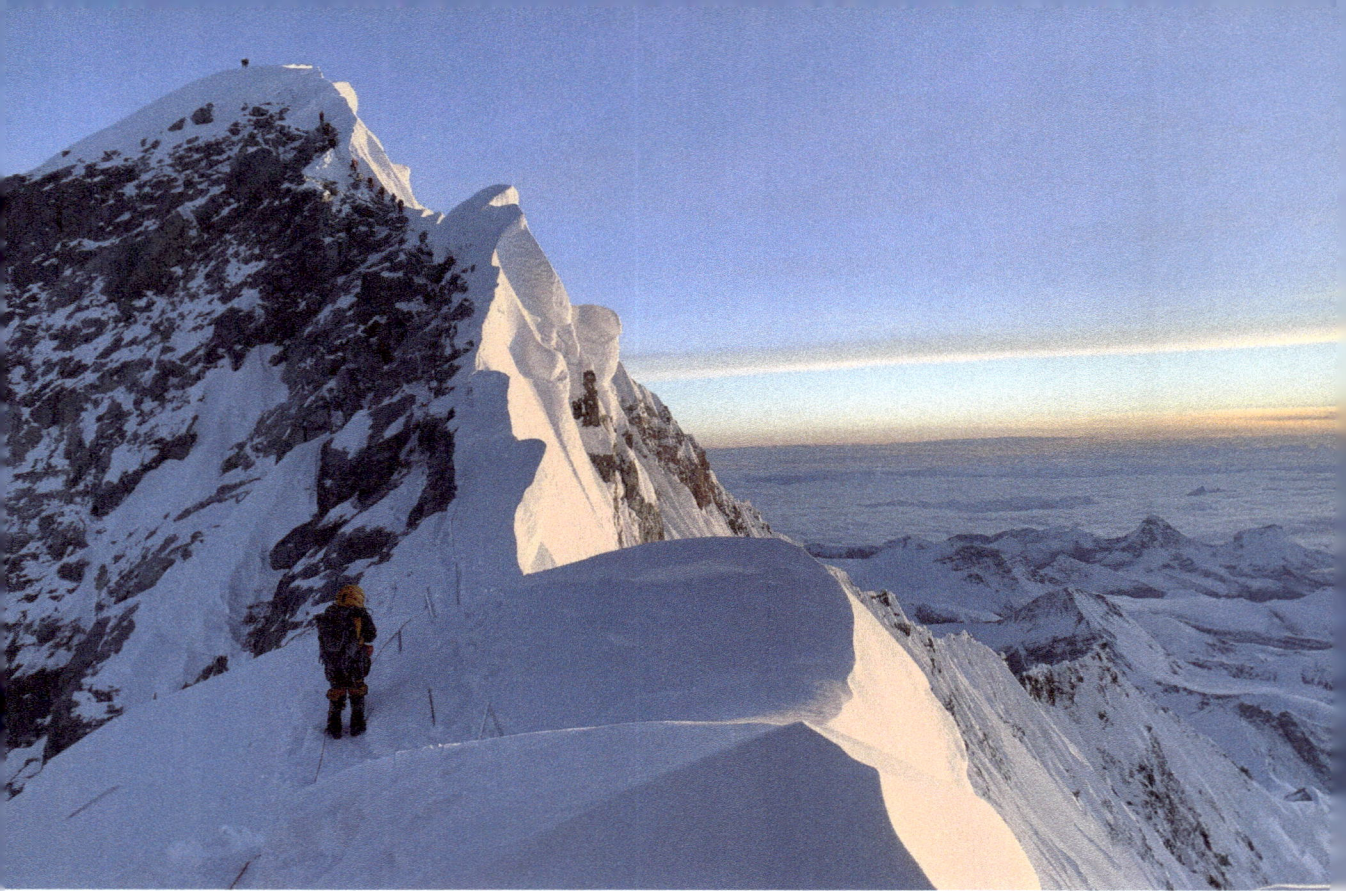

from its resting place. The task was so taxing that the film crew stepped in to assist. Sadly, the recovery attempt was unsuccessful.

I have a near full bottle of oxygen to trust in, which offers an abstract glimmer of hope.

I can see the summit, I'm nearly there!

It's like treading water and I don't want to be defeated now. Exhausted, I push on. The lack of fluids, the lack of food, the lack of oxygen mean my body is struggling. I'm literally slowly killing my body.

Move forward ... the end is so close.

It's around 8:40 am. The few people in front of us are stationary, celebrating. There is no further to go. Here is the

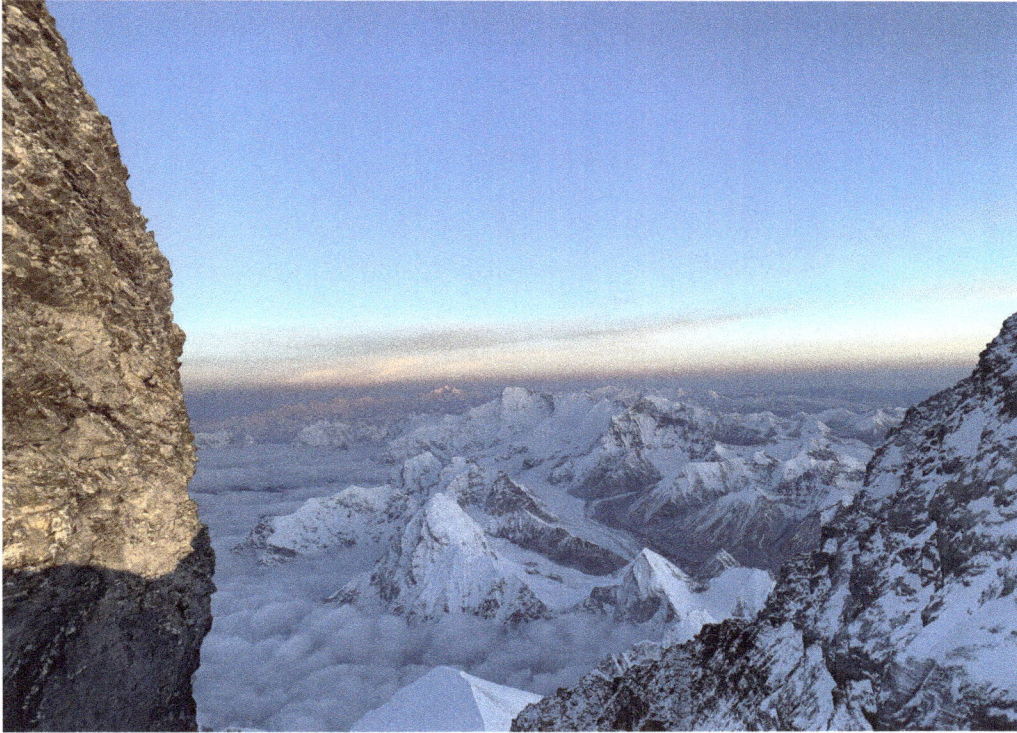

summit—the last steps to the very top. Too exhausted to celebrate on the side of an ice-clad hill, I clip my bag to the last
guide stake and simply sit. Here on the ridge that is the border
between Nepal and China, I stare at a whole new climbing
route and a whole new country from my humble seat. The
area on my immediate left is surrounded by Buddhist prayer
flags, a small statue and more people now frequently arriving.

That abstract concept, time, with its man-made seconds
and minutes, floats past without much thought.

All the unsaid pressure, doubts and fears don't exist here.

The views of these rugged, snow-covered mountains and
these peaceful moments will be remembered long after I depart.
Once distant, intimidating impressions of the biggest, highest

above High above...
everything

opposite Traversing
the ridgeline

mountain on Earth are no more. Now those impressions are reality. Sitting here—'on top of the world'—is truly a privilege.

Mt Everest captures the human imagination like no other mountain, and rightly so. Both triumphs and tragedies are part of its captivating story.

It's already 9:15am. The arrival of new summiteers is an opportunity to ask a nearby alpine worker to assist with my summit photo. Removing my mask to engage in strained communications, I have to persevere past the language barrier. The photo I'm trying to stage isn't one of myself in some hero pose. Standing in a state of exhaustion, I'd like my Sherpa, Cherry, to hold my cherished Diabetes Australia flag with me. We got here together. It's what feels right in the moment, and I wouldn't be here without this individual's respected effort.

I feel proud, if only for a few moments. I hope Cherry feels the same way.

My phone freezes for the exposure shortly after we get in position.

'Did you get the picture?' I gasp, receiving my phone back. 'Yes, yes, yes.'

We'll see, and, now that's done, I have nothing but contemplation as I sit back and absorb.

Caught in my own fatigue, just to be present here, I'm so grateful.

I'm surprised and a little deflated by the sight of the now growing crowd's antics. Not all, but a few offenders are littering, throwing sponsor banners and engaging in ever-competing cheers, seemingly trying to be better than the last. I'm trying not to judge, as I know their stories are varied and often compelling, but the moment didn't match the reality of what I'm witnessing.

It's going to be a hard journey down too. More people die descending from the summit than trying to reach it. I reach for more gummy sweets.

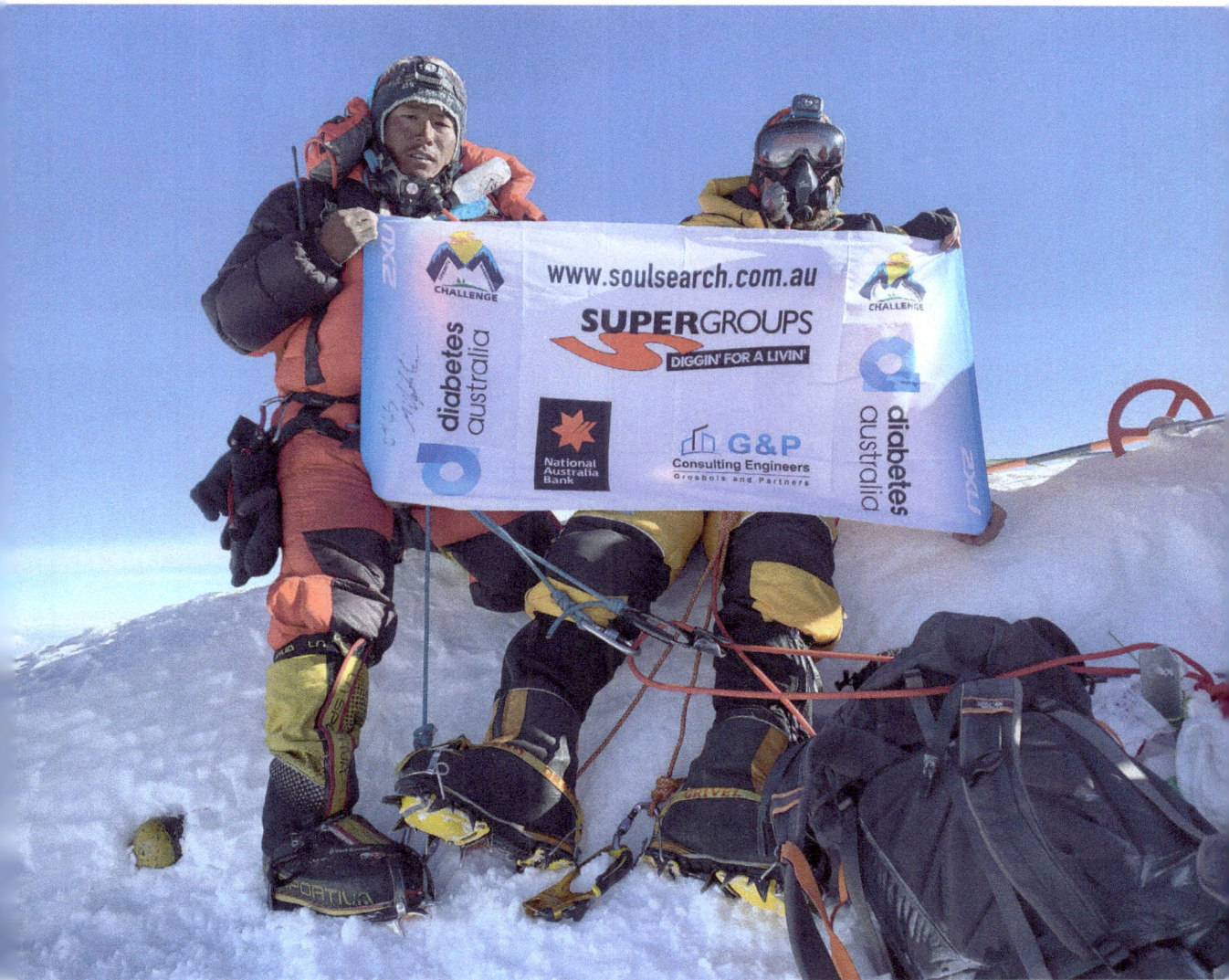

above My cherished
one Summit photo

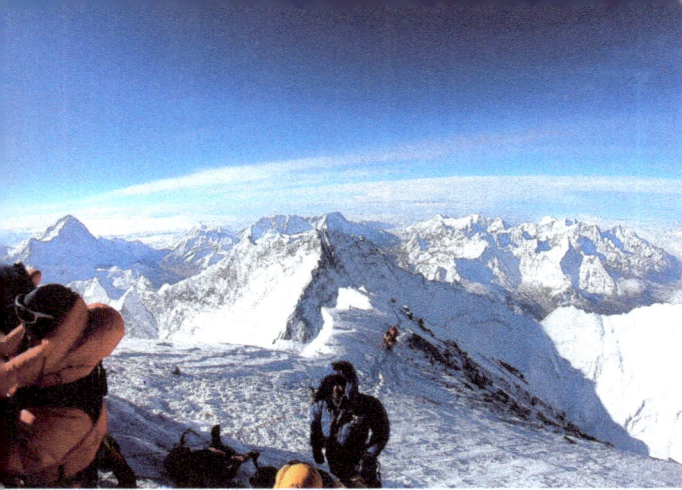
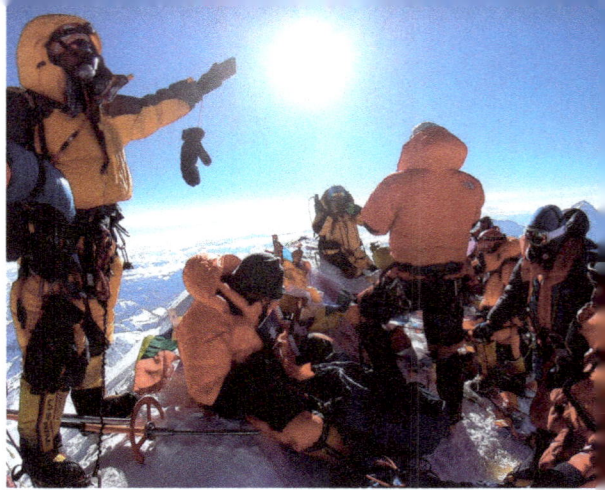
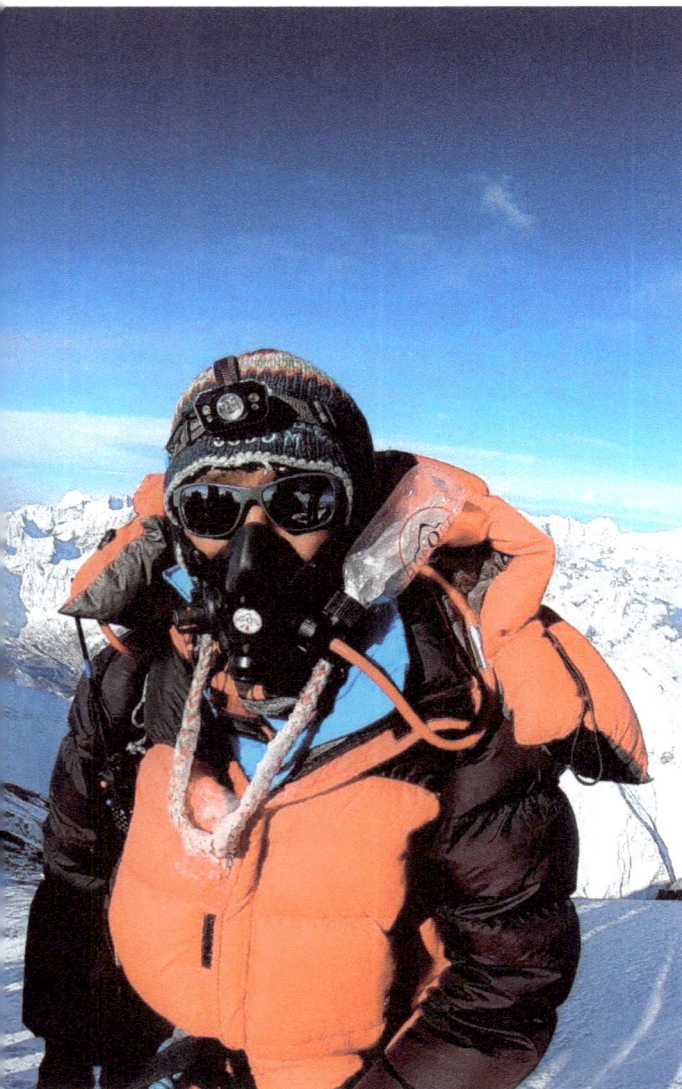
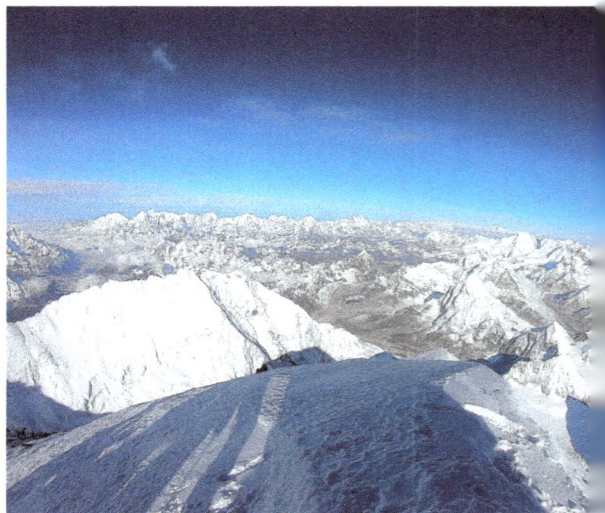
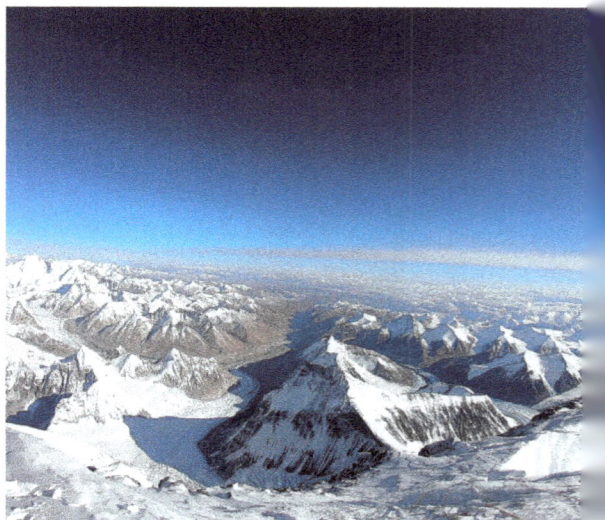

Motivation finds me, and I can finally stand again to take in the 360-degree view.

I'm ready to go, but now the Sherpa have fired up to take pictures of each other. I assist them with their flag holding and self-portraits. I have oxygen, I can wait.

It's so beautiful up here.

It's about 9:30 am ... time to go.

Wrestling my backpack on once more, I take a deep breath as I gaze over the horizon in every direction.

Let's do this ...

Hi Heidi,

He made it! Just got word from Base Camp, David is standing on the summit of Everest right now!

Our hearty congratulations go out to him and all of those who have lived through this journey with him. It's been one heck of a season, but the hard work has paid off, truly a huge feat to accomplish the summit of Everest.

We wanted to reach out and let you know in real time as it's not uncommon for climbers to stay focused and not get on the sat phone until they are back at the South Col several hours from now. The descent can easily take 5–8+ hours, so if you don't hear from him for a while, no news is still good news.

Our best wishes and congratulations to David, what a day!

All best,

ROBERT JANTZEN
Program Manager
CTSS

opposite, top left
Summit approach

opposite, top right
Summit Celebrations

opposite, bottom left
Thanks to the Sherpa

opposite, middle right
Top of the world view

opposite, bottom right
Taking in the
360 degree view

ACTUAL EVEREST SUMMIT ITINERARY—2021 EXPEDITION—DAVID MORGAN

Apr 3	TEAM ARRIVES	Apr 26	Hotel Moonlight
Apr 4	KTM Day, Team Meeting	Apr 27	Hotel Moonlight
Apr 5	Fly to Lukla/Phakding	Apr 28	Hotel Moonlight
Apr 6	Trek to Namche	Apr 29	Hotel Moonlight
Apr 7	Rest	Apr 30	Kathmandu to EBC
Apr 8	Trek to Tengboche	May 1	Pumori HC (5700m)
Apr 9	Rest	May 2	Everest Basecamp to Camp 1
Apr 10	Trek to Pheriche	May 3	Camp 1 to Camp 2
Apr 11	Rest	May 4	Touch Lhotse Face
Apr 12	Trek to Lobuche base camp	May 5	Rest
Apr 13	Rest/Hike	May 6	Camp 2 to Camp 3, return to Camp 2
Apr 14	Move to Lobuche High Camp	May 7	Camp 2 to EBC
Apr 15	Acclimatise	May 8	Rest
Apr 16	Summit and descend Lobuche BC	May 9	Everest Basecamp to Camp 2
Apr 17	Trek to EBC	May 10	Camp 3
Apr 18	Rest/Puja	May 11	Camp 4
Apr 19	Pumori HC (5700m)	May 12	SUMMIT! Back to Camp 4
Apr 20	Train/acclimatise	May 13	Camp 2
Apr 21	Rest	May 14	Camp 2 to Everest Basecamp to Kathmandu (medical Evac)
Apr 22	Rest	May 15	Marriott Hotel
Apr 23	Khumbu Icefall	May 16	Marriott Hotel
Apr 24	Pumori HC (5700m)	May 17	Depart Nepal
Apr 25	EBC to Kathmandu	END ITINERARY	

PART 3

THE SEVENTH SUMMIT

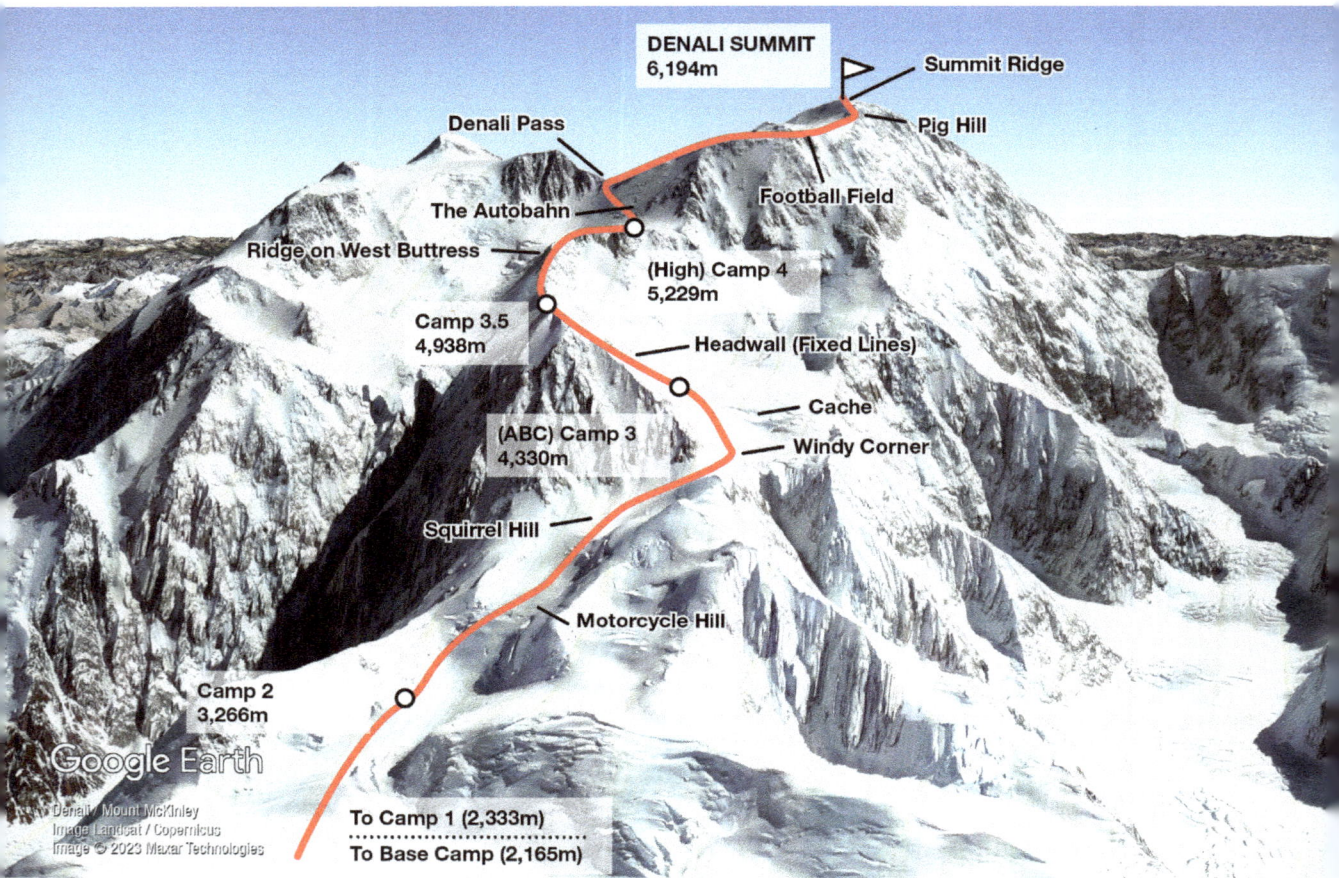

DENALI SUMMIT
6,194m

Summit Ridge

Denali Pass

Pig Hill

The Autobahn

Football Field

Ridge on West Buttress

(High) Camp 4
5,229m

Camp 3.5
4,938m

Headwall (Fixed Lines)

Cache

(ABC) Camp 3
4,330m

Windy Corner

Squirrel Hill

Motorcycle Hill

Camp 2
3,266m

Google Earth

Denali / Mount McKinley
Image Landsat / Copernicus
Image © 2023 Maxar Technologies

To Camp 1 (2,333m)
To Base Camp (2,165m)

DENALI (MT MCKINLEY)

12,540km from Home

ELEVATION: 6,194m

COORDINATES:

N 63 06.908

W 151 00.632

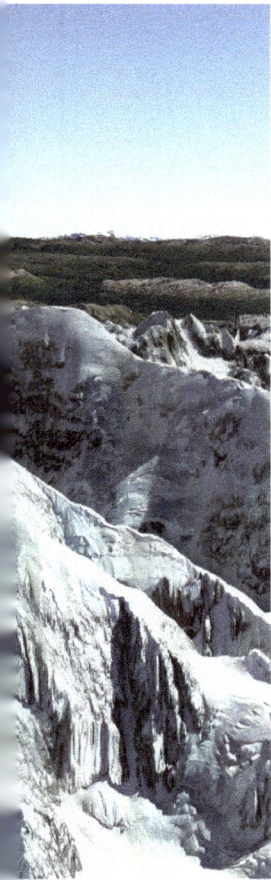

DENALI

7 JUNE—22 JUNE 2021

IN THE MODERN ERA of risk aversion, we are losing the ability to persist so that we can survive. Decision-making in the mountaineering industry is now largely in the hands of commercial operators. At least on the big mountains. While medical professionals and insurers play their part, the businesses that sign you up retain unprecedented rights to cancel your expedition at any moment for reasons that are many and varied. Ironically, these same businesses can contribute to, or even manage, your success.

Certainly some individuals do themselves no favours, their ambitions being greater than their abilities. Policies can and will be altered circumstantially. With eyes wide open, I accept that my expedition company has several reservations about my participation this season. It's not unusual for climbers to finish an expedition with frostbite, but I suspect it's highly unusual for a climber to start an expedition with a frostbite diagnosis.

While I had made it down Everest in one piece, it was touch-and-go for a while. My enthusiastic Sherpa, Cherry, flew down the mountain and got us to Camp 4 in just three-and-a-half hours. It was there that I took my boots off for the first time, and was not happy with what I saw. Tenji, Ryan, April and I stayed overnight at Camp 4—in the death zone. We shouldn't have, but we did. People died on the mountain that day.

Leaving Camp 4, we found many of our oxygen bottles were frozen. My pace was slow. I knew I had frostbite.

Depleted of oxygen, I endured hallucinations and black-outs. I also met saviours—incredible people who gave me the life-saving gift of oxygen and their shoulder to lean on as I struggled to descend.

At Base Camp the ER doctor looked at my feet and swiftly ordered the helicopter. I was evacuated to Kathmandu.

Three days later I left Kathmandu on a Turkish Airlines flight, which was one of only two flights departing. Due to the ever-deteriorating Covid-19 situation in Nepal, it was officially designated a humanitarian charter. In anticipation of our arrival from the mountains and need to leave the country, Gobinda had the foresight to book a block of ten tickets while they were still available. At our hotel, foreigners were considering paying 23,000 euros to exit the country, if the opportunity could be confirmed. I will be forever grateful to Gobinda, my Sherpa guides and all the friends and strangers who helped me get down from Everest and leave Nepal.

So here I am in Alaska, not exactly the best place for keeping frostbitten toes warm. But it is the home of Mt Denali, the final mountain in my challenge. And call me crazy, but, if they let me, I'm going to climb it.

Aside from my frostbitten feet, another concern is that I remain the only unvaccinated participant in our Mt Denali climbing team, although I continue to receive negative Covid-19 PCR results.

The approval of Dr Peter Hackett, an expert on Denali medical concerns who established the medical camp at 14,200 feet, was also required before I could join the planned expedition. I was eventually permitted to climb, and Peter had these recommendations and comments on my condition:

> The pics tell it all. His surgeon was correct, not much to do at this point. But, he should be on ibuprofen 400 mg three times a day. I have to admit, not a lot of data on that, but most experts recommend it based on animal studies.

He will certainly lose his toenail, might lose the end of his toe as well. It will be more clear in a couple weeks.

I would not want to climb Denali with this frostbitten toe. On the one hand, all the experts would recommend against that, for a couple reasons. His toes will be cold sensitive and he risks making that one and some of the others worse. Another is what can he do in the field if the wound breaks down, or starts weeping instead of staying dry, or gets infected?

On the other hand, if he can keep his feet/toes warm, and he is lucky, he might get away with it and be no worse off. It's a gamble.

I have one more mountain to climb. Here comes my attempt at a push to the summit of Denali, which means 'The High One', and is the Koyukon Athabascan name for North America's highest peak. North America's highest mountain has a summit elevation of 6,190 metres above sea level, and is renowned for its extreme cold, harsh weather and severely thin air. This will be a challenge.

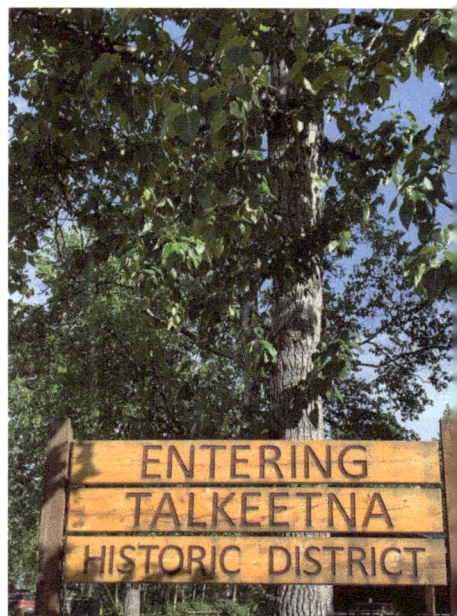

above Talkeetna

Talkeetna—Day 0

Here we are, four strangers, standing at the Anchorage Airport shuttle shelter. Nothing in common other than our distinctive travel duffels. So distinct are these worn-out duffels that I confidently call out to the tall, thin man nearby, 'Are you Bob, by any chance?' He is. With a handshake, Bob approaches with his wife, Nicky. Varun, another American, joins us, and we're now a united team. Who else would be carting heavy duffels but us, the Denali expedition team?

A taxi from Talkeetna—a small town at the gateway to Denali National Park—arrives as our transportation. Relieved of our luggage, we can relax and get acquainted on our way to pick up Julie, the missing member of our small climbing team, from a nearby hotel. Julie is a breath of fresh air and straight to the point: 'You just climbed Everest, didn't you?' In the climbing world, everyone knows somebody who knows somebody who knows something about someone else.

Among this group there's plenty of climbing experience, which is a good start. Nicky has climbed Denali four times and reached the summit once. Bob has been here on three expeditions, but he has yet to reach the top. The drive to Talkeetna, 190 kilometres northeast of Anchorage, takes a couple of hours. Upon arrival at the Swiss Alaska Inn, our little group are strangers no more. And we'll certainly get to know each other even more in the coming weeks.

Day 1—Preparation

The new day brings new opportunities to explore this quaint town and the banks of the Talkeetna River. One thing I won't forget about Talkeetna is the mosquitoes... they are savage and outnumber us by millions.

Just after midday it's time to haul our gear over to the headquarters of Alaska Mountaineering School (AMS), which has been guiding people on Denali and throughout the Alaska Range for thirty-five years. On arrival we're introduced to our guides—Jeremiah, Hannah and Naomi. These are the people who will make or break our Denali experience.

'Tomorrow we fly' always comes with a disclaimer: 'If weather permits.'

It's time for final preparations and a chance to dial in our gear for the upcoming twenty-one days. I haven't even fully unpacked my climbing gear since it was stuffed in my duffels on Mt Everest, nor have I been anywhere near my home, which means I've been living in hotels, on couches, and even in a tent since departing Nepal. Stuff is strewn everywhere as the manic search for my go-to gear begins. No doubles, no back-ups, just one set of layers that work.

Minimalist.

Soon my backpack is loaded and ready for business, and the afternoon is rounded out with sled rigging and loading. I think we're mostly ready to roll. But where's my lip balm? There's always something to stress over at the last minute!

Day 2—Waiting

We're picked up early and taken to the small airstrip, as we're expecting to fly at some stage today. I'm buzzing, probably from caffeine overload, but also because it's all happening; we're in final preparations to catch our small aeroplane out to the Denali mountain range.

A ranger from the National Park Service is here to deliver our first briefing. We're enthusiastically educated on Denali National Park and Preserve, which was established in 1917. Rangers have a permanent presence on the mountain during the climbing season, but it's mostly an oversight tenure for environmental protection. They will only assist in the event of immediate danger to life or limb. The areas we focus on in the briefing include the 'leave no trace' mountaineering policy, established in the late 1970s. Climbers remove all their garbage from the Alaska Range, with the aim of allowing the generations after us to enjoy the mountain as it is now. Everything we take up must come down. An equally important part of our discussion leans into planning and preparing for the journey ahead. It can be a hostile environment at times out there, we've been warned. The most common issues reported are altitude sickness and frostbite.

I should still be somewhat acclimated, and I already have frostbite.

Drizzling rain has begun to fall while Jeremiah, our lead guide, gives an update: 'They're socked in at Base Camp.' Translation for the non-Americans—weather isn't good enough to land. Denali is the third most prominent, and also the third most isolated, peak on Earth, after Mt Everest and Aconcagua, so we'll just have to wait. Meanwhile it's off to lunch.

Covid-19 rules are in place, so I eat outside. I'm the only unvaccinated individual here, as Australia was yet to have vaccines available before I departed the country and I've been in transit since I left for Everest. Of course there are vaccines available in the US, but there is no available data on how any side effects might present at altitude. I have enough medical concerns currently, and the medical advice is that I now have some natural immunity to Covid as a result of being infected. Where we are going is remote—really remote, so I'll accept the medical professionals' advice and decline vaccination for the moment.

But we're not flying today. The weather has turned through the ranges.

Day 3—Still waiting

Peering out the window of our hotel, I see there's nothing to get excited about—the skies are grey, everything looks wet, and it's spitting raindrops.

According to the whiteboard at the rangers' federal building, there are 988 registered climbers this year. Currently 435 are on the mountain. So far 165 climbers have made the Denali summit this year, making the summit success rate fifty-one per cent thus far.

Back at AMS headquarters we're advised the next update: 'Pilots have run some sightseeing around the area. It's improving, but they can't land yet. We need to hang here and they'll call it at 5pm.'

Familiar story, and I'm guessing I know the ending.

Five o'clock arrives and the call is confirmed—we're not flying today.

Day 4—Talkeetna to Base Camp

ALTITUDE: 2,165m
PULSE OX: 92%

Sticking my head out the door reveals sunlight and even a patch of blue sky. That gives me enough confidence to change into my climbing gear for our 7:15am pick-up.

Greeted by our guides at AMS, our schedule is confirmed—we're to make our way to the Talkeetna Air Taxi runway. Bob, Nicky and I head to the plane.

'Anybody here not flown over this area?' asks Paul, the pilot.
'I haven't.'
'Okay, you can ride up front,' says Paul.

So here I am in the cockpit next to the pilot. Talk about striking it lucky. Best view in the house.

The mountain range is clear in the distance, and the rivers flowing from them are light grey in colour from all the glacier silt they move. Flying across vivid green plains, the Denali mountains are soon upon us. First it's just patches of ice at the foot of the mountains, then within minutes there are glaciers to our right and left. Patchily covered mountains are replaced with a fully snow-covered landscape and sheer rock faces appear.

The plane barely lifts altitude as we fly over One Shot Pass. As the name suggests, it's the best shot you have for flying a direct route to Denali Base Camp on the south-east Fork Kahiltna Glacier. Just below the weather, Paul makes the shot for the open passage. Thick fog rises to both sides of the plane, following the contours of the land, giving the pass a sense of drama.

Winding into the mountains, from here I can even spot people below. We must be close. Descending, the snow runway comes into view. We're landing on giant skis fitted under the plane, which is a new experience for me. Slowing significantly,

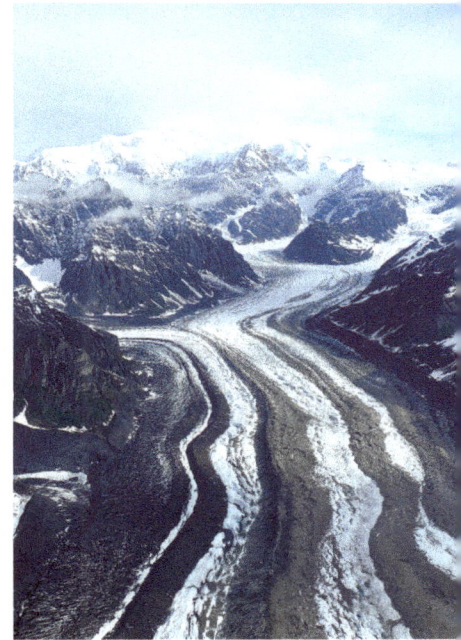

above Remote Alaska

plumes of snow lift around us as we touch down. People are surrounding the airstrip, eager to depart. We're relieved, happy to have finally arrived.

Disembarking, I take my first steps towards completing the last of my Seven Summits.

Nervously stepping back into my climbing boots, they feel tight, and pins and needles are more noticeable. Circulation will be an issue. But for now I get the pleasure of gazing upon new sights from this tiny camp, and become immersed in this completely new environment, the incredible vistas of the Alaska Range, and the amazing peaks of Foraker, Hunter and Denali in full view.

The sky turns greyer, and Jeremiah confirms we won't move from Base Camp until our other teammates arrive. Seems like that could be a while.

I take a lap around camp, and I'm surprised at the frequency of rock avalanches I can hear somewhere in the distance. The sound of falling rocks is distinctive, but, while we can hear the avalanches, we can't see them. Apparently they're caused by the amount of sun blazing on the mountains, even though it's early in the climbing season.

Although the weather hasn't improved, in the distance we hear a plane, which soon emerges from the dense, grey clouds. Julie, Varun and Naomi arrive. We pitch a tent for them, and we're all ready to roll out as hoped. An open kitchen will suffice for one night, and steps, seats and a table are built into the snow with shovels.

We'll be getting up at 1am so that we can try to navigate the crevasses at the coldest point of the day. As snow has been falling consistently for five days, there are heavy, wet snow bridges that haven't frozen properly, making travel especially dangerous, Jeremiah explains. We'll gear up and travel with another expedition to try to stay as safe as possible, but a question mark remains as to whether the area is passable. We'll see.

opposite Setting off once more

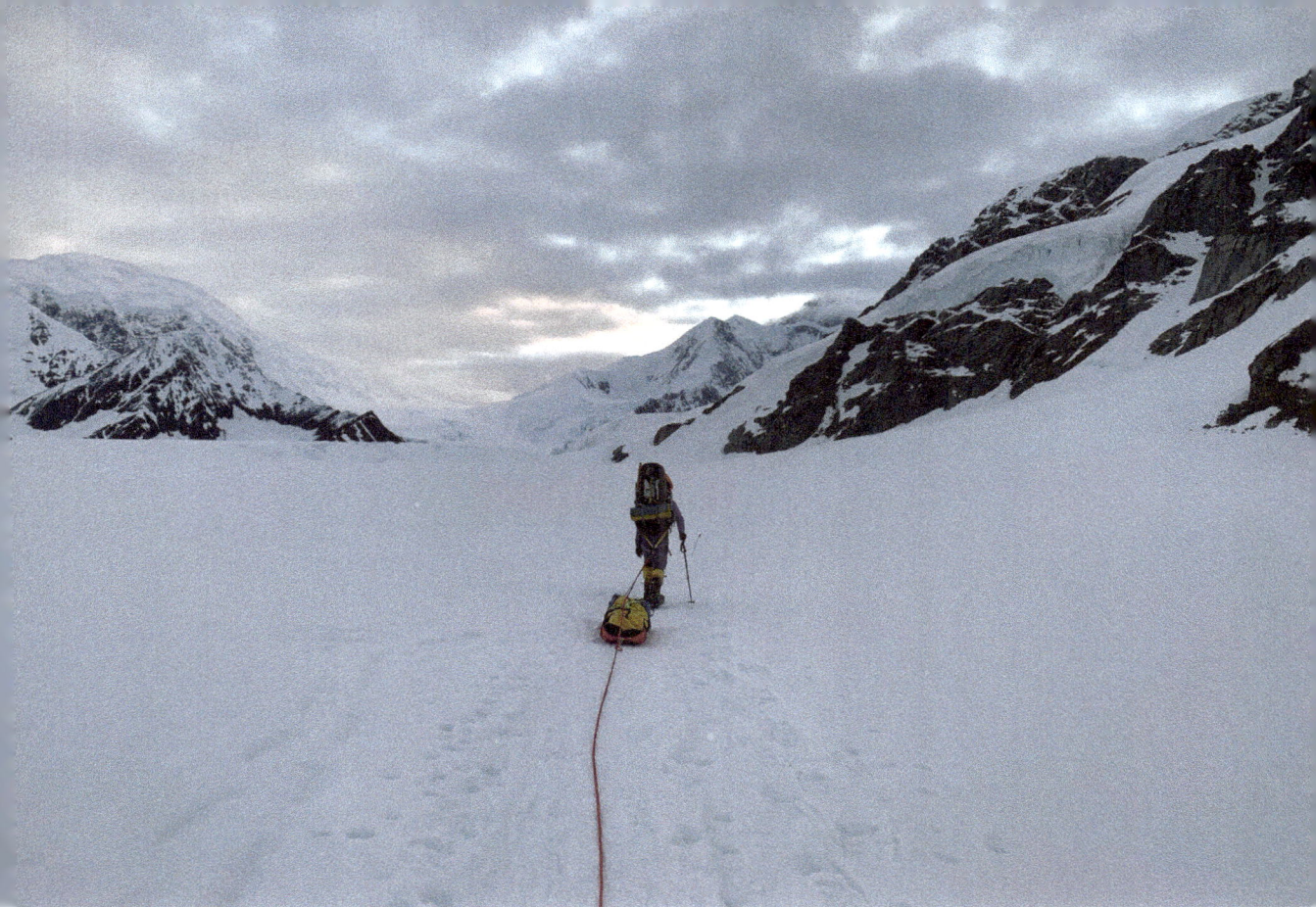

Day 5—Base Camp to Camp 1

Our 1am wake-up is pushed to 2am to allow the snow extra time to ice in the freezing cold morning air. Overnight both my hands went to pins and needles at various times. Unfortunately, my toes are always like that and there's nothing I can do about it.

Weighing my bags is not one of the morning's highlights. I'll be lugging thirty kilos in my backpack and pulling a further 20.5 kilos in a sled connected to my hips. More than fifty kilos, plus I'm wearing heavy cold-weather climbing gear and

DISTANCE: 8.75km

TIME: 4:48 hrs

ASCENT: 337m

DESCENT: 155m

ALTITUDE: 2,333m

PULSE OX: 93%

a harness with all my rigging, while snowshoeing, which I've never done before.

Should be interesting.

I cart my gear over first to our team rope, opting to go behind Jeremiah, who leads. After rigging, I go to help Julie, who is clearly struggling. She'll be directly behind me on the rope, and Varun will be the last member of our nimble rope team to the rear.

With snowshoes strapped over my climbing boots and my backpack secured to pretty much everything else, it's time to try walking. I'm sure I can hear my body creaking.

It's not a pleasant start. The snowshoes are somewhat cumbersome, and we never really stop except for a crevasse warning or one of our regular breaks taken on the hour. Although, when the sun causes a huge, heavy avalanche off Mt Foraker, everything stops as we watch the massive spectacle, which starts high on the mountain and takes its time to roar to the bottom.

It's backbreaking just lowering and re-loading my backpack. I've already worked a sweat up and my shoulders ache. It doesn't help that I lost ten per cent of my body weight, probably mostly lean muscle mass, to the demands of the Everest expedition.

A rope-gang descending the mountain in the opposite direction look every bit the fatigued mountaineers. They place one foot in front of the other, slogging it out. 'Embrace it …' one of the climbers says before returning his gaze to his feet.

There's not really a track to speak of here; it's more a pack-hardened route climbers have taken before. You can see puncture footprints where snowshoes have broken the top section and people have gone down, probably knee and waist deep in snow. Big crevasses are everywhere, and just punching the snow a little has made Julie apprehensive. 'Slow down, I'm freakin' out a little,' she says. All we can do is keep good rope tension and try navigating the hard sections.

'Sorry guys, I'm going to need a longer break,' calls Varun. 'I need to take my boots off to tape my feet.' He already has blisters, big ones. Unfortunately, it takes Varun a long time to tape his feet. More than double a normal break, and everyone is getting very cold. It takes a lot of patience to be cold and just wait, and longer to warm up after that break. At least we're not struggling for views of Mt Crosson, which is majestic amid clear skies on our left.

My hands are numb, so I swing them as I walk. Breathing deliberately to cope with the pronounced pain in my feet while suffering is the new norm. All I can do is focus on the next break, take it moment by moment, and just get the next hour done.

Coming into the next break, where we pull a few steps off the route, Julie collapses. The snow hasn't compacted here, so is less supportive. She's unable to get up, so has to disconnect and crawl to the side.

It's weird, but I just don't think about my frostbitten toe once I start moving. The short sharp pains tend to remind me, but I've purchased battery-heated socks, which I hope will be my saviour.

Over the last rise, we're walking towards tents; not many, but this is Camp 1. Finally.

The process here is to probe the perimeter first, then probe the internal space in a sequence to check for any crevasses or dangers before we can begin setting up camp. Then the pack comes off, but there's no rest. In fact, the opposite. We've got to stomp the area in our snowshoes first, then level it off with shovels before pitching tents. It takes time, but we work together and get it done. The guides meanwhile build a toilet and a kitchen, and pitch their own tent. Now it's time to sort our gear, return the communal gear and move into tents. I check my feet and dig out the ibuprofen.

The day is heating up. To lie in some sort of shade, I've clipped my sleeping bag on the outside roof of the tent, and can now nap. With sunshine and heat like this, I shouldn't be

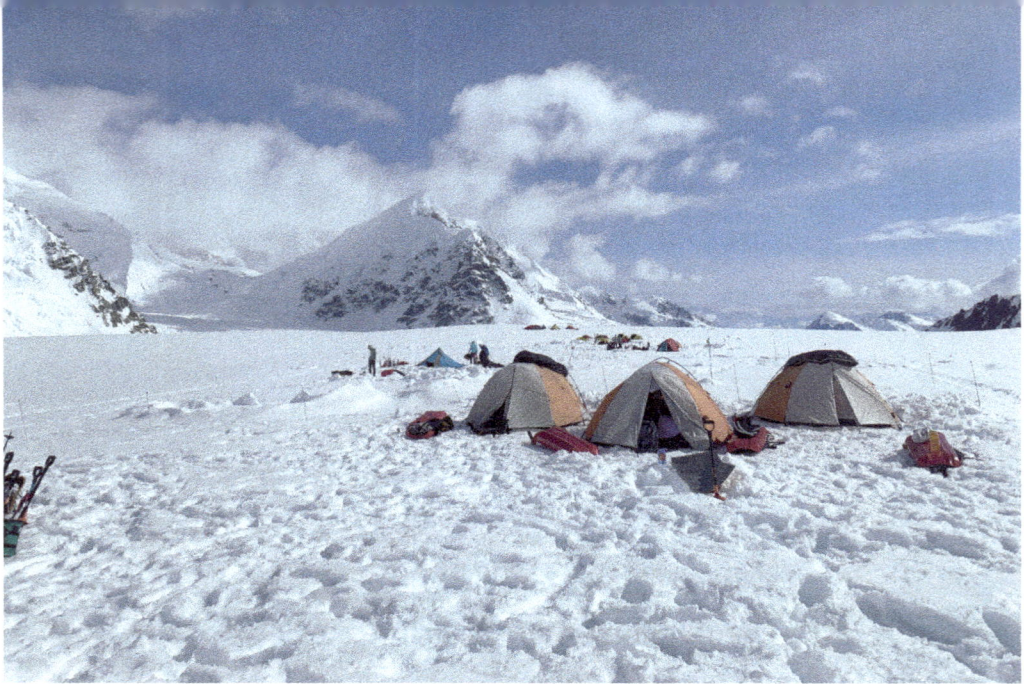

shocked that the mountains continue to shed glaciers, and the roar of snow often pounds down the mountainside.

Suddenly there's a massive announcement—Bob and Nicky are pulling out, explaining they don't have the fire to execute this challenging climb.

Day 6—Carry day

DISTANCE: 9.78km
TIME: 7:36 hrs
ASCENT: 732m
DESCENT: 780m
CACHE ELEVATION: 3,065m
PULSE OX: 90%
BACKPACK: 23 kg

'Varun and Julie, you're going to have to work at getting on the line quicker in the mornings.' We're well past the hour allocated to leave and the same people are holding back our departure.

Everyone has opted for sleds to lighten their backpacks and split the weight. But I've looked at the long hill in front of us, 'Ski Hill', and opted to ditch the sled and put all the weight in my backpack. It's not as heavy as yesterday, and I believe I can manage it. However, Ski Hill is deceptive and requires more effort than it appears to from the base.

'Can we slow the pace down a whisker?' asks Varun. It's the same request as yesterday, which is a little frustrating when combined with all the complaints about the cold.

Mt Hunter is on our right, while we trek in the shade of the mountains. Sunlight fully drenches many notable features. It's a nice contrast, the sunny mountain against our shadowy route. Only a narrow section of our route is pack hardened, with soft snow off to both sides. As the wind moves the light snow around, snowdrifts look like grains of sand in ever-changing forms. The path also makes overtaking other teams near impossible if they don't have the spatial awareness to let you do so. Today we're the ones stuck behind the slow traffic of other climbers.

The sun moves higher in the sky, bathing the mountains in light. We're approaching the line where we step out of the shadows and into the sunlight. I imagine it'll be nice for about ten minutes, then we'll be hot and complaining about the glare.

As soon as we stop at the site Jeremiah has selected for our cache, a small area is probed out and everyone comes together. Here, of all places, Varun surprises us. 'Jeremiah, I think I'm done. I think this is a good spot to call it so I can take my gear back down. I'm just not coping with the cold, and the blisters could stop me anyway.'

Now it'll just be Julie, me and the guides.

Our cache needs to be dug six feet deep into the snow so the ravens don't interfere with it. Time to start digging. Meanwhile Hannah and Jeremiah re-prioritise our group gear and sort out the logistics of what has just transpired. This is a carry day. We'll now descend lighter and tomorrow we'll walk straight past here to build Camp 2, returning the following day to pick up this gear.

I thought descending would be easy, but in reality it's the opposite. With these snowshoes you can only walk square down the mountain, which smashes my toes. Painfully, I

opposite Tents up—
Camp 1

wriggle them to try to help circulation while the pain increases. At least with crampons you can have the side of your foot going downhill to reduce the pressure.

Varun breaks any rhythm as the line stops and asks, 'My blisters are sore. Can we go slower?'

The sun is really beating down on us—it's hot. Everything looks different on our descent from the way it looked earlier; shadows are replaced with crisp detail, and panoramas stretch clearly into the valleys far below.

My feet are hurting like hell as we finally come into camp. Bob and Nicky greet us with positive enthusiasm that even the weary appreciate. In a way I'm relieved Varun is departing with them, even if I'm still slightly surprised his decision came so early in our expedition. Sometimes I feel it just takes time in the mountains to appreciate that nothing comes easy.

Day 7—Camp 1 to Camp 2

DISTANCE: 5.03km
TIME: 6:51 hrs
ASCENT: 926m
DESCENT: 1m
ELEVATION: 3,266m
PULSE OX: 90%
BACKPACK: 23 kg
SLED WEIGHT: 15 kg
DIAMOX COMPLAINTS BY
GUIDES: Face tingling, hands
tingling, even ears tingling

I'm determined to help get Julie prepared and ready for the day's climbing on time, minus the accompanying stress. My layering works and my gear is minimal but efficient—after so much time in the mountains, I can help others and take comfort that my personal systems are dialled in.

As Julie starts packing, I drop the tent—I'm already ready. I'll carry most of it, for today anyway. The tent fly, caked with ice, is the worst. Even after a shake it feels heavy. Group gear is split into two piles. After I get my share, it's time for the scales, then to help rig Julie's sled. I'm not putting more than I carried yesterday on my back, so the sled becomes slightly heavier than ideal.

Heading out of camp, now on time, it's soon apparent that yesterday was tough on my feet. As we ascend, the pins and needles in the front of both feet are intense. I try to look at the scenery, focus on making the next hour, but it's painful and I can't do anything but struggle. I hate these snowshoes. They necessitate an unnatural stepping sequence; wide steps, toes always pointed forward. Yet they're definitely required in this soft snow. The first stop can't come soon enough. I don't know what I can do differently. My feet are killing me. Although surrounded by beautiful scenery, I just stare at my feet as we join other teams in a slow turtle race up the mountain. One in front of the other—small steps.

Staring out at the mountains on a break, I'm grateful for how far I've come. The snow glistens, and the sparkles look like something out of a fairytale. It's captivating and reminds me of our daughters and their love of anything with sequins.

Julie is starting to really suffer beneath the weight of her pack and is struggling with her breathing. It has been a long day and it's not over yet as we push on to the cache.

Passing the cache, now armed with shovels, we're off to build the next camp. Here we go again, slogging upwards, dragging this burden of a sled in snowshoes I'd like to throw off the mountain. It's taxing, and we take a standing break to hydrate and shed unnecessary layers. I'm down to a base layer, and keep a bandana over my face and ears to prevent frying my skin in this blistering sun. If it's not cold, it's really hot!

This brutal section is a continuous 200 metres of elevation gain. Julie is so exhausted that she has called to stop three times. All we can do while she curses out loud is tell her to save her energy, take deep breaths, and press on. Needless to say, when we crest the final section that leads us into camp and the tents, I know I'm not the only one who feels a huge sense of relief.

We're finally here—Camp 2. Hannah and Naomi have arrived before us and started to level some platforms. It's not time for rest; it's time to work. But just getting this load off motivates me to move freely and help build camp. Straightaway I fall a foot deep on the platform where our tent will sit, so I have to compact the snow before I can level it off with a

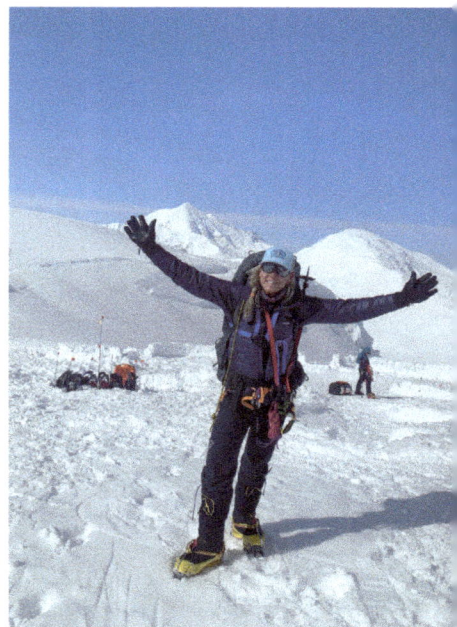

above Julie—Camp 2 arrival

shovel, clear a path and dig some steps. It takes me over an hour of solid digging, but I've created a passage you can stand in with bench seats either side—our newest dining room.

Our guides have had a sleepless twenty-four hours. As well as just getting to this remote place, they've had to deal with the logistics of the others departing. Julie, who is exhausted, is game enough to ask the guides how they think she's going.

'I think you have a lot of suffer in you. You're really lucky to have David patiently helping you. You're doing better, but you're going to struggle up higher. Breaks need to be shorter— we can't do delays up there. You just need to keep working,' Jeramiah tells her in response.

opposite Hanging out in the kitchen tent

Day 8—Back-carry day

It's back-carry day. We're taking empty backpacks down the mountain to grab the gear we cached a couple of days ago. Also known as the active rest day, the best thing about today is no snowshoes.

After morning coffee, the five of us jump on the rope again and make tracks. The sun is still behind the mountains, and it's so cold the ice is hard enough to walk on, at least downhill. Our crampons are in the cache bag, so from here we can employ those. We're also thankfully done with hauling the sleds, and they stay here too. I'm so relieved to be back in crampons. Well, I say that now. As insurance I've taped up my big toe. It's tender to the touch and looking suitably painful. Poor abused toes.

Downhill we go. The scenery is dramatic, awe-inspiring. The rugged Alaska Range is spectacular to gaze upon beneath blazing blue skies with the merest wisps of light cloud passing overhead.

We move downhill quickly, and I'm happy to volunteer to dig up our gear when we arrive. Digging gets me really

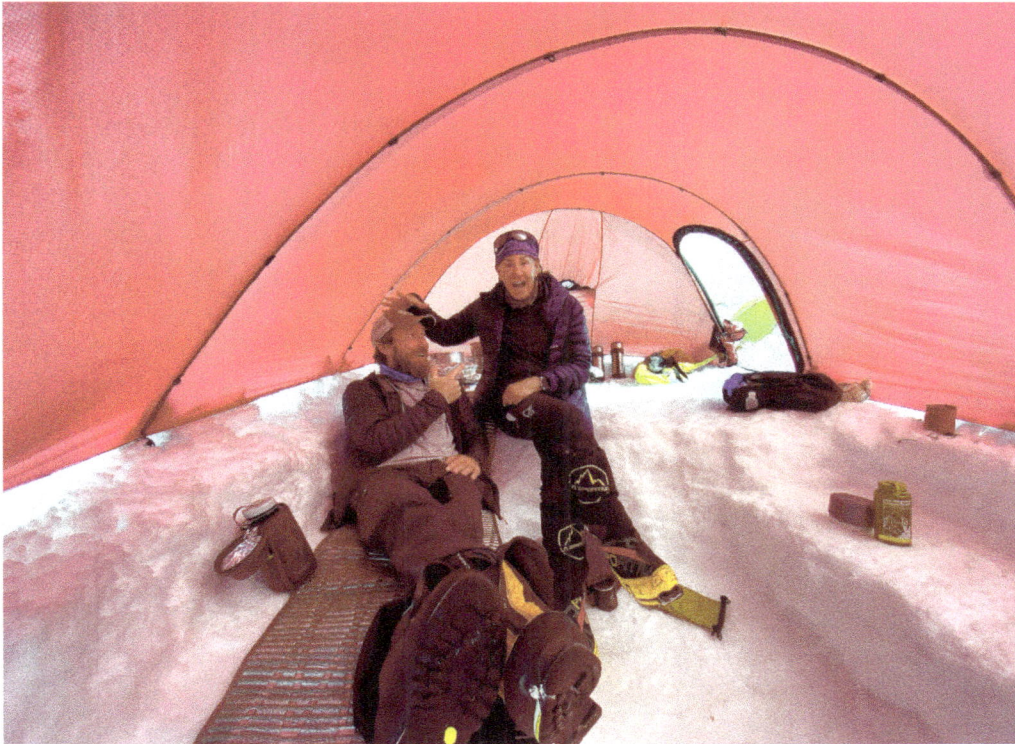

warmed up, as opposed to getting cold watching somebody else do it. The guides just think I like to dig.

An avalanche starts roaring spectacularly on the ridge just above our camp when we arrive, which is an immediate reminder of the dangers to consider. Jeremiah comments briefly, 'That's not a sound you want to hear from here.' It looks impressive though, and I wonder if it sets a precedent for more avalanches on that mountain face today. They're certainly heard frequently enough in the surrounding area.

When you're rigged into the rope system, you don't get too much conversation, so it's nice to have a chance to chat with Hannah while we have an afternoon off the ropes. She's twenty-six years old, and this is her first gig on Denali as an assistant guide. Her boyfriend, Matt, is also an assistant guide for AMS. When she's not climbing mountains, she works for the park service and lives in Stewart, Alaska.

When 4pm rolls around, Naomi comes to start dinner. I offer assistance, but filling the snow bag for water is all she's got. Naomi lives in a place called Juno in Alaska, but is originally from Northern California. She has completed a three-month University of Alaska south-east internship with AMS, for which only two people are generally selected each year. An internship recommendation must first come from a professor at the college they have attended. The internship was awarded to both Naomi and her roommate, and after she completed that she helped with an AMS training course before staying on with AMS and landing the job here as an assistant.

The meals our guides produce on this trek have been phenomenal, and dinner brings us all together.

Day 9—Carry day

WEIGHT: 19 kg
DISTANCE: 5.77km
TIME: 6:44 hrs
ASCENT: 654m
DESCENT: 754m
CACHE ELEVATION: 3,970m
PULSE OX: 90%

The morning is cold, the skies are clear, and we're spoilt for views. The most difficult part of the morning is getting my boots on—damn toes. Julie and I are super-organised this morning. On the line ready, on time—again. She's getting the systems down pat, and says she is feeling better every day.

There's no easing into the morning's climb. It's out the gate and straight up the mountain. Our first challenge out of Camp 2 is Motorcycle Hill, which is directly in front of us. At 180 metres, it's the steepest part of the mountain where we'll be pulling sleds.

Unfortunately, Julie needs coaching when we start climbing, as her crampon skills are not quite up to the grade. Even with instruction, she still seems to be lifting her left foot from the ball of her foot only. Here a steady footing is required, and it hasn't gone unnoticed. There's only Jeremiah up front and me behind Julie on the rope team. It's not apparent to me why she can't get her footing sorted, but it's holding us up. I frequently stop to wait, but I'm not too fussed, for the incredible vista across the mountains is worth embracing—you can see for miles.

At the top we pause to break. My toes are doing better in the crampons, much better than the snowshoes. I can angle my foot, protect the big toe and still climb effortlessly. Pain is now the companion I greet with a grimace and embrace through my days. It took a few days for my muscles to wake up and adjust to these new stresses, but now I'm at least climbing well. The pace for me is casual, and I can take some photos.

To our right we now have Squirrel Hill to climb. As we incline, I can see the exact location of yesterday's avalanche and the leftover debris still scattered about. It's awesome to see it from this aspect after witnessing it from below at Camp 2. After Squirrel Hill it gets easier; the gentler Polo Field feels like a good break after two hills in a row.

Soon the famous Windy Corner is in sight. Funny thing is, it's not windy—not even a breath of wind. But that's just today—Windy Corner is regarded as one of the most dangerous parts of the mountain, where extreme winds can rush past high rock formations and make it a dangerous place to spend time. Denali climbers have been killed here by falling rocks and boulders, and it's best to pass by as fast as possible.

Jeremiah raises his concerns with Julie's climbing, or at least that's what I thought was being discussed. But the reality is he's trying to gently tell her she can't climb any higher.

'I'm sorry, Julie, this is the worst part of my job,' he says.

Julie isn't pleased. 'Are you kidding me? You're calling it now?' she shrieks.

Around and around the argument goes, but Jeremiah's points are valid: although Julie's climbing has improved, this is not the environment for learning. Her systems aren't 'dialled'. Throughout today's climb Jeremiah has felt unsafe, he says, because Julie's climb has been shaky at times. I leave Jeremiah and Julie to thrash it out. She's so upset, and I can only

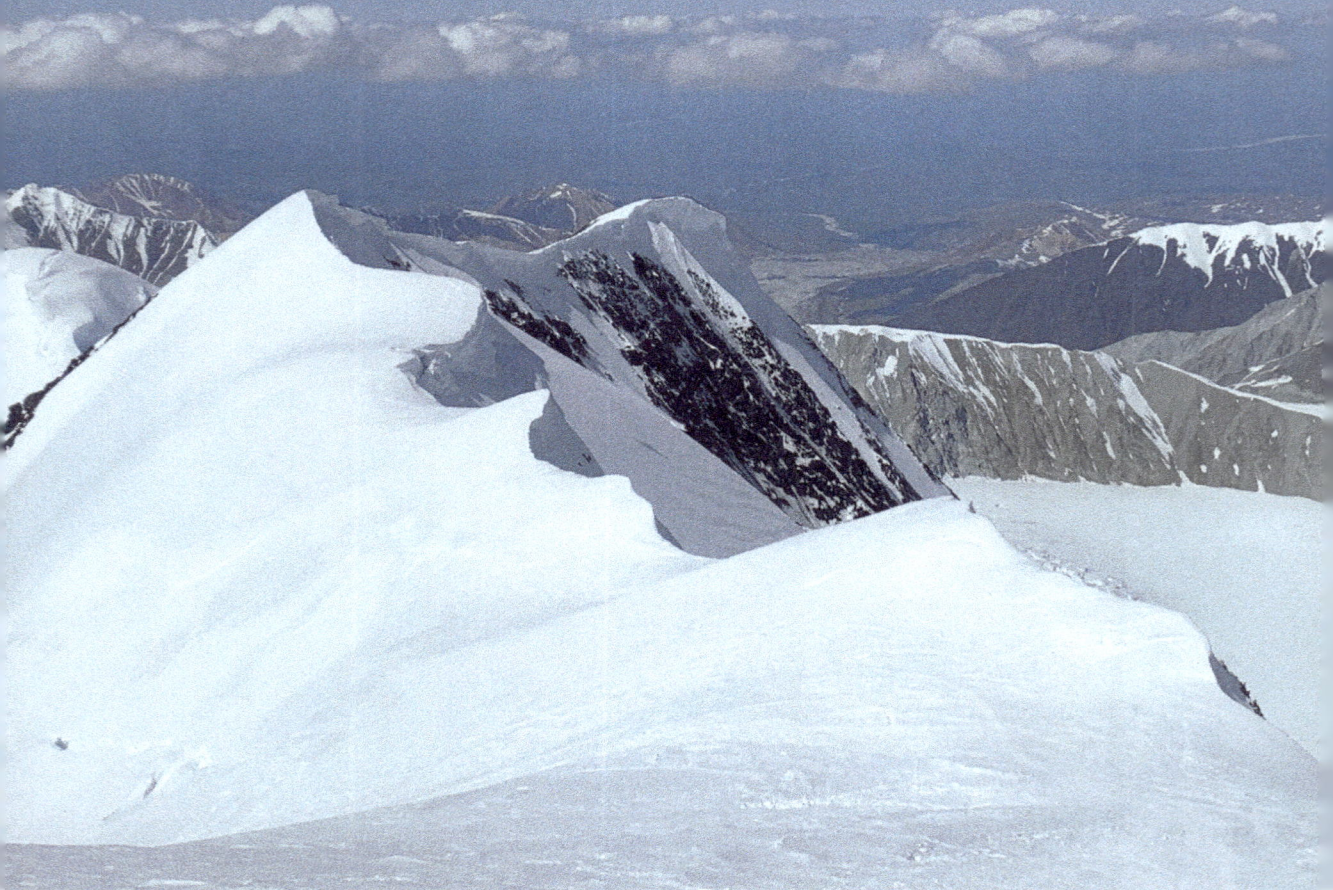

above Moving on up

imagine what this means to her. Finally, everybody simmers down and common sense takes over. We're back on the rope and continue on, burying our cache after another half hour of climbing.

It's a sober mood on the rope back down to Camp 2.

Motorcycle Hill is a very steep descent, and on the way Julie comes clean. Her feet are in pain, she admits, and we need to slow. This explains her poor footing. So on we tramp—slowly.

Back at camp, Julie seems more accepting of Jeremiah's decision. She's suffering real pain in her feet and her left ankle is swollen, which poses a huge risk here. Jeremiah's experience had picked up on it earlier.

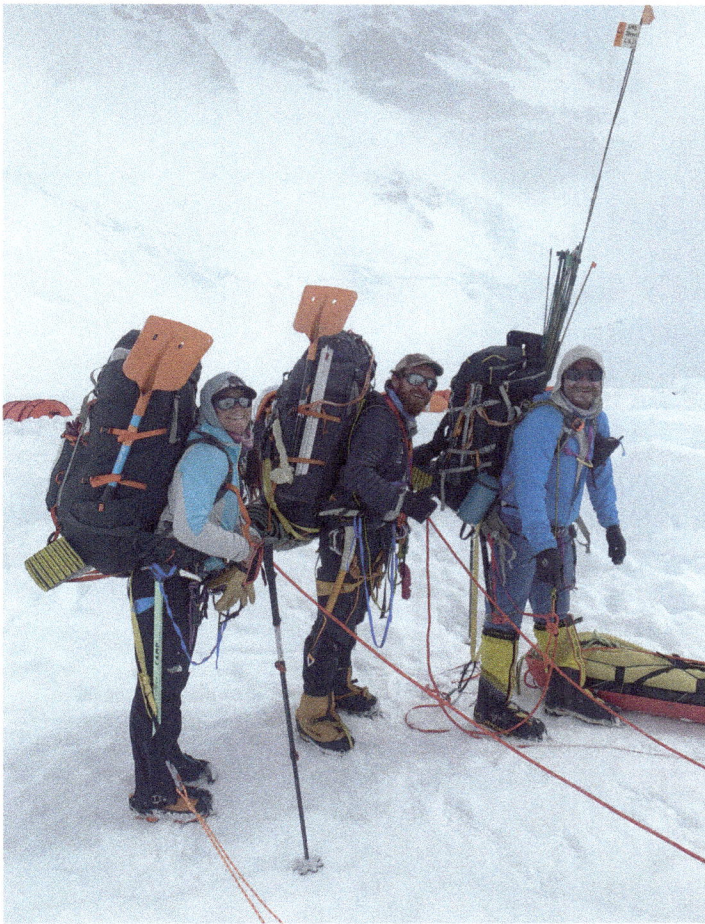

left Away we go . . .

Day 10—Camp 2 to Camp 3 (Advanced Base Camp)

Camp 3, also known as Advanced Base Camp, or simply ABC, is at 14,200 feet (4,330 metres) and is today's destination. We'll be leaving both Julie and Naomi here at Camp 2. They'll descend with the next team heading off the mountain. But fewer people equals more weight to carry up, which I'm not overly excited about. My pack is already full, but now I have to cram in group gear too. On top of that the weather has closed in, with periods of snow.

Although we hit the trail with even heavier packs, our pace is substantially faster. Jeremiah leads, I'm the middle child,

CAMP 3 ALTITUDE: 4,142m

DISTANCE: 4.35km

TIME: 5:48 hrs

ASCENT: 813m

DESCENT: 3m

ELEVATION: 4,142m

PULSE OX: 90%

BACKPACK (START): 24.5 kg

BACKPACK (FINISH): 35 kg

and Hannah is at the rear of our new, small rope team. From here on, it's just the three of us.

No time to rest, no micro breaks; we're headed straight up Motorcycle Hill at the fastest pace we can sustain and in almost half the time we completed yesterday. And the faster we get up this mountain, the quicker I can get down.

Snow is softly floating down against a backdrop of sheer rock face. It's more breathtaking than I can begin to describe.

opposite Camp 3 weather day

The guide I'm passing has been talking to Jeremiah and says, 'I hear you're the last man standing?'

'Unfortunately, yes,' I reply.

'Go kick some ass!' he calls as I trudge past.

Across the Denali Flats we trek, and continue on to Windy Corner, where we've arrived back at an elevation of 3,965 metres—and our cache site. Digging up our stash is a reality check. There's lots of gear here. Food, fuel and our personal belongings all add to the weight. Shedding a layer of clothing, I have to re-pack my whole backpack to even have a chance of fitting in my portion of the evenly distributed weight.

'Do you think you can manage that?' Jeremiah enquires.

'Let's weigh it.'

It's 37.5 kilos.

'Yikes,' says Jeremiah. Hannah's load is lighter, so we move some weight onto her sled.

Still, at thirty-five kilos I have to sit down in the snow to strap on the backpack, and use my climbing pole and axe to pull myself up. Wow, this is really heavy. The first few steps aren't easy, and I can't say it gets any easier.

It takes an hour to climb to an altitude of 4,091 metres. We'll stop here before the last climb into camp. Or possibly collapse here. I'm sucking in big gasps of air, trying to calm myself, dumping my pack on the ground. That was tough. My body is quivering a little as I try stretching my shoulders. My feet ... well, let's just say they don't like this one bit. Indeed, camp can't come fast enough.

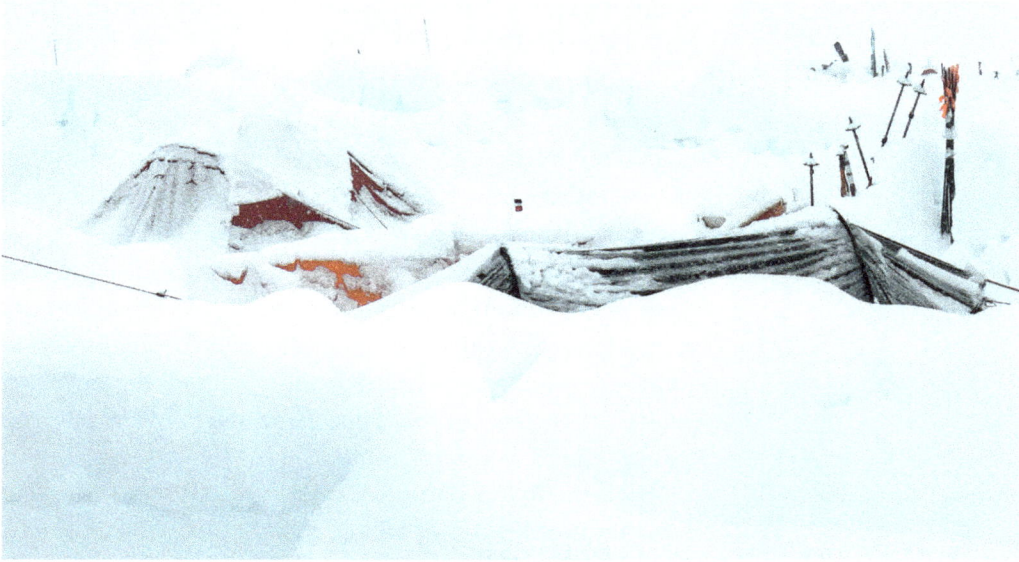

Soon we're off again, and as we crest the last rise I can see tents—an end is finally in sight.

In camp, I try to compose myself, regain my breath, and let the relief settle in. Finally, I can sit directly on the Clean Mountain Can (CMC—a portable loo), do my business, and wave to those who walk past. Modesty is gone. You get used to it, but it's chilly with ya pants down and the snow falling.

Day 11—Rest day

Twelve hours' sleep! That's virtually unheard of.

It's warm in the tent with the remainder of our climbing team—Jeremiah, Hannah and me. Outside is a different story. The view is non-existent, just white and snowing. It's difficult to distinguish the ground from the horizon at first. There's work to be done shovelling snow from tents and gear, but first I need a coffee.

Unfortunately, I need to use the CMC again. Not my favourite activity in these snowy conditions. I struggle to see the path to it in these whiteout conditions, but at least there won't be too many spectators today. Trudging to the loo with my boots deep in snow has made my feet cold. Something I'll have to address immediately. Obviously, getting frozen toes more frozen could be the end of the climb.

Back to the tent, where I put on my heated socks. Self-care is essential; nobody will do it for you. While I'm at it, I dig out my long johns and change underwear for the first time. It's a weight issue to have fresh underwear all the time. My batteries to the heated socks die. Time to deploy the back-up strategy—hand warmers go into my socks.

This is the first real rest day we've had. Most days have an element of back-carry or hiking, but not today. There's nothing at all planned, except to get oneself ready for tomorrow. If, weather permitting, we move. After six inches of snow, and the tracks buried, some sun is needed to make the traverse safe.

We have plenty of food and fuel, so for now we'll just chill out on the mountainside. And eating is a good idea. Over the last few months I've not only continued to lose weight, but I've lost lean muscle mass as well. My pants are fixed to the smallest setting and my harness adjusted to the minimum on its clips. Everything will fall off me soon.

By mid-afternoon the skies have turned bright blue, and it's hot. This mountain is one of extremes—whiteouts and snow one minute, sunshine and warmth the next. Sticking your head outside the tent is the only way to get the weather forecast.

Day 12—Waiting

In direct contrast to yesterday, the skies are clear and I can see for miles. But there are other, more subtle signs that indicate it's safe to move higher that only experience can detect. This morning's story is all about the wind. It's calm here at camp, though cold. My heated socks are invaluable in the chill of the ice before I get moving.

At 5,304 metres, Mt Foraker is the second highest mountain in the range and the most prominent in the view from here. Stacked clouds show wind on her upper reaches, which must be considered. Mt Hunter, at 4,445 metres, is also a view to admire. Messner, the mountain directly behind our camp, seems to have fast-moving cloud peeling off its summit.

Reports are that winds have been increasing at Camp 17 (17,000 feet). Initially everyone was packing to leave, but after breakfast the hive of activity has ceased. Clouds that weren't present when we got up are building. Jeremiah calls timeout to pack up camp; the situation requires re-evaluation, he says. Better to be strong at Camp 14 than withering away and colder at Camp 17.

The weather continues to deteriorate, so the decision becomes obvious. We're staying here. And the forecast for tomorrow isn't any more favourable. All there is to do is stay healthy, active and keep occupied.

Day 13—Camp 3 to Camp 3.5

The mountain peaks are clear, indicating that the winds have died down, but, below our altitude, the clouds look dense. Some clouds remain above nearby Mt Messner, but they're not moving with the intensity of yesterday. Looks like a good climbing day to me, but I'm not the expert.

We're all well rested, which helps morale, and it's decided— we're moving up. The sun is just breaching the surrounding mountains, giving the tents a chance to dry before we pack them up. Our loads are heavy, heavier than expected or ideal, but I've sacrificed everything that could possibly be left behind. The only luxury I insist on taking is coffee. Dragging

BACKPACK: 32 kg

CAMP 3.5 ALTITUDE: 4,900m (16,076 feet)

DISTANCE: 1.24km

TIME: 3:32 hrs

ASCENT: 411m

DESCENT: 1m

PULSE OX: 77%

my pack to the rope, I stretch and hope for the best. This body has held up well, just a few more days—please. There's no looking back.

In no time I've worked up a sweat, and my lungs are reminded what a workout is. The weather isn't extremely cold, or at least I'm not feeling it too much, but it's starting to snow. Soon I'm sweating profusely; the mountain is like a never-ending staircase that I have to climb. Stomping one foot at a time through the snow, with so much weight on my back, I wonder, again: how long can an hour drag out?

But eventually the break comes, and I can catch my breath. From here, looking up the fixed lines, I can see other climbers slowly moving up this brutal section. Then, as I reload my backpack burden, heavier snow starts to fall. It's wet, and visibility becomes poor as the weather further deteriorates.

There's a massive fracture line in the ice that needs to be ever so gently traversed before we can catch up to the climbers on the fixed lines, who are slowly filing up the mountain. One guy is pulling himself up with an ice axe because his ropes have tangled.

It's a long, lung-busting ascent up the fixed lines to Camp 3.5 at 4,938 metres. I'm in the pain cave; this is where I live now.

While the route continues to the right, Jeremiah has a small campsite that's around to the left. There's only enough room for one tent to be perched here, and it's a long, pretty much completely vertical drop down. We level the tent platform, careful with our footing as wet snow continues to dump on us, raise the tent, and get out of the elements. A new sanctuary in the middle of nowhere to get dry, warm and comfortable.

The weather forecast has proved to be wrong again; these mountains provide extreme changes at will. But at least we're here. Weather-wise, we can't stay at this spot too long, so hopefully tomorrow it's onwards and upwards. After a warm, instant, rehydrated meal, it's time to retreat to the comfort of one's sleeping bag.

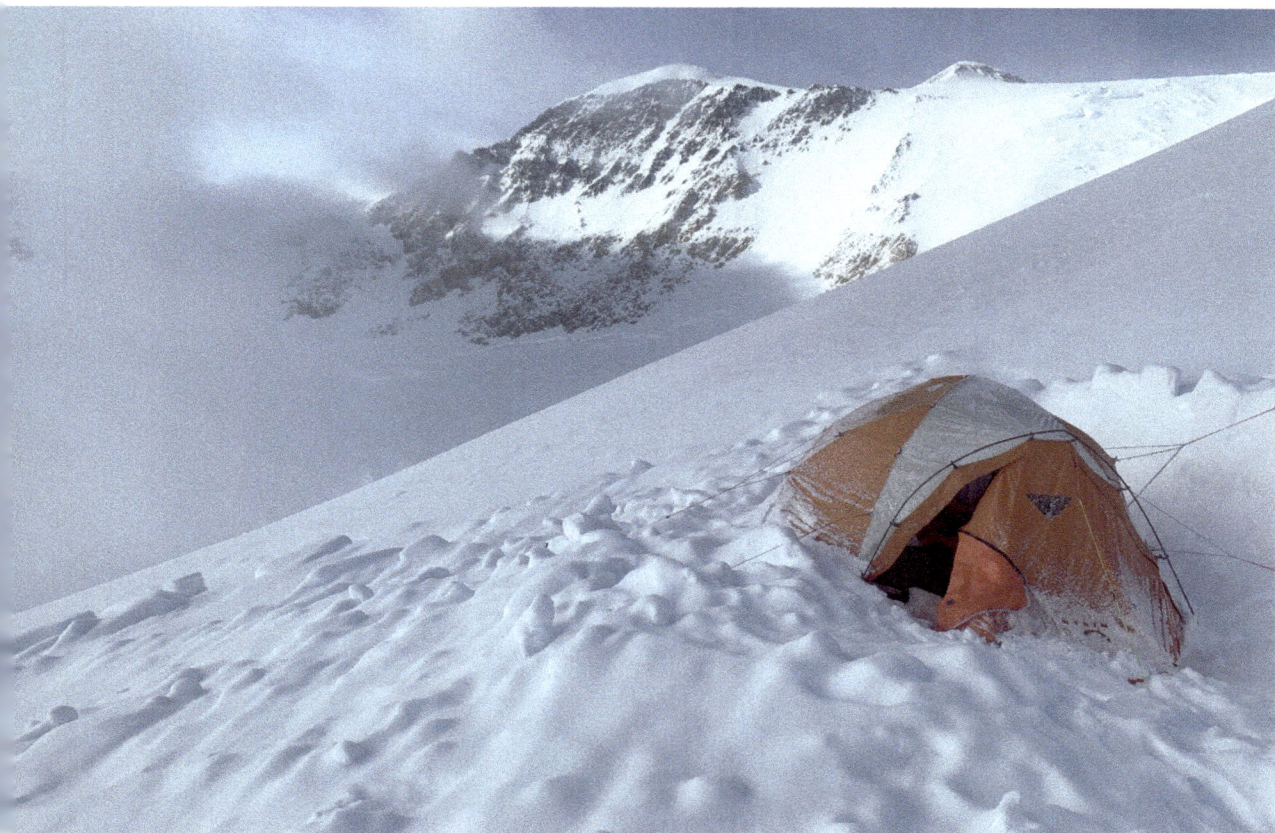

Day 14—Camp 3.5 to Camp 4 (High Camp)

No doubt about it, we're moving off this ridge: everything is wet, the tent is iced over, and nothing has dried. Although the snow has stopped for now, and the skies are clear.

In the pre-dawn light, I leave the comfort of the tent, tramp across fresh snow while being careful not to slip off the edge of the mountain, and use our makeshift bathroom facilities. The CMC sits in the open overlooking the best view I've ever had on the john. No walls, no privacy, no worries. Just me and the can on the side of this mountain.

The sun hits the tent, and it's time. Out we crawl again, one by one, to start the packing up process. Everything is a little

BACKPACK: 32kg

CAMP 4 ALTITUDE: 5,229m

DISTANCE: 0.86km

TIME: 2:35 hrs

ASCENT: 343m

DESCENT: 15m

PULSE OX: 83%

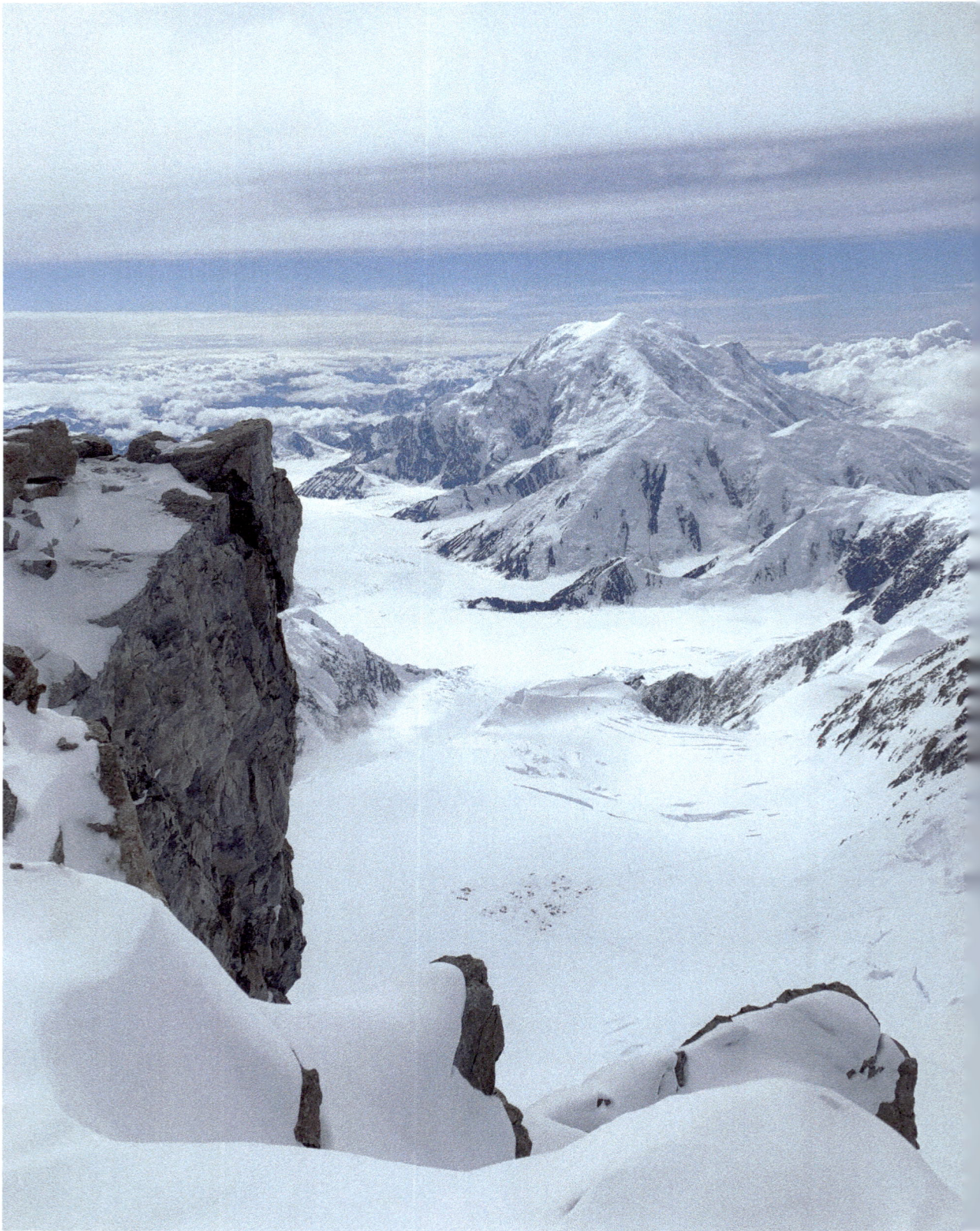

heavier, damper and more difficult, but we smash it all in our packs, swing our arms and legs for circulation, and depart.

We're straight onto fixed points as we scale steep terrain. You can't be afraid of heights here—it's either up or down. The sides of the snow-hardened track are soft and uncomfortable to walk on, requiring even more effort. After climbing a couple of hundred metres, my focus shifts from the precarious footing to the views, which are spectacular.

Finally, we move out onto the infamous '16 Ridge'. While climbing the ridge is not technically difficult, the consequences of a single misstep on the narrow route are potentially catastrophic. This is certainly when one gets the sense that the serious climbing has begun.

It's almost warming up as, after almost three hours of solid slog, we crest the last rise and can finally see the tents of Camp 4—High Camp. Snow walls have already been built around a compound with a spare tent site inside, meaning less work for us to get set up. Once the wet tent has been pitched, I check out the views. I can see all the way from a sheer edge down to Camp 3. It is beyond breathtaking.

Here the priority is always to get out of the elements, get in a tent, and then attend to my feet. I haven't taken the bandage off the big toe for a couple of days, and, looking at it, maybe I should have left the bandage on. The big toe is shedding thick layers of skin and is an unhealthy blue colour. I don't even want to touch it, yet dry socks have to go back on with a hand warmer for insurance. Not sure what else I can do except keep this same routine.

opposite On the edge—what a view

Day 15—Summit Day

'We don't remember well, but we have good memories,' says Jeremiah on why he keeps returning to the mountain after twenty-one expeditions and fourteen summits.

We're up at 5:30am to see if we can undertake our summit bid. The skies look clear, so we start to go through the motions.

The other climbing group rolled in here overnight after a seventeen-hour summit trek. It could be called successful, I suppose, but one of the three clients has a frostbitten finger and the other two have concerning coughs.

While the glaciers, mountains and alpine tundra provide motivation and inspiration, they also deliver harsh experiences to the underprepared. Self-care is vital; any expedition demands it. Though we all share the goal of reaching the summit, listening to your body is what will get you there. Numbers on digital displays reading personal metrics are only part of the decision-making; it's what happens in that six inches between your ears that matters most.

Once out of the tent, I instantly recognise that my layering is all wrong. It's incredibly cold. Even during the climbing season, the weather near Denali's summit can be punishing. In May this year, temperatures recorded at High Camp hovered around minus twenty-five degrees Celsius. After shuffling around trying to warm up, I'm unsure how this morning will pan out.

'Lenticular clouds are developing, and it's windy up there.' Jeremiah's mountain sense is one I've come to trust.

Back in the tent, the wind howls around us as I dig out my heavier layers. Looking outside at the terrible weather, decisions must be very considered. The stakes are high and the consequences could be dire. I'll rely on Jeremiah's expertise for this call.

And just when I think we'll adjourn—we're going!

There's no rush while the three of us go through the now well-known preparations. Leaving camp, back on our rope, other climbers watch us from their tents, formulating their own summit plans. While grateful for the decision that we'll attempt the summit, I'm also nervous. We're the first team to make the call and exit camp, with many well wishes.

Fresh snow makes any previous path unrecognisable. Certainly, if you've not climbed here before, the direction to take would be completely obscure.

The first part of the climb we approach is the Autobahn, which is the snow and ice slope leading from High Camp at 17,200 feet (5,242 metres) to Denali Pass at 18,200 feet (5,547 metres). Conditions on the Autobahn can vary from deep snow (avalanche danger) to hard ice. This section of Denali has been the scene of more fatalities than any other part of the mountain.

Jeremiah digs the hidden leash out of the snow, which is anchored by a stake, and then attaches a carabineer to the end of it. Different climbing tasks require different types of carabineers—different shapes, gate type, size or weight, and strength. Strong, durable and easy to use carabineers are the best. The leash location is marked by a thin wand. Once uncovered, we can use our carabineers to clip onto these leashes, which act as an anchor point to prevent a fall. As each climber transits, they leave carabineers exposed for the next climber. But to clip in the first time, Jeremiah has work to do to find these piton points in the fresh snow. A stake and a leash can be found at most of the wand points. But sometimes there's no indicator where the wand should be, and the work of digging in the snow is in vain.

Being the first to cut a track through the snow is a huge energy-sapper, particularly for Jeremiah as he's in the lead. I'm in the middle, so I can follow his steps, sort of, but nothing is solid underfoot. Safety is your own responsibility. Stomping my feet as the grade gets steeper, I just hope for some solid footing. Our progress is slow; it's going to be a long day. But at least we are making progress.

Jeremiah starts having coughing fits. I watch, listen, and become concerned. Without him, it's game over. Each mountain continues to teach valuable lessons and the struggles are real. Here a copious amount of snow remains on a path that is anything but defined, hindering our way forward.

We progress in silence as an icy wind whips down from above and the air becomes thinner.

Rounding the top of the Autobahn, out of the wind, we eventually arrive at Denali Pass, at 5,547 metres, and our first break. The silence is broken after ice axes firmly secure us, buried to their heads in the snow, connecting us together by tether.

Awesome rock formations surround us as we continue climbing. An hour out of Denali Pass, the unique Zebra Rocks are to our right. These migmatites—literally 'mixed rocks'— typically contain alternating lighter layers (leucosomes, comprised of light-coloured minerals such as quartz, feldspar and muscovite) and darker layers (melanosomes, comprised of dark-coloured minerals such as amphibole and biotite).

Soon, smaller rocks give way to bigger, even more impressive variations of migmatites. Sections are steep, and our approach winds uphill consistently. Sheltered behind some large formations, we take a standing break at Zebra Rocks. I'm starting to really feel the cold, and icicles are forming on my beard. Then, when we get moving, I start to get hot in this bizarre freezing-to-sunny climate. I think I can persevere to the next stop, but my mind is drifting to thoughts of dehydration.

For the first time on this trip, I call it: 'Jeremiah, can we stop for a sec? I'm cooking here!'

On a rope team, nothing happens without everybody doing it in unison. We stop on the rise, and I take off my hot balaclava. I feel guilty for the stop, but we're quickly underway. Now hatless, I can feel my face burning from the sun within minutes. But I don't want to make a habit of stopping our progress, so it will have to wait.

Farthing Horn, just before cresting the summit, is our next break stop. Out comes the balaclava again. We're not too exposed here and pass the Archdeacon's towering rock

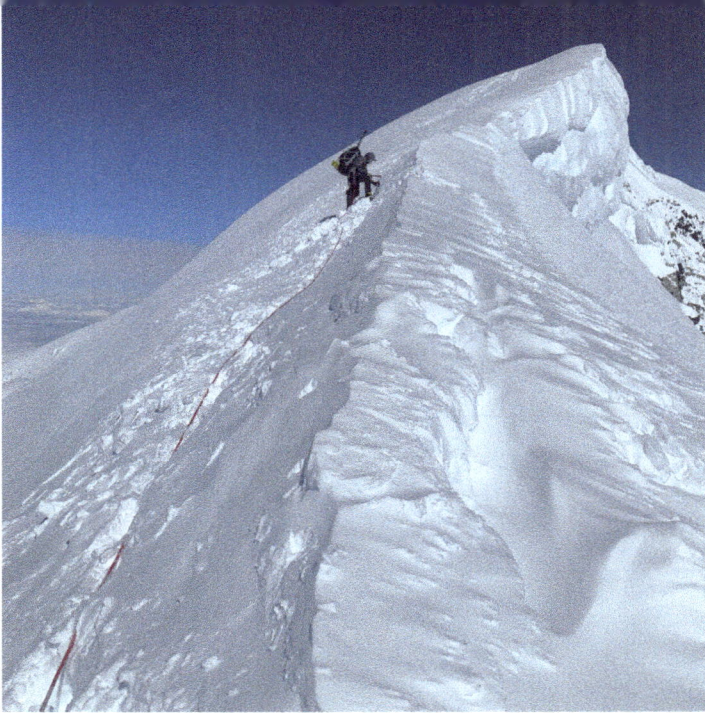

formations on our way to a new milestone, the Football Field, and our first bit of downhill trekking. It's a huge relief on the legs and feet, not to mention morale.

In the middle of the flat Football Field plain it hits me—I'm getting tired. My ears are ringing. This is just so hard. But I can't turn back now. There's no way I want to come back and climb this mountain again. In this moment I can't give up and I can't keep going. It's emotional, and I think of Fin, my family and all the struggles that continue to compound. How could I tell my kids—I nearly made it? I have to finish what I started.

My personal motivation isn't about me at all. Human nature is such that we naturally want to help. I want to help find a cure for type 1 diabetes, and life is better when triumphs are shared. But what about failure? Who wants to share that? This is no time for a pity party.

We have a mini-break while Hannah passes all our aluminium stakes to Jeremiah. Why he needs so many isn't obvious at first.

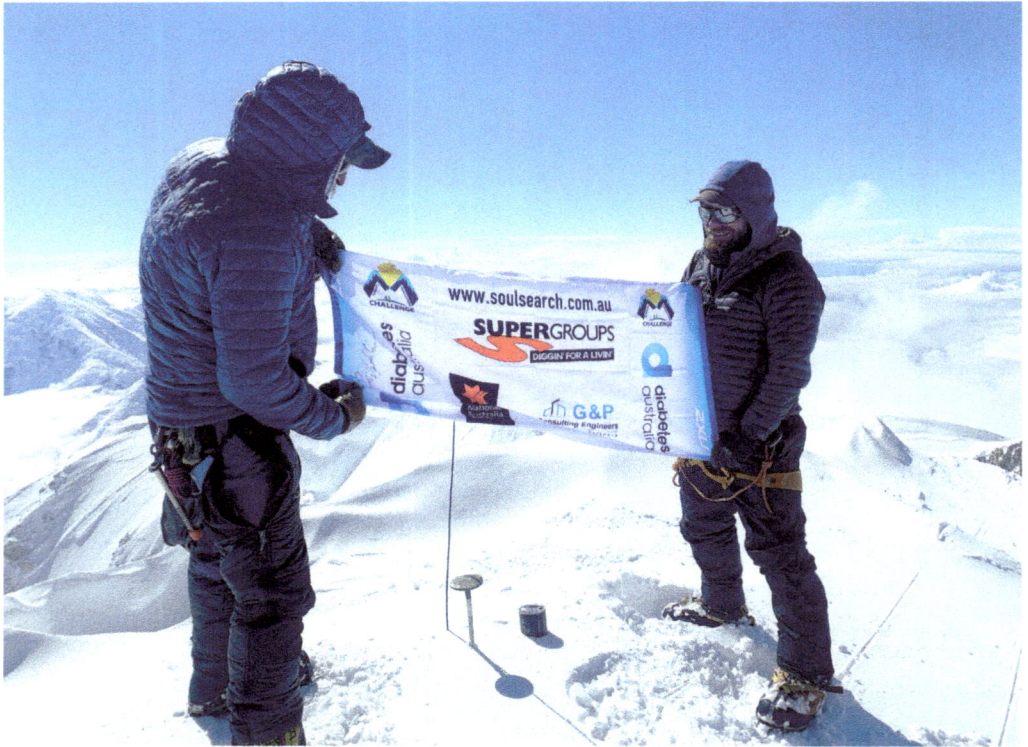

above Pure relief

I can see Pig Hill, roughly resembling the shape of a pig, which has a long ascent including plenty of switchbacks. Pig Hill is the intimidating last climb that is now in front of us. It has been an extremely challenging expedition due to the unpredictable weather and moments like these. Slogging through the snow, I keep telling myself, over and over: dig deep, keep walking, you'll get there.

At the top of Pig Hill we hit the cold wind of the south side of the summit ridge. And here, something changes. For some reason, my terrible fatigue falls away, and something feels different. I'm actually excited about reaching the summit.

It was on 7 June 1913 that three climbers became the first verified people to reach the summit of Denali. Now here I am,

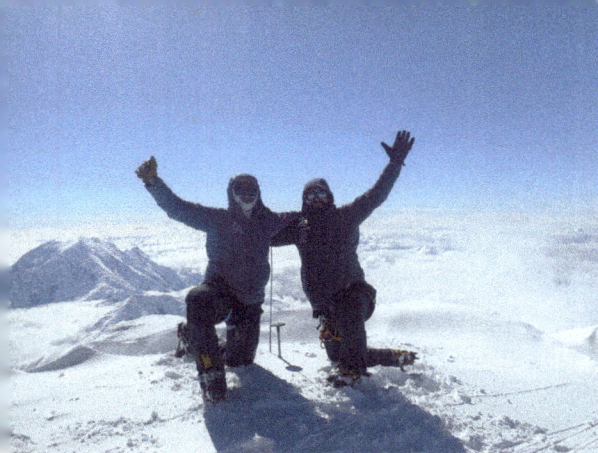

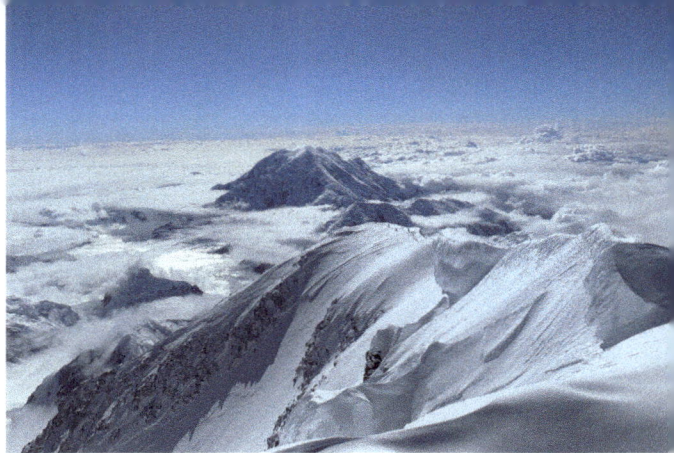

more than a century later, making the same pilgrimage. On this dramatic ridge there's no safety whatsoever, no tracks, no-one who has been before us—well, at least today. Jeremiah forges ahead through the virgin snow, staying as central as possible, because there are perilous, near-vertical drops on either side. I follow behind.

'Stop,' he shouts every now and then as he bashes a stake in as a safety measure should we slip and fall. I use these pauses to quickly snap a photo. Any distraction helps. Then the three of us proceed, bit by bit, up the rope.

Wow. Wow. Just wow. This moment, this view up here, is one of the most spectacular I've witnessed on our amazing planet.

After an eight-hour grind up the mountain, we've arrived.

Right where we stand is the centrepiece of Denali National Park, the Denali summit. In the background Mt Foraker, southwest of Denali, tops out at 17,400 feet (5,304 metres) and is the third highest mountain in the USA. What a back-drop for our summit views. While there have been epic views along the way, this is something else. This is pure satisfaction. I'm proud to have made it here, and at this moment I feel so alive, in awe of my surroundings. I've been both physically and mentally challenged during this climb, but relief has finally arrived. This is the moment to cherish, to capture, to wish to emulate. This is what will remain as an unforgettable mem-ory. To make this moment even more special, there's nobody

left Denali summit— 6,194 m

right Time to go home...

else here, just three climbers on the top of North America. So remote, so pure.

It's an accomplishment years in the making. Once the euphoria settles, I need to undertake one final task to complete this accomplishment—roll out my Diabetes Australia flag. My Seven Summits are now complete, and I can make my way home, satisfied.

The relief is like a burden lifted that I've been carrying for too long. It has been harder than I ever could have imagined. After half an hour of summit bliss, humbled by the sheer magnificence of the mountains, the inevitable task arrives—we need to descend.

STANDING WAITING at the baggage claim at Melbourne Airport, I see my two large, red expedition duffels slowly come around the bend of the luggage carousel. Those duffels were my constant companion as I travelled the globe. They're dirty, worn and no longer the vibrant red they once were. It's an effort to heave them, one at a time, from the progression of clean suitcases that fill the conveyor belt. With effort and a thud, each hits the floor at my feet.

I feel the way my bags look. Scruffy, grubby and with visible signs of wear and tear. I tend to forget how a stranger might judge me, but am quickly reminded of how observant humans can be.

'Wow, you look like you've been on an amazing adventure!' a friendly stranger says.

'It's been an adventure, that's for sure,' I politely reply.

'Well … welcome home.'

Home was indeed welcoming. Seeing Heidi and the kids after being away for months was the tonic I needed to begin healing from the ravages of my final two summits.

And they had a surprise for me.

My family sat me down in our living room and presented me with a list of the names of donors who had contributed to

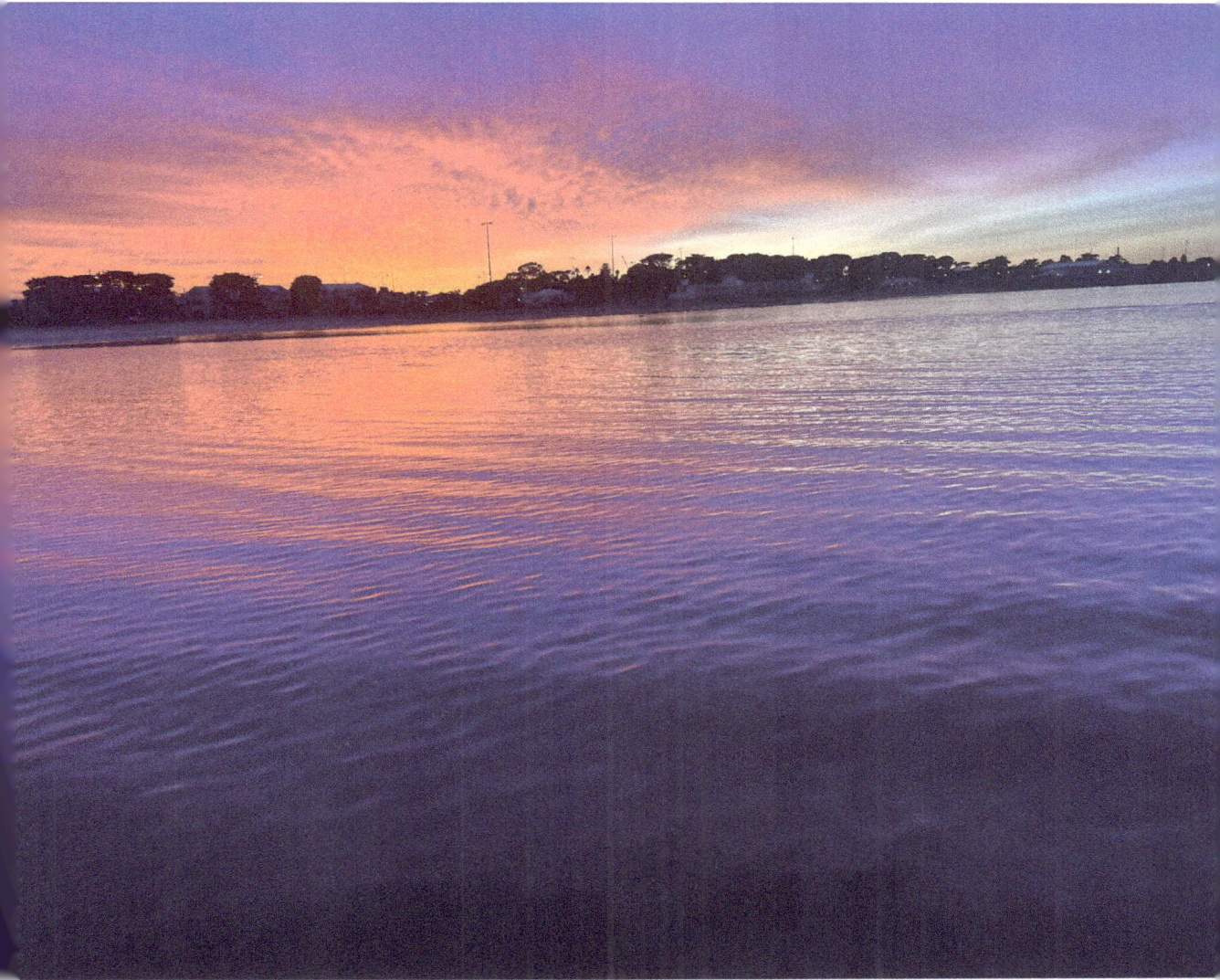

above Home at sea level

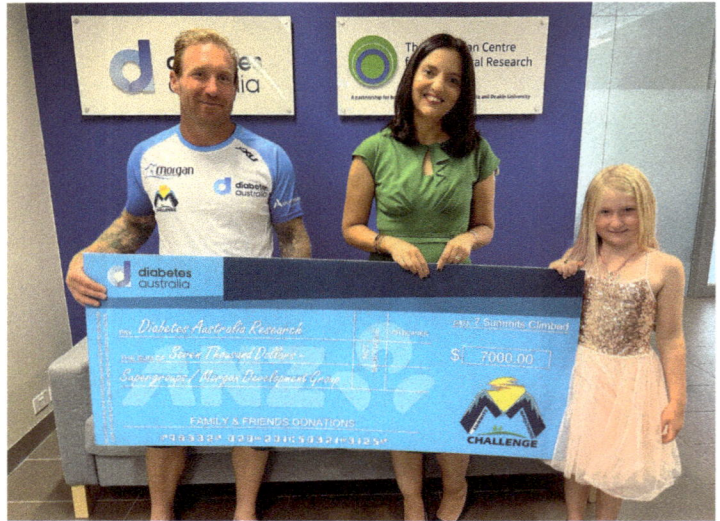

above Giving back...

the cause while I had been away. I didn't even know they had been fundraising on my behalf. The donations had been gathered on their own initiative. It was emotional to recognise that my family too were a part of this undertaking.

Heidi had personally coordinated community donations from friends and family who wanted to contribute while I was on Mt Everest. This was on top of the pandemic forcing her to intermittently undertake the home schooling of our kids, and came as a complete and delightful surprise. I discovered that our local school rang the school bell to signify my reaching that summit (which, happily, occurred between Victorian lockdowns), and excitement filled the school rooms. The local kindergarten that my younger daughter, Arlo, attended had a map on the wall with the local newspaper clippings about my adventures. It became part of their discussions and was actively followed. Throughout the challenge, while school kids raised money, strangers gave proceeds from their poker nights and a few regular contributors provided monthly donations.

Fin made a little speech: 'Dad, we are so very proud of you for climbing all the mountains to raise money for diabetes. We wanted to do something to help while you were gone, so Mum set up a secret fundraiser.'

Kai added, 'Lots of family and friends donated to the secret fund, as they think you are as amazing as we do. So, Arlo would like to give you something . . .'

Arlo then gave me a novelty cheque for 7,000 dollars. I was completely taken aback.

Later, Fin and I presented a 7,000-dollar novelty cheque (and a real one) to Diabetes Australia at its offices, which we named the 'Friends and Family Cheque'.

CONCLUSION

I̓T TOOK me three years to complete the Seven Summits challenge, a challenge that was entirely self-funded. I gave my time, money and energy with the intention of spreading awareness and furthering interest in the diabetes sector. Over the course of the challenge, 68,439 dollars was raised for Diabetes Australia. This money was raised despite a pandemic being thrown into the mix. At times we had great traction and at other times we stalled. Diabetes Australia didn't publicise the later stages of our campaign, given that Australian borders were closed at the time, and many, many citizens were compelled to stay at home via government orders. In Melbourne and Sydney, all everyone talked about was 'iso'—self-isolation. There was a concern that if Diabetes Australia was backing an individual who was able to leave the country, a public backlash might overshadow the good intent of the campaign. But privately, from individuals within the organisation, I received many thanks and congratulations for completing the challenge and for my efforts to raise donations. I'm forever humbled and grateful to everybody who contributed.

The pandemic stalled my efforts, but in a way it also provided hope. The rapidity with which a vaccine for Covid was developed is astonishing. This is what happens when money, effort and urgency combine. The globe could not ignore Covid. My hope is that by creating greater awareness of diabetes, greater effort will follow.

The Seven Summits challenge gifted me physical and psychological exhaustion, and it took time to heal from that experience. I'm finished now, and it feels right. I gave everything I had to the challenge in mind, body and spirit. After three years, it was the right time for its natural conclusion. Right for me, right for my family.

Upon finishing the challenge, I was invited to and attended the Diabetes Australia Supporters Morning Tea at New South Wales Government House, hosted by Her Excellency, the Honourable Margaret Beazley AC KC. I spent the morning talking with Her Excellency, researchers, and many people who've led long lives with type 1 diabetes.

Her Excellency eloquently delivered a speech in which she told the story of Phyllis Adams, who in 1923, as a six-year-old, became the first Australian to be treated with insulin. Phyllis weighed less than ten kilograms when she received her first injection of insulin, which arrived in Sydney on board a P&O ship from Vancouver wrapped in cotton wool. It was just two years earlier, in 1921, that four Canadian researchers had discovered how to isolate insulin from the pancreas and then refine it, with the first injection of insulin administered in 1922. A medical breakthrough like no other, it prevented diabetes from virtually being a death sentence.

When the P&O ship carrying her first dose of insulin arrived in Australia, Phyllis Adams had survived for eight months on just a teaspoon of peanut butter, a lettuce leaf and a glass of junket per day. At the time starvation was often advised to prolong a child's life so the family could have just a little longer with their child. Insulin was the game-changer. Phyllis went on to live a full life, dying at the age of eighty-one and even making *The Guinness Book of Records* for her longevity.

The story of Phyllis struck a chord with me. She was so young, like Fin, but unlike my daughter her chances of survival were slim. Her family went to great lengths to try to help her, and I could relate to the urgency they must have felt.

Our kids are not born with type 1 diabetes. Rather, they lose their ability to make insulin because their immune system attacks the insulin-producing cells in the pancreas for reasons that are not clear. The work modern researchers undertake, the technological advances, are all brilliant—but there is still no cure. Is the next medical breakthrough just around the corner? As a father, I hope so.

It is also my hope, by completing and writing about a challenge few people dare to attempt, that you will understand why someone would go to such lengths. Climbing the Seven Summits might seem impossible, as can finding a cure for type 1 diabetes. I have proved to myself that the Seven Summits can be conquered. And I believe that, together, we can eventually find a cure for diabetes.

By holding this belief close, I dare to dream.

I began this adventure knowing almost nothing about mountaineering. Counterintuitively, I both wish I had learnt more about the demands of the Seven Summits challenge from experienced mountaineers before I began, and am glad that I didn't. For if I'd known exactly what I was up against, I might not have started. I discovered a whole new version of myself through this challenge, and that self can see that, initially, I wasn't prepared.

Prior to these challenges, I didn't consider myself an athlete (far from it). I'd say I was somewhat naïve about what was actually required to stand atop the highest mountain of each of the world's continents. I'd certainly never met anybody who had climbed any of them. Except Jim, a friend who'd walked to the top of Mt Kosciuszko in Australia with his family—the smallest of the Seven Summits.

Each stage in the Seven Summits challenge was initially something I was not capable of doing. With the support of my family, I put together the best plan I could to become the kind of person who would complete that challenge and arrive at the end of a long journey. It took burning candles at both ends, commitment to the training, time management in both work and family obligations, overcoming setbacks and a whole lot of sweat and tears.

But through this challenge I discovered that being an athlete is a mindset, not what you look like or what your race result is. It's a way of thinking and a series of actions you take. An athlete formulates a plan and takes responsibility for the outcomes. Once I started, every day, every step forward, and even every setback, was an opportunity to progress towards the next summit. A little luck helped. Surely the same mindset can help us find a cure for diabetes.

It's been a humbling experience, but the achievement isn't important. For all my many faults, ego wouldn't be one of them. To seek simplicity and fresh air is a privilege and luxury many people don't have. I take with me from this experience many memories and friendships that I would otherwise never have acquired, and personal growth that would otherwise not have occurred.

I've had some losses. The circulation in my feet remains poor, and the big toe on one foot turns purple when it's cold. My toes cramp often and there's limited sensation and mobility, but I kept them against the odds—well, for now. And even if I lose a toe or two, it's a small burden compared to the burden that Fin carries.

I've climbed each of the highest mountains on the world's seven continents to contribute in my way towards research into type 1 diabetes. But there is still work to do ... I'm currently contributing towards the 'Families Project Expert Community Consultation Group'. Our collective shared experiences and challenges will help Diabetes Victoria provide quality support and services, tailored to children living with type 1 diabetes.

Meanwhile, I continue to hope for a cure.

Cultivated perseverance is the only way forward.

To break through our perceived limits takes hard work—never quit.

I've faced the reality of what it takes to climb geological wonders that are spectacular icons of the nations and global

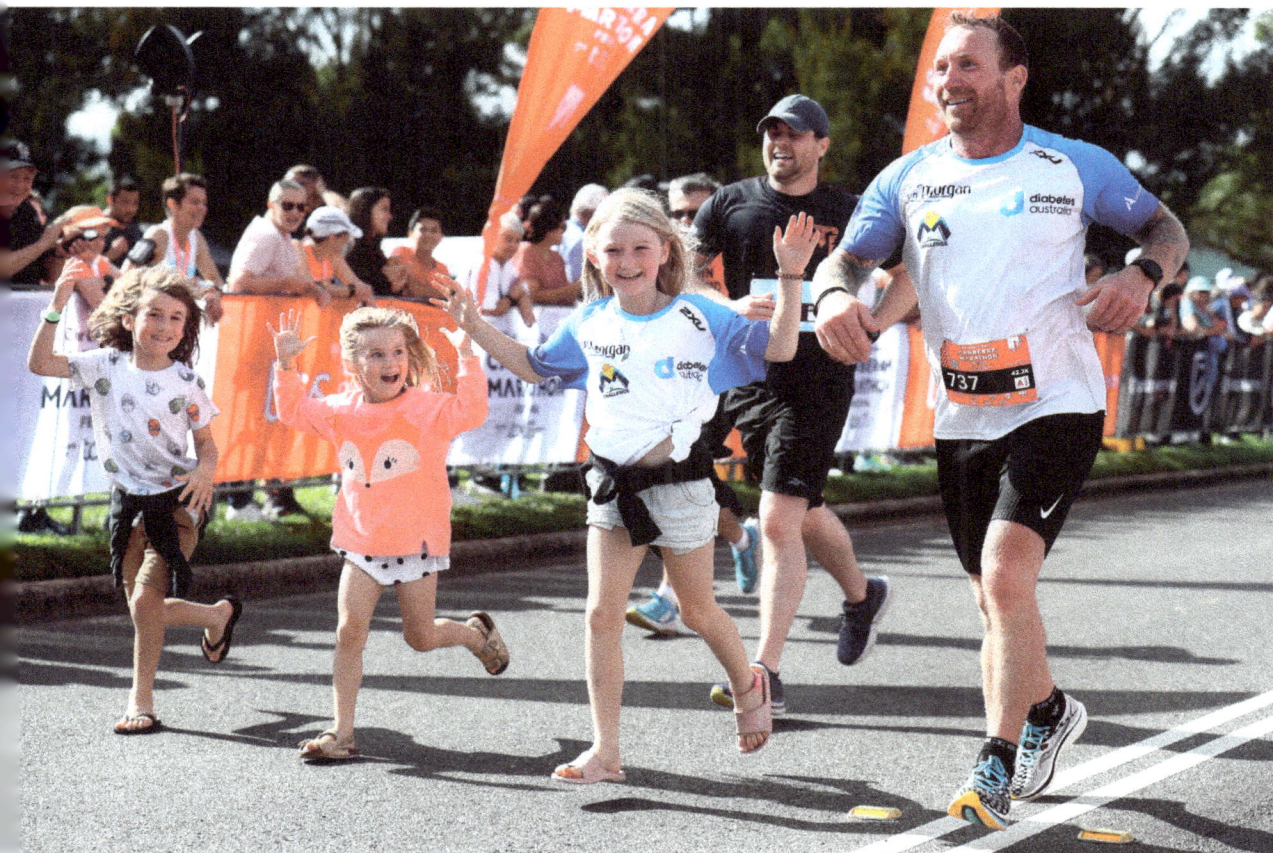

citizens that treasure them. I highly recommend taking time to look at the world around you and marvel at the diversity within nature. There's something about the outdoors that stirs the soul and occasionally takes your breath away. No words can describe the experience of witnessing the interplay between light and snow, seeing the first light of dawn as the sun begins to rise or taking in the view that a clear night and full moon can offer on a mountain.

The forces that smash tectonic plates together below the ground and push huge slabs of rock into the air give us mountains. Other forces push magma to the surface and give us volcanoes. I never appreciated that the world is full of incredible rock formations until I started to climb them. We can evolve to a higher potential just like two sections of the ground can break down before they break through. Nature favours what thrives—our lives can follow a similar pattern.

If you can't get out in the mountains, hopefully I've brought them a little closer to you.

To all my children—almost anything is possible. Have fun, smile, be healthy. Have courage in the moment, be brave enough to change what you can. Along the way your memories are the reward, the obstacles you overcome will fall away—you're stronger. Nothing worthwhile comes from instant gratification. Go outside and play.

ACKNOWLEDGEMENTS

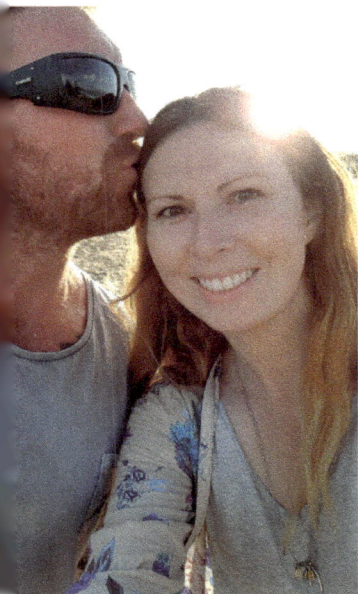

above Home again

THERE ARE MANY people I wish to thank and acknowledge— in helping my family navigate Fin's diabetes diagnosis, in helping me achieve the Seven Summits challenge, and in assisting with the publication of this book.

From the Royal Children's Hospital staff, Diabetes Australia, JDRF, Diabetes Victoria, researchers, representatives and fundraisers, my family has received all the help our daughter needs to adjust to a life living with type 1. I couldn't imagine handling the diagnosis without these supports. The whole fundraising challenge was a chance to give something back to the type 1 community, which has been so generous in our family's education and support.

I could not have climbed the seven highest mountains on the seven continents without the help and technical expertise of the companies that I chose as my expedition partners. Particular gratitude goes to CTSS, which was my expedition partner for Mt Vinson and Mt Everest. Navigating the difficulties that Covid threw into the mix while attempting Everest may have been impossible without its assistance.

I'd like to thank, in no particular order, all the generous people who contributed to the 7,000 dollars my family raised while I summited Everest:

Nora, Chris, Billie & Bridgette O'Connor; Kristine Jeremiah; Nadia & Steve Nitschke & family; Brad & Maile Edwards & family; Wendy & Tilly Liversidge; Bek & Jenna Ralph & family; Melanie & Lili Bentley; Rachael & Dean Stanley; Jacqueline; Peter & Sue Lawler; Lu Lefranc & family; Lauren Edwards;

Trent & Anni Morgan & family; Brent & Stacy Szalay; Michael & Janis Rodwell; Jan Edwards; Lee Thurley & Aitken Ruen; John Wegner; Ryan & Julie McQuitty; Shaye, Andrew, Byron & Liam McQuitty; Dane & Amanda McQuitty & family; Kim & Ruby Wilson; Courtney Pinwell; Darren, Emma, Cooper & Hudson Wright; Jan & Mark Schiffer & family; Brett Fitzpatrick; Justin Brown; Sharon, Peter, Darcy & Stella Flaherty; Carl & Veronica Haworth & family; Renee Cox; Chris Browne; Rosie Bennett & family; Andrew & Michelle Mammerella & family; Julie & Andrew Edwards & family; Joel Rahtin; Jodi, Christian, Evelyn & Sebastian Pevez; Denise Porter & Rob Pearson; Lora, Paul, Sam & James Winter; Amy Richards Kane, Jason Kane & family; Sam & Mike Hunneyball & family; Jasmina & Sash Kacevski; Kim Hinte; Ebony Walgers & family; Tanya Bowen; Lisa & Lyndon Watson & family; Brooke & Felix Bentley; Amy, Adam Baldacchino & family; Jason Delphone; Loren & Kyle Eagan & family; Catherine Yaraisantos; Emma & Dan Sumner & family; Hug & Yeel Hailu; Kellie Delaney; Carrie, Stewart, Alexis & Nick Burhop Keller; Melissa & Mark Bisby; Rochelle White; Jacqui, Peter, Zara & Mya Skrekovski; Tracey & Brett Waldelton; Adele Chivers; Heidi Wegner, Finlay, Kai & Arlo Morgan; Kelly Keeshan & Troy Johnson; Tammi Wegner; Justin Hughes; Tracey Reginald

Many businesses also supported the initiative. Thank you to:

- Superkub Pty Ltd t/a Super Groups
- G&P Consulting Engineers
- Aughtersons Insurance Brokers
- Morgan Development Group
- National Australia Bank (NAB)
- SJD Homes
- Macdonald Estates
- Drew Robinson
- Peake Real Estate
- My Expert
- Optimal Strength Coaching

I'm forever humbled and grateful to everyone who supported my family and donated. Thank you.

Turning the Seven Summits challenge into a book was a challenge in itself. Writing, re-writing, editing and writing again has allowed me to enjoy these memories and brought me a lot of joy from this project.

From day one, freelance journalist Sandy Guy supported the Seven Summits challenge for the benefit of Diabetes Australia and contributed to the many blog posts that followed. Further, Sandy showed me her love of writing and encouraged me to write further of my travels. I came to enjoy the process thanks to her support.

This book just wouldn't be in its published form without the contribution, help and support of Carolyn Jackson, the project's lead editor. With an intuitive flare and professional approach, Carolyn has provided the genuine care and guidance my manuscript required.

RESOURCES

Can I help?
Email me at:
challenge@soulsearch.com.au

Want to donate?
https://www.diabetesaustralia.com.au/donation/

Support services
Diabetes Australia
diabetesaustralia.com.au
T: 1800 177 055

JDRF Australia
jdrf.org.au
T: (02) 8364 0200

ABOUT THE AUTHOR

DAVID MORGAN is an adventurer who has sailed from Australia to America via Vietnam and China and run marathons in various destinations, from New York to Tokyo. He has also hiked the Kokoda Trail and Great Ocean Walk in the pursuit of adventure.

In just over three years, with purpose and determination, David climbed the famed 'Seven Summits', the highest peaks on each of Earth's seven continents, following in the footsteps of Richard Bass.

Upon finishing, he rebuilt his depleted body and went on to finish a full Ironman.

By living life and fulfilling his optimal potential, David's story proves that no challenge cannot be overcome if the motivation is great enough.

David is the founder of Morgan Development Group and Morgan & Co, and continues to occupy diverse roles within the construction and real estate sectors.

He is also always on the lookout for a new adventure, whatever that may be.

First and foremost, however, David is a father to four precious children. He lives with his partner and children in Williamstown, Victoria.

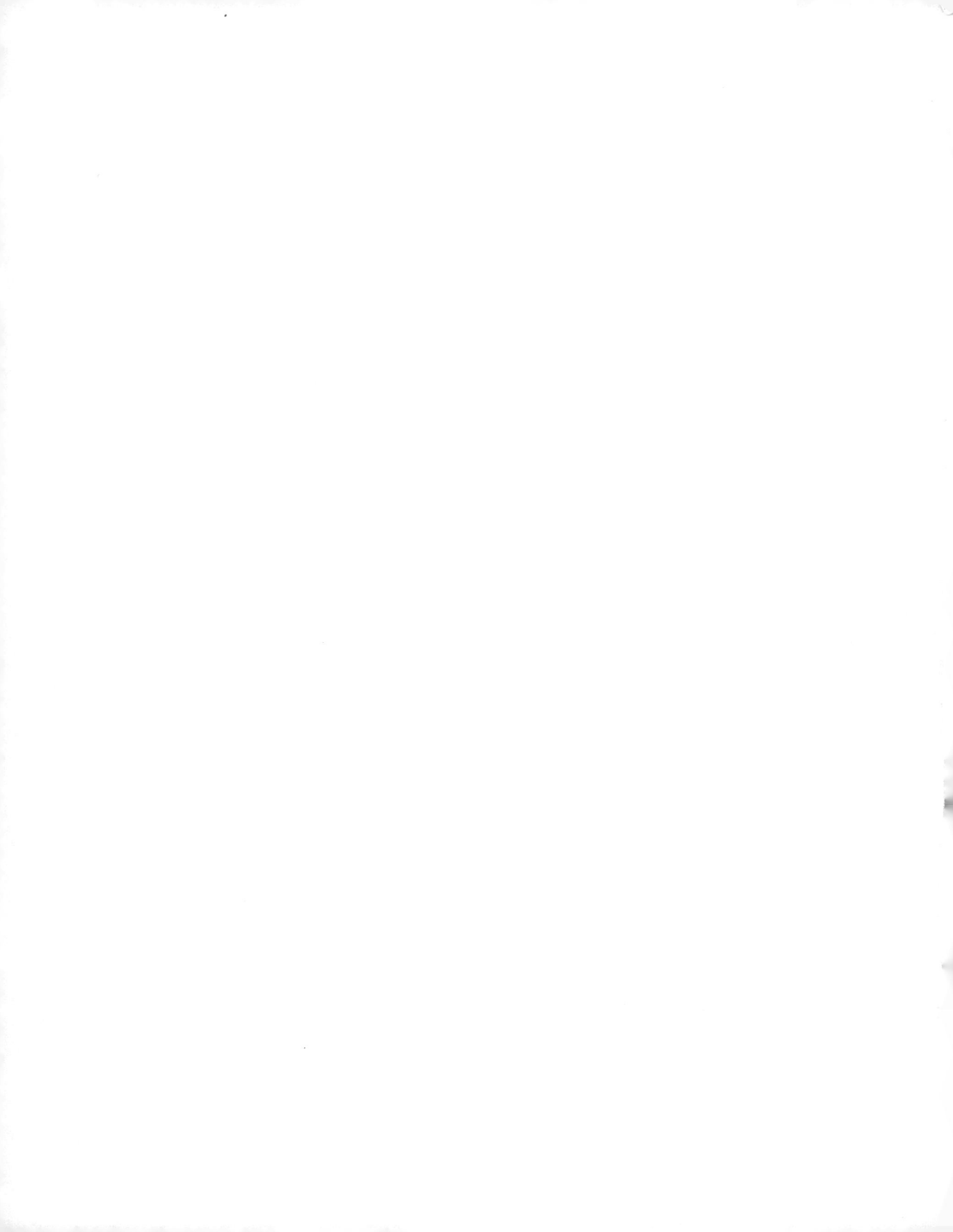

www.ingramcontent.com/pod-product-compliance
Lightning Source LLC
Chambersburg PA
CBHW042332030426
42335CB00027B/3309